THE HISTORY OF HEALTH SERVICES IN MISSOURI

The History of Health Services in Missouri

By John C. Crighton

1993
BARNHART PRESS
Omaha, Nebraska

Table Of Contents

The Founding of St. Louis
Early Medical Services
Medical Aspects of the Lewis and Clark Expedition
Slow Growth of St. Louis Under the Spanish Regime
Changes Produced by American Immigration
The Movement of American Doctors to St. Louis
Municipal Development

St. Louis as a City
The Cholera Epidemic of 1832
The Improvement of St. Louis's Water Supply
The Development of a Medical Profession
A Center for Medical Education
St. Louis as a Hospital Center
Public Health Legislation
The State of Medical Science
Sectarian Medical Systems
Problems of Disease Classification and Identification
Medical Journals
State Non-Intervention in Medical Matters

St. Louis in the 1840s
The 1849 Cholera Epidemic
The Beginning of a Sewer System
Shortages at the Waterworks
Health Department Matters
The Crisis of the Medical Profession
Hospital Expansion
Progress at the Medical Colleges
Care of the Insane: From Local to State Control

Importance of Missouri to the Union Cause
St. Louis as a Military Headquarters
St. Louis as a Military Hospital Center
Regional and National Activities of the Western Sanitary Commission
Influence of the War on the Provision of Health Services
Emergence of the "Social Evil."
Dispersion and Reunion

Preface

Medical history has emerged as an important new area of historical research and writing. A list of significant works in this field would include the following: *Medicine and Society in America, 1660-1860,* by Richard Harrison Shryock; *The Cholera Years,* by Charles E. Rosenberg; *History of Medicine in the United States,* by Francis R. Packard; *Conquest of Epidemic Disease*, by Charles-Edward Amory Winslow; *The Social Transformation of American Medicine,* by Paul Starr; and *A History of the Rockefeller Institute 1901-1953*, by George W. Corner. Strong faculties of medical history are found at Johns Hopkins, Harvard, Pennsylvania, and Wisconsin universities.

In Missouri this field has been generally neglected, except for Max A. Goldstein's *One Hundred Years of Medicine and Surgery in Missouri,* published in 1900, and E. J. Goodwin's *A History of Medicine in Missouri,* issued in 1905. These two volumes contain valuable photographs and data regarding hospitals, medical schools, and physicians of the state, particularly of St. Louis. Goldstein's book has reminiscences of early St. Louis medical history by a number of doctors still practicing near the turn of the century.

The problem of how to organize the data of my proposed history of health services in Missouri arose early. I realized that it would be impossible to investigate and relate the history of each community in the state of Missouri. I finally decided to tell the story of the development of health services in St. Louis, as representative of what happened in the state as a whole.

St. Louis was the state's largest city. As the "Gateway to the West," it experienced in severe form the major epidemics of the nineteenth century, including cholera, smallpox, typhus, and yellow fever. For St. Louis the state legislature developed the forms of health administration, i.e., quarantine, a board of health, and health commissioner, that were applied later to other cities at various stages of development. St. Louis physicians took the lead in the advocacy of a state board of health and in promoting medical practice legislation, including strict licensure laws. St. Louis since its founding has enjoyed a high quality of medical care. As an important station of the French colonial establishment, it always had a post surgeon as well as French civilian physicians. Its early American doctors, many trained in Philadelphia and abroad, were of top quality. St. Louis received another important influx of foreign scientific talent in the German emigrations of 1848 and 1849.

It was decided to make this book comprehensive in scope, to cover the history of medical science, medical education, the medical profession, hospitals, nursing, major epidemics, and the treatment of the mentally ill. With extensive footnotes, an index, and a table of contents, it should be useful to scholars who wish to study and write on more specialized topics.

This volume is based upon first-hand sources, particularly St. Louis newspapers. Enough political and social context is provided to illuminate the discussion of health problems.

It was not until 1883 that Missouri established a state board of health. Prior to this time the city of St. Louis acted on its own in establishing quarantines against epidemics introduced by its river traffic with New Orleans. This belated action of the state was due in part to the existence of strong medical sects, e.g., homeopathy and Eclectic medicine, which feared that a state board would discriminate against them. At first the state board was very grudgingly funded by the legislature and for several years not at all. Its function was minimal, mainly the operation of a bureau of vital statistics and the licensing of doctors. It was not until the 1920s that the board became fully operational, with nurses and sanitarians working in the field to combat disease.

As the twentieth century nears its close, the problem of providing Missourians with adequate medical services remains unsolved. With the failure to establish a national health insurance system, thousands of citizens are without any protection, whether from Medicare or Medicaid. Rising medical costs accentuate the problem. Medical corporations, for profit as well as non-profit, threaten the continued operation of voluntary and public hospitals. The state's care of the mentally ill has come full circle, from its original policy of non-intervention, leaving their care to the discretion of the county courts, to its present deinstitutionalization, without providing an adequate safety net for thousands of former custodial cases.

JOHN C. CRIGHTON

Acknowledgements

The proposal that I write the history of health services in Missouri originated in a conference with Dr. Herbert R. Domke, director of the Division of Health, and Dr. H. Denny Donnell, state epidemiologist, at the University of Missouri Medical School in 1975. They had read and liked several articles on early Boone County medical history, which I had written as Sunday feature stories in the *Columbia Daily Tribune*. I, at that time, was completing the newspaper series on Columbia and Boone County and was interested in undertaking another major writing assignment. I want to express my thanks to Drs. Domke and Donnell for suggesting the health services project and encouraging me at various stages to complete it. Dr. Robert Harmon, who succeeded Dr. Domke at Jefferson City, also lent his strong support to the undertaking. For this I express my deep appreciation.

Before starting my specific research on the development of health services in Missouri, I spent two years becoming acquainted with the general history of medicine beginning with the Greeks and Romans. The epic account of the discovery by careful research of how the human body functions, of the nature of disease, and of the means to overcome it has greatly enriched my general education. This has been one of the fringe benefits for which I am grateful.

My research for the health services project was accomplished at the State Historical Society of Missouri library, particularly in the journalism section. Over a period of ten years I read the St. Louis newspapers from 1808 through 1980. I want to express my special thanks to the newspaper library staff for their generous assistance in helping me find references and in copying a lengthy list of source materials. The staff in the general reference library were equally helpful.

I want to thank Dr. James W. Goodrich and Joseph Webber, former president of the State Historical Society of Missouri, for the grant of the 1989 Richard S. Brownlee award. This has been of great assistance to me in preparing my typescript for publication. Dr. Dorothy L. Rodgers suggested that I get in touch with the state's medical societies for assistance in publishing my book. Lee Gibson, executive secretary of the Boone County Medical Society, willingly took on the task of contacting the St. Louis Medical Society and also the Missouri State Medical Association in an effort to establish a coordinated plan to sponsor and subsidize publication.

My daughters, Nancy Botts and Florence Olsen, and my wife Rebecca lent support and encouragement during the long preparation of the book. My son-in-law, Rodney Olsen, from his wide knowledge of the literature of medical history, selected for me a number of the most significant books in my research field.

Mary K. Dains edited the typescript. The designing of the book was performed in expert fashion by Dr. Paul Fisher. Dr. Alan Havig and Lynn W. Gentzler performed a much appreciated service by reading and editing the printer's proofs. Wyeth-Ayerst Laboratories generously gave me permission to reproduce in color the Dean Cornwell painting, "Beaumont and St. Martin," and to use it on the cover of my forthcoming book, *The History of Health Services in Missouri.*

Charles Lockwood, manager of the Missouri Bookstore of Columbia, made available the resources of his organization and of its parent company.

Chapter I

The Colonial and Territorial Period

1. The Founding of St. Louis

THE SITE CHOSEN by Pierre Laclede in 1763 as a trading post for the conduct of the fur trade on the west side of the Mississippi River gave promise of developing into a healthy as well as prosperous settlement. The spot was about eighteen miles south of the mouth of the Missouri River. Here the ground rose from the bank of the Mississippi River to a summit known as "the Hill." The incline included two gentle ascents and two plateaus or terraces about 300 feet wide. The terraces were heavily wooded. The distance from the water's edge to the summit was about 1,000 feet.

A wide ravine, which followed the course of present Walnut Street, offered an easy route from the river to the first plateau. Boats could be landed at the foot of the ravine. A second gully reached the river several hundred yards to the north. Sinkholes in the limestone bedrock of the site provided additional drainage. Limestone bluffs, in places thirty-five feet high, stood at the water's edge. The river current was strong near shore and deepened rapidly offshore. West of the hill stretched a prairie.[1]

Timber for building, abundant farm land, excellent drainage, an adequate water supply, a deep approach for boats and a swift current to carry away the settlement's refuse and wastes – all of these were available at the site which grew into the city of St. Louis.

The early French population of St. Louis arrived in three contingents. A group of thirty workers under the direction of Rene Auguste Chouteau, Laclede's stepson, early in 1764 cleared the site chosen by Laclede and began the construction of buildings. Anticipating the surrender of Fort Chartres to the British in 1765, as part of the transfer of the French territory east of the Mississippi in accordance with the terms of the Treaty of Paris (1763), a considerable migration to St. Louis of settlers from the vicinity of the fort and other settlements of the Illinois country occurred. Several families from Ste. Genevieve and New Orleans joined in this movement. They were followed on October 10, 1765, by the commandant at Fort Chartres, Captain Louis St. Ange De Bellerive, with the troops under his control.[2] The captain, in the name of Spain, the new sovereign power, which by the Treaty of Paris had gained all French territory west of the Mississippi, established rule over St. Louis and the Upper Louisiana Territory.[3].

In their new home the French settlers followed a variety of occupations. Many were farmers, tilling their assigned strips in the spacious enclosed common fields. The farmers lived in the village of St. Louis and went out each morning with their carts and implements to perform their chores.[4] Fur trading, the major reason for the founding of the settlement, occupied the efforts of a select company. Boatmen comprised another important category. Various craftsmen applied their skills to satisfy the community's needs for food, shelter, and clothing. A small garrison provided protection for the post. The military cadre usually included a post physician.[5]

Captain Amos Stoddard, who on March 9-10, 1804, as representative of the United States government, accepted the transfer of the Louisiana Territory from France (the territory had been ceded by Spain to France by the secret Treaty of San Ildefonso 1800) thus described these new American citizens[6]:

Perhaps the levities displayed and the amusements pursued on Sunday may be considered by some to border on licentiousness. They attend mass in the morning with great devotion, but after the exercises of the church are over they usually collect in parties and pass away their time in social and merry intercourse. They play at billiards and other games, and to balls and assemblies the Sundays are particularly devoted. To those educated in regular and pious protestant habits such parties and amusements appear unseasonable, strange and odious, if not prophetic of some signal curse on the workers of iniquity. It must, however, be confessed that the French people, in these days, avoid all intemperate and immoral excesses, and conduct themselves with apparent decorum . . . When questioned relative to their gaiety on Sundays, they will answer that men are made for happiness, and that the more they are able to enjoy themselves the more acceptable they are to their creator.

A majority of the original settlers were of middle age[7] and married. Being of French, especially of Canadian-French background, they formed a homogeneous group. The influence of their Catholic priest was strong, not only in forming their religious beliefs but also their life style.[8] They were generally sober, law-abiding, and inclined to settle their differences by peaceful means.

The early settlers enjoyed an Arcadian existence and were rarely visited by sickness.[9] Their physical isolation on the frontier of civilization protected them from disease introduced by European immigration. The absence of low, swampy areas in the vicinity minimized the incidence of malaria, and a wholesome water supply furnished insurance against cholera. The most common ailments were of a respiratory nature,[10] probably from outdoor work in all kinds of weather.

2. Early Medical Services

The first physician in St. Louis was Dr. Andre August Conde, a native of Aunis, France, and a surgeon – or military physician – in the French establishment. He was a member of the garrison at Fort Chartres before moving over to St. Louis with St. Ange de Bellerive in 1765. His military responsibilities did not interfere with his building up a large private practice. His account books, when he died on November 28, 1776, indicated that 233 of his patients were indebted to him for professional services. Frederick L. Billon, the analyst of early St. Louis, described Dr. Conde as "a gentleman of fine education . . . and a prominent man in the village in his day."[11]

The second doctor in St. Louis was John B. Valleau, a native of La Rochelle, France, who had transferred his allegiance to Spain. He was surgeon of the military detachment, which Don Antonio de Ulloa, the first Spanish governor of Louisiana at New Orleans, sent late in 1767 to build forts at the mouth of the Missouri River as protection against the British. His care for the health of the troops required him to make frequent trips to Bellefontaine on the Missouri River where the fortifications were being constructed. Exposure to the hot sun during the summer of 1768 brought on an illness from which he died on November 24.[12]

Dr. Antoine Reynal lived and practiced in St. Louis from 1776 to 1799, when he moved to St. Charles. [13] Other doctors who lived in St. Louis for varying periods of time but apparently did not practice there were Bernard Gibkins, Claudio Mercier and Philip Joachim Ginger.[14]

The memory of these early doctors did not outlast their generation. To St. Louis, in 1800, however, came a young doctor whose influence is still felt. Scientist, physician and philanthropist, he embodied the talents and concerns that made him a role model for his successors and won for him the title of the father of the medical profession of St. Louis.

Antoine Francois Saugrain was born in Paris on February 17, 1763, into an educated and prosperous family, which on his father's side was distinguished as librarians, editors, and booksellers.[15] His youthful years coincided with the most creative period of the intellectual movement known as the Enlightenment. In 1751, the first volume of the French *Encyclopedie* appeared, a series designed to "collect under one roof all the active writers, all the new ideas, all the new knowledge, that were then stirring the cultivated strata of society."[16] The pursuit of science engrossed the attention of many of the ablest minds, including young Antoine Saugrain. Although his major interest was in

chemistry and mineralogy, it is obvious from his later career he must also have studied the life sciences, which are the basis of the discipline of medicine.

Saugrain quickly established a reputation in his professional field and about 1784-1785 traveled in the service of the king of Spain to Mexico to examine the processes involved in mineral production. In 1787, he came to the United States, in company with two young Parisian friends, M. Raguet and M. Pique, the latter a botanist. Saugrain brought with him a letter of introduction to Benjamin Franklin, who in 1785 had returned to America after almost a decade of diplomatic service in France. During that time, Franklin had won acclaim not only as a diplomat but also as a scientist. Dr. Franklin in Philadelphia graciously received Saugrain and promised to render him any services within his power.[17]

In the spring of 1788, Saugrain and his two friends and an American named Pierce left Pittsburgh in a flat boat to descend the Ohio to the vicinity of the falls, now Louisville. The purpose was ostensibly to conduct a pioneering botanical survey. En route the party was attacked by Indians, who killed Raguet and Pique. Pierce and Saugrain managed to escape after being captured and found their way to an American fort at Clarksville, Indiana.[18]

Saugrain returned to France in the summer of 1788 and remained there through the eventful year 1789 in which the French Revolution began. Discouraged, perhaps regarding his professional prospects in the new revolutionary society, he left France in April 1790, with a group of French emigrants bound for a new settlement at Gallipolis, Ohio. Later he married Genevieve Rosalie Michau, whom he had met on the vessel which brought them to America.[19] In Gallipolis, he displayed his sign as a physi-

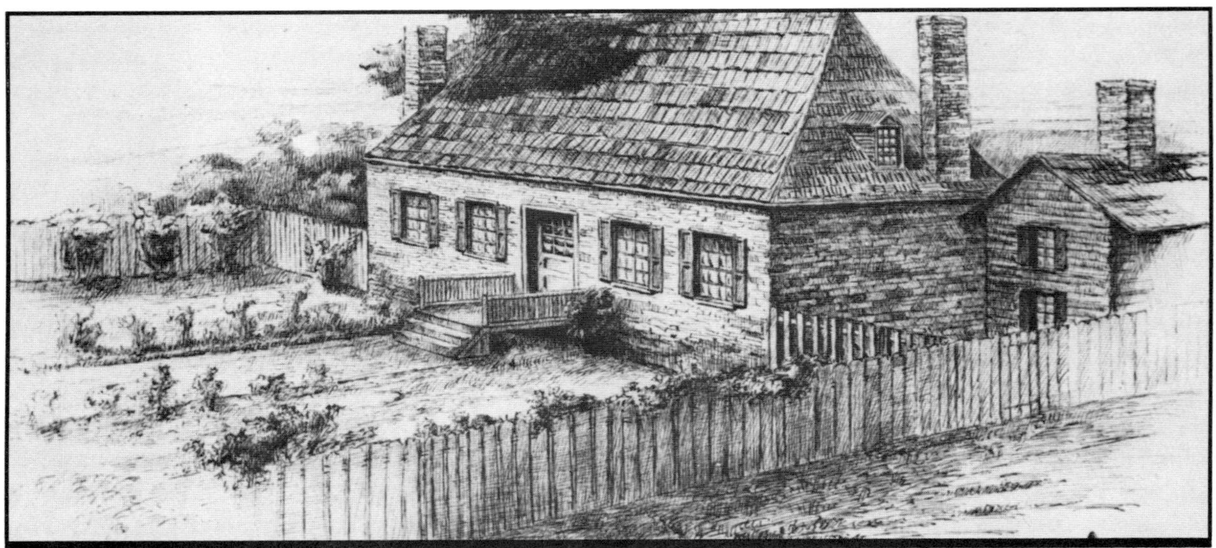

Missouri Historical Society, Saugrain residence. Ink drawing by C. Hoblitzelle, 1887, 22, 29.
Saugrain residence

cian. Two years after his arrival in town, he and the other local doctors were busy combatting an epidemic of malaria, which claimed a number of lives.[20] From Gallipolis, the Saugrains moved to Louisville and then to St. Louis in 1800.

The Spanish administration at New Orleans in 1801 decided that St. Louis had reached the importance justifying a hospital and a government physician. Dr. Saugrain was appointed physician at a salary of $30 a month.[21] The twelve-bed hospital was for military personnel exclusively. The exact location is not known. It did not survive the transfer of the Louisiana Territory to the United States, and it left no immediate successor.

3. Medical Aspects of the Lewis and Clark Expedition

In 1804, Dr. Saugrain had an opportunity to place his knowledge and skills at the service of the American government. President Thomas Jefferson had for some time been considering the exploration of an overland route to the Pacific coast. The transfer to the United States by France of its vast trans-Mississippi territory made this project timely and essential. Careful planning, of a quality perhaps not equalled until the moon voyages of the 1960s, preceded this ambitious venture into an unknown world.

The exploring party, in going out and returning, would have to traverse almost 5,000 miles of unmapped territory, including two lofty mountain ranges. Whether the Indian tribes they would encounter would be friendly or hostile was an unknown factor. The party would have to carry with them a minimum stock of food and medicine, counting on supplementing this supply from natural sources. Once past the Mandan villages in present North Dakota, the expedition would lose contact with its base of operations; thus there would be no possibility of correcting planning errors.

To lead the expedition, President Jefferson chose Captain Meriwether Lewis, who picked as his co-leader Captain William Clark. Both were professional army men. Many of the rank and file members were selected at various army posts. The maintenance of the health of the men was a major planning concern, in which President Jefferson personally took a hand. The president was well informed on medical matters, as on other scientific subjects, and had an excellent medical library.[22] For two years prior to the start of the trip, he had instructed Lewis, who had been brought to the White House to serve as his private secretary, in medical science. Both Lewis and Clark had enjoyed some practical experience in health care, since as army officers they had been responsible for the well-being of the troops under their command in the absence of an assigned physician.

The president also arranged to have Lewis spend some time in Philadelphia in order to receive from Dr. Benjamin Rush, America's leading physician, instructions for preserving the health of the men, and suggestions of medicines and medical equipment to be used on the trip.[23] Dr. Rush summarized part of his instructions in a list of ten simple rules which he prepared.

A supply of an emergency ration, consisting of meat and other ingredients, boiled down to a thick consistency and packed in cans, was ordered.[24] This was an early version of the "C" ration of World War II and was to be used only when game was unobtainable.

While the exploring party in May 1804 was encamped at Wood River, Illinois, opposite the junction of the Missouri and Mississippi rivers, in final training for the trip, Captain Lewis visited in St. Louis with Dr. Saugrain.[25] With the doctor, Lewis undoubtedly talked about health problems that would likely arise among the men. He would want to know also

what vegetation that he might find on the trip had medicinal value. Since St. Louis was the headquarters for the government of Upper Louisiana and the base of operations for fur trading and exploring parties, it was the logical place for Lewis to acquire the desired information. Dr. Saugrain, who served as post physician under both the Spanish and American regimes and had made a specialty of using local plants and herbs in his practice, was the best qualified person to assist Captain Lewis.

The medicines which Lewis and Clark received from Philadelphia upon Dr. Rush's recommendation, with the theory governing their use, comprised a compendium of standard American medical practice in the first decade of the nineteenth century.

The ideas of Dr. Benjamin Rush dominated medical thinking of his time. Rush held that disorders of the vascular system were the causes of febrile diseases, and that the universally effective remedy was depletion of the blood supply by artificial blood-letting. Expressed in Rush's own words, the theory was that

> the higher grades of fever depend upon morbid and excessive action in the blood-vessels. It is connected, of course, with preternatural sensibility in their muscular fibers. The blood is the most powerful irritant which acts upon them. By abstracting a part of it, we lessen the principal cause of the fever.[26]

In addition to blood-letting, Rush advocated other depleting measures such as sweating, vomiting and purging. His mode of treatment called for the restoration of the body's resources by the use of stimulants, following the elimination of the morbid agents.

The medical supplies from Philadelphia comprised some forty-seven separate items,[27] falling into three main categories: medicines, flavoring agents and medical accessories. The initial item on the medical list was fifteen pounds of Peruvian bark, also known as cinchona. The bark contains many alkaloids; one of these, quinine, is effective in fighting malaria.[28] Ample provision was made for the possibility that the restricted diet of the men might promote constipation. Besides fifty dozen bilious pills, concocted according to Dr. Rush's prescription, each with ten to fifteen grains of calomel and jalap,[29] the expedition's medicine chest contained sizable quantities of jalap, rhubarb, cream of tartar, Glauber's salts, magnesia, calomel, ipecacuan, and asafetida.[30] Two pounds of sal nitri or saltpetre were available for treating fevers and possibly gonorrhea.[31] Mercury, the standard remedy for syphilis, was stocked in the form of calomel and also as a mercurial ointment.[32] A quantity of white vitriol (zinc sulphate) and sugar of lead (lead acetate) was brought along to be used in a solution for treating the various eye ailments of Indians encountered along the route.[33] Balsam traumat (or compound tincture of benzoin) was used to cure abrasions and other surface wounds.[34]

A pocket set of surgical instruments and a set of instruments for dental work were carried in the medicine chest. The stock of equipment also included three lancets for artificial blood-letting and four syringes for irrigation of venereal infections.[35]

With this meager stock of old-fashioned drugs and a few plants garnered from the countryside, Lewis and Clark, serving as physicians as well as expedition leaders, were able to bring back their whole party safely, with the exception of a single member.

Although Dr. Saugrain assisted in planning the medical aspects of the Lewis and Clark expedition, it should not be assumed that he agreed with the Rush method of treatment. Dr. Saugrain had an unfavorable opinion of bleeding.[36] The tradition is that Dr. Saugrain relied heavily on medicinal herbs, which he grew in his own garden; however, he also used the traditional chemical drugs.[37]

Dr. Saugrain is remembered for his role in introducing the practice of vaccination in St. Louis. A case of smallpox had appeared in St. Louis the year after Dr. Saugrain arrived[38] and from that time on the dreaded disease paid occasional visits to the city. While practicing previously at Gallipolis, Ohio, he had treated smallpox with inoculation. In an advertisement in the St. Louis *Missouri Gazette* of June 7, 1809, Dr. Saugrain informed "such physicians and other intelligent persons as reside beyond the limits of his accustomed practice, that he will with much pleasure, on application, furnish them with the Vaccine infection." He generously stated that persons "in indigent circumstances, paupers and Indians will be vaccinated and attended gratis." He gave a comparative description of the effects of smallpox, inoculated smallpox and vaccination. Regarding the advantages of the latter he declared:[39]

> Vaccination is an infallible preventive of the Small pox, always mild, free from pain or danger, never fatal; not contagious. No eruption but where vaccinated. No confinement, loss of time or expense necessary. No precaution — no medicine required. No consequent deformity. No subsequent disease. It is passing over a safe bridge.

4. *Slow Growth of St. Louis Under the Spanish Regime*

The village of St. Louis grew very slowly during the forty years of Spanish administration. A major migration to St. Louis of French settlers from the Illinois country had occurred in 1765; other French habitants on the east side moved to New Orleans. As a consequence, the former French villages were abandoned, thus extinguishing this source of possible enlargement of St. Louis's population.

It was not until the end of the eighteenth century that the western movement of American settlements passed through Illinois and Kentucky and reached the Mississippi.[40] While there was abundant land east of the river, Americans were reluctant to expatriate themselves by becoming Spanish subjects. Since the official Spanish policy barred the conduct of non-Catholic church services or the performance of marriages and baptisms by Protestants,[41] American newcomers would have had to forego freedom of worship. Frederick Billon estimated that by 1804, St. Louis had grown into a village of 925 residents, mostly French, and contained 181 buildings.[42]

5. Changes Produced
by American Immigration

With the transfer of sovereignty over Upper Louisiana in March 1804, the tide of American immigration to St. Louis mounted. The new citizens were mostly from Kentucky and Illinois. Their life styles were vastly different from those of the French Creoles. Under the impact of this influx, important changes were wrought in the customs of French St. Louis with its medieval land system, its union of church and state, and its cooperative system of life.

Gradually the common fields system of agriculture was abandoned. The American farmer preferred to own and live on his individual piece of land, and did not greatly mind the isolation this often entailed. Land, which under the common fields system had been valued solely because of its use in the production of food, became a species of wealth, subject to widespread speculation. The union of the Catholic church with the government administration under the Spanish regime was replaced by religious pluralism and freedom of worship. Commercial and professional pursuits rose to predominance over farming and handicrafts as major occupations.

The French emphasis upon gracious living and the enjoyment of such simple satisfactions as music, dancing, good food, fashionable clothes and social intercourse was outmoded by the new quest for wealth, power and prestige. The quest was conducted in a congenial society which encouraged freedom, individualism and competition.

The Americans brought progress and many social improvements. Among the less desirable characteristics introduced was the tradition of military action and violence, established during the long period of Indian warfare. This was exemplified in the gentleman's code of honor, the observance of which spawned frequent duels, which took the lives of some of the city's leading citizens.

6. The Movement of
American Doctors to St. Louis

One of the first American physicians to establish a practice west of the Mississippi River was Dr. Bernard Gaines Farrar, who was born in Goochland County, Virginia, July 4, 1785. His family moved to Kentucky shortly after his birth. At fifteen years of age, Farrar commenced his medical studies in Cincinnati in the office of a physician preceptor. He attended medical lectures at the University of Pennsylvania in Philadelphia during 1804. Farrar began his career as a physician in Frankfort, Kentucky, at twenty-one years of age.[43] Influenced by his brother-in-law John Coburn, one of the judges of the Superior Court of the Louisiana Territory, he moved to St. Louis in 1807.[44]

The location of his first office in St. Louis is unknown. In June 1809, he had his shop in Joseph Robidoux's house on Second Street; in October of that year he moved to General William Clark's residence on Main Street. In these two quarters, it is likely the doctor had only a room, which served during working hours as his office and at night as his bedroom. A chair or two, possibly a couch for examination of patients, a few books, and his medical and surgical instruments comprised the major furnishings of his room. Water had to be hauled up by cart from the nearby Mississippi River. Hot water regularly was available only in the kitchen.

Dr. Farrar made house calls in St. Louis and the surrounding country on both sides of the river.[45] To reach his patients, he rode horseback over the forest trails, his medicines and instruments in saddle bags. Traveling thus required considerable riding and path-finding skills. Particularly hazardous was the crossing of the Mississippi River during winter in a rowboat, when the stream was swift and filled with ice floes.

A young bachelor of excellent Virginia background with a growing medical practice, Dr. Farrar was one of the town's most eligible matrimonial prospects. He chose as his bride Sarah Christy, eldest daughter of Major William Christy, a former justice of the Court of Quarter Sessions and a trustee of the newly incorporated town of St. Louis.[46]

Dr. Farrar had the unfortunate distinction of being a principal in the first duel fought in the St. Louis area. In December 1810, he was the bearer of a challenge to a young lawyer, James A. Graham. Graham refused to accept the challenge, claiming that the challenger, a junior army officer accused of cheating at cards, was not a gentleman. According to the established code in such cases, Dr. Farrar then became the substitute challenger and

principal. In the exchange of fire, Graham was severely wounded and died within a year. The outcome was particularly tragic for Dr. Farrar, since Graham was a close friend.[47]

In January 1812, Dr. Farrar, in partnership with Joseph Charless, editor and publisher of the St. Louis *Louisiana Gazette,* opened an apothecary shop in a building adjoining the newspaper printing office. However, the doctor continued to practice medicine, surgery and midwifery.[48] An advantage of owning a drug shop was that it provided him a more satisfactory place for seeing his patients than a room in a boarding house. The drugstore also would give him a second source of income, supplementary to his medical fees.

In August 1812, he entered into a partnership in the practice of medicine with Dr. David V. Walker, who had just arrived in St. Louis. Dr. Walker married Matilda, the third daughter of Major Christy.[49]

Dr. Farrar's account book for 1811-1812 lists the price of venesection at fifty cents.[50] This would indicate that his medical treatment was in the tradition of Dr. Benjamin Rush. Dr. Farrar's skill and success as a surgeon were legendary in St. Louis medical circles. He performed an amputation at the thigh on George Shannon, a member of the original Lewis and Clark party, who was shot by Blackfoot Indians while on a later expedition to discover the sources of the Missouri River. Dr. Farrar also was credited with performing a pioneer bladder operation.[51]

During the War of 1812, he acted in the capacity of surgeon and soldier in the territorial volunteers during the Indian warfare in the St. Louis vicinity.[52] He served as a member of the house of representatives of the First Territorial Legislature of Missouri from 1812-1814.[53]

After more than forty years of service in St. Louis, Dr. Farrar died in the cholera epidemic of 1849. He was generally regarded as the dean of the St. Louis medical profession. Dr. Charles A. Pope, in a eulogy pronounced before the St. Louis Medical Association, declared that Dr. Farrar's acts of charity and benevolence were "unparalleled."[54]

The second war with England stimulated the growth of St. Louis. Since it was the westernmost military station, a sizable force was maintained in the area as protection of the frontier settlements against the British and Indians. After the war, many of these soldiers, both officers and men, became residents of St. Louis and the surrounding country.[55]

Indian titles to the lands north of the Missouri River were extinguished. During 1818, the government opened offices for the sale of these public lands in St. Louis and Franklin, Missouri. Thousands of families from Virginia, Kentucky and Tennessee migrated in covered wagons to this new frontier. They crossed the river by ferry at St. Louis. Some remained to make their homes in the city; more pushed on to the Boon's Lick area in the central part of the Territory of Missouri. The human tide increased when the Missouri Compromise of 1821 established the right of Southerners to take their slave property into the newly admitted state of Missouri.

The growth and prosperity of St. Louis after the war attracted additional doctors.[56] The list of newcomers and the dates of their arrival follows: Dr. Pryor Quarles, 1815; Dr. Edward S. Gantt, 1816; Dr. George P. Todsen, 1817; Dr. Arthur Nelson, 1818; Dr. Paul M. Gebert, 1819; Dr. Herman L. Hoffman, 1819; Dr. Robert Watt, 1819; Dr. Louis Beck, 1819; Dr. William Carr Lane, 1819; Dr. Richard Mason, 1820; Dr. Samuel G. J. Camp, 1820; Dr. Zeno Fenn, 1820; Dr. Samuel Merry, 1820.[57]

At first, Main Street was "Doctor's Row." Later offices were opened on the east-west streets. Two-member partnerships were frequent. Several of the doctors held foreign medical degrees. Dr. Watt was a licentiate of the Royal College of Edinburgh; Dr. Gebert held a diploma from the Faculty of Medicine at Paris.[58]

The St. Louis directory for 1821 indicated that there were thirteen physicians in active practice in the city.[59] Several, who had arrived in the previous decade, had ceased practice or moved away. With a population of approximately 5,500, this would make one doctor for 423 persons.

In a series of articles concerning the Missouri Territory, the St. Louis *Missouri Gazette* of May 24, 1817 gave the following information, which would be of particular interest to the medical fraternity:

> The diseases incident to this country are the same as in other countries of similar latitude; sudden changes of the weather are most complained of. In the low lands, contiguous to ponds and marshes, intermittents and agues prevail.[60]

The susceptibility of St. Louis to diseases of its latitude had been demonstrated two years previously when an influenza epidemic, sweeping rapidly from the east, reached St. Louis and the adjacent villages.[61]

In addition to drug shops operated by physicians and other retailers, wholesale drug firms made an early appearance in St. Louis. David W. Tuttle offered for sale, besides a general assortment of drugs, medicines and surgical instruments, a stock of shop furniture, fine dry paints, oil paints, gunpowder, paper, ink, sealing wax, shotguns, beads, knives, blue cloths and other articles.[62] J. J. Smith, Jr., and Co., in September 1821, advertised an extensive list of drugs and patent medicines, stocked in large quantities, e.g., 100 pounds of calomel and 20 pounds of mercurial ointment.[63]

By 1821, St. Louis had established a strong position as a regional health care center and as a well-stocked market for the purchase of drugs and medical supplies.

7. *Municipal Development*

On November 9, 1809, upon petition of two-thirds of the inhabitants, the village of St. Louis was incorporated as the Town of St. Louis by action of the Court of Common Pleas.[64] As a town, St. Louis was governed by five trustees. The board established a schedule of rates to be charged by ferries crossing the Mississippi River on the eastward trip. It provided for the construction of a new market house with twelve stalls at La Place d'Armes on the river front.[65] It also passed an ordinance, effective as of October 1, 1819, calling for the appointment of a clerk for the market, with broad powers of supervision, including the responsibility "to prevent all blown, unsound and unwholesome provisions from being sold or exposed for sale" within the market place.[66]

Some citizens thought the new government was not doing enough. The St. Louis *Missouri Gazette,* coincident with the choice by the Missouri legislature of St. Charles as the capital, declared editorially in its December 6, 1820 issue:

> Neither paved, nor lighted, nor cleansed, St. Louis presents to the stranger, accustomed to the order of European or Eastern towns, no inducement to remain, and to those who are its permanent inhabitants offers no comfort out of the verge of their own habitations . . . It is time that this state of things should be changed, that greedy speculation and

penurious egotism should give way to the more generous and sound policy of public improvement.

The provision of a water supply was a problem for which the trustees had no quick or easy solution. The spring-fed Mill Creek would have provided an ideal water source. But it entered the river approximately a half mile south of the original town, too far away to be tapped. Efforts to sink wells were frustrated by the thick limestone bedrock just below the surface. Auguste Chouteau, one of town's wealthiest citizens, at great expense drilled two wells through the rock; one produced no water, the second a scanty amount.[67]

To utilize the Mississippi River water, it was necessary to quarry a road along the route of present Market Street, from Main Street to the river's edge, through the high bluffs which lined the stream. The first water distribution system was privately operated. The water merchant hauled water up from the river, a barrel at a time. Customers were provided with large earthen jars in which to receive their supply.[68] The jars served as household water tanks and also as settling basins. The water generally was regarded as wholesome and potable, but it retained the telltale coffee color of its river origin.

Chapter I

The Colonial and Territorial Period

1   Walter B. Stevens, *St. Louis, The Fourth City* 1764-1909. Vol. 1 (St. Louis, The S. J. Clarke Publishing Co., 1909), pp. 20, 23.

2   Frederick L. Billon, *Annals of St. Louis in Its Early Days Under the French and Spanish Dominations* (St. Louis, 1886), pp. 15, 20-21.

3   Walter Williams and Floyd C. Shoemaker, *Missouri, Mother of the West.* Vol. 1 (Chicago, The American Historical Society, Inc. 1930), p. 66.

4   David D. March, *The History of Missouri.* Vol. 1 (New York, Lewis Historical Publishing Co., 1967), pp. 103-104.

5   Stevens, *opus cit.*, pp. 585-586; Billon, *opus cit.*, pp. 58-59.

6   Walter B. Stevens, ed., *The Building of St. Louis From Many Points of View by Notable Persons* (St. Louis, Lesan-Gould Co., 1908), p. 10.

7   Williams and Shoemaker, *opus cit.*, p. 70.

8   March, *opus cit.*, p. 114.

9   Stevens, *St. Louis, The Fourth City*, Vol. 1, p. 586.

10 Louis Houck, *A History of Missouri.* Vol. 2 (Chicago, R.R. Donnelly and Sons, 1908), p. 28.

11 Billon, *opus cit.*, pp. 389-390.

12 *Ibid*, pp. 58-59.

13 *Ibid*, p. 392.

14 *Ibid*, pp. 392-393.

15 *Ibid*, p. 476.

16 *The Encyclopedia Americana.* 1953 edition. Vol. 9. "Denis Diderot", p. 91.

17 Billon, *opus cit.*, p. 476.

18 *Ibid*, p. 476-477.

19 *Ibid*, p. 478.

20 Eldon G. Chuinard, *Only One Man Died, The Medical Aspects of the Lewis and Clark Expedition* (Glendale, California, The Arthur H. Clark Co., 1979), p. 196.

21 Stevens, *St. Louis, The Fourth City*, Vol. 1, pp. 585-586.

22 Chuinard, *opus cit.*, p. 165.

23 *Ibid*, p. 111.

24 *Ibid*, pp. 160-161.

25 Although there is no absolute proof of the meeting of Capt. Lewis and Dr. Saugrain, a mass of circumstantial evidence and a continuing tradition in the Saugrain family have persuaded Dr. Chuinard, in his recently published study, *Only One Man Died, the Medical Aspects of the Lewis and Clark Expedition,* to accept it as a fact.

26 Chuinard, *opus cit.*, p. 72.

27 The list of drugs purchased from Philadelphia was as follows: 15 lb. Pulv. Cort. Peru; 1/2 lb. Pulv. Jalap; 1/2 lb. Rhubarb; 4 oz. Pulv. Ipecacuan; 2 lb. Pulv. Crem. Tart; 2 oz. Gum Camphor; 1 lb. Gum Assafoetic; 1/2 lb. Opii Turk. opt; 1/4 lb. Tragacanth; 4 oz. Laudanum; 2 lb. Ung. Basilic Flav.; 1 lb. Ung. e lap Cailmin.; 1 lb. Ung. Epispastric; 1 lb. Ung. Mercuriale; 1. Emplast. Diach. S.; 1. Set Pocket Insts. small; 1 Set Teeth; 1. Clyster Syringe: 6 lbs. Sal Glauber; 2 lbs. Sal. Nitri; 2 lbs. Copperas; 6 oz. Sacchar. Saturn. opt; 4 oz. Calomel; 1 oz. Tartar Emetic; 4 oz. Vitriol Alb., 1/2 lb. Columbo Rad., 1/2 lb. Elix.

    Vitriol; 1/2 lb. Ess. Meth. pip.; 1/4 lb. Blas. Copaiboe; 1/4 lb. Bals. Traumat.; 2 oz. Magnesia; 1/4 lb. Indian Ink; 2 oz. Gum Elastic; 2 oz. Nutmegs; 2 oz. Cloves; 4 oz. Cinnamon; 4. Penis do.; 3. Best Lancets; 1. Tourniquet; 2 oz. Patent Lint; 50 doz. Bilious Pills to Order of Dr. Rush; 6 Tin Canisters; 3 8 oz. Gd. Stopd. bottles; 5 4 oz. Tinctures do; 6 4 oz. Salt Mo.; 1 Walnut Chest; 1 Pine do. (Chuinard. *opus cit.*, pp. 153-154).

28 Chuinard, *opus cit.*, pp. 156-157.

29 *Ibid*, pp. 155-156.

30 *Ibid*, pp. 158-159.

31 *Ibid*, p. 156.

32 *Ibid*, pp. 153-154, 158.

33 *Ibid*, pp. 157-158.

34 *Ibid*, p. 159.

35 *Ibid*, pp. 153-154.

36 *Ibid*, p. 205.

37 *Ibid*, p. 202.

38 Stevens, *St. Louis, The Fourth City*, Vol. 1, p. 586.

39 St. Louis *Missouri Gazette*, June 7, 1809, p. 3:2-3.

40 Billon, *opus cit.*, p. 257.

41 Duane Meyer, *The Heritage of Missouri, A History* (St. Louis, Mo., State Publishing Co., Inc., 1973), p. 105.

42 Billon, *opus cit.*, p. 76.

43 Frederick L. Billon, *Annals of St. Louis in Its Territorial Days From 1804 to 1821* (St. Louis, Printed for the Author, 1888), p. 240.

44 *Idem.*

45 St. Louis *Missouri Gazette*, June 7, 1909, p. 1:4.

46 Billon, *Annals of St. Louis in Its Territorial Days From 1804 to 1821*, p. 241.

47 Louis Houck, *A History of Missouri*, Vol. 3 (Chicago, R R. Donnelly and Sons Co., 1908). pp. 75-76.

48 St. Louis *Louisiana Gazette*, Jan. 18, 1812, p. 3:2.

49 Billon, *Annals of St. Louis in Its Territorial Days From 1804 to 1821*, p. 240-241.

50 Chuinard, opus cit., p. 75.

51 Stevens, *St. Louis, The Fourth City 1764-1909*, Vol. 1, pp. 587-588.

52 St. Louis Missouri Gazette, Sept. 26, 1812, p. 3:3.

53 Billon *Annals of St. Louis in Its Territorial Days From 1804 to 1821*, p. 44.

54 Stevens, *St. Louis, The Fourth City 1764-1909*, p. 588.

55 Billon, *Annals of St. Louis in Its Territorial Days From 1804 to 1821*, p. 24.

56 Prior to the ending of the War of 1812 the following physicians joined Drs. Saugrain and Farrar in practice in St. Louis: Dr. J. M. Read, 1811; Dr. Robert Simpson, 1812; Dr. David Walker, 1812. The following towns were served during the first three decades of the nineteenth century by the physicians mentioned: Ste. Genevieve, Drs. Walter Fenwick, Aaron Elliott and Lewis F. Linn; Cape Girardeau, Drs. Zenas Priest, Thomas Neale, John C. Duncan and Dr. Blumenau; New Madrid, Dr. Robert A. Dawson; St. Charles, Dr. Andrew Wilson and Drs. Wheeler and Stoddard; Franklin, Drs. Hardage Lane, J. J. Lowry, D. P. Wilcox, Jabez Hubbard, Charles Kavanaugh, J. B. Benson and David Woods; Columbia, Drs. James H. Bennett, William H. Duncan, William Jewell, James W. Moss, William Provines, Alexander M. Robinson and D. P. Wilcox. A number of these doctors were active in

politics and served in local, state and national legislative bodies. (Houck, *History of Missouri,* Vol. 3, pp. 80-83).

57 Billon, *Annals of St. Louis in Its Territorial Days From 1804 to 1821,* p. 164.

58 St. Louis *Missouri Gazette.* Jan. 1, 1819, p. 3:5; *ibid.,* March 24, 1819, p. 3:2.

59 St. Louis *City Directory 1854-55,* With 1821 Reprint (St. Louis, Chambers and Knapp Printers, 1854), p. 261.

60 Intermittents and agues were contemporary names for malarial fever.

61 St. Louis *Missouri Gazette,* Jan. 13, 1815, p. 3:4.

62 *Ibid.,* May 26, 1819, p. 1:3.

63 *Ibid.,* Sept. 21, 1821, p. 4:2.

64 Billon, *Annals of St. Louis in Its Territorial Days From 1804 to 1821,* p. 21.

65 *Ibid.,* pp. 21-22.

66 St. Louis *Enquirer,* Sept. 25, 1819, p. 2:4.

67 Billon, *Annals of St. Louis in Its Early Days Under the French and Spanish Dominations,* pp. 83-84.

68 Henry Shaw, "St. Louis 1819," Missouri Botanical Garden *Bulletin,* Vol. 14, No. 6, June 1926. p. 89.

Chapter 2

Foundation of Health Services in St. Louis, 1821-1848

1. St. Louis as a City

IN DECEMBER 1822, the newly-organized state legislature enacted a law incorporating St. Louis. The population of the city at this time was approximately 5,500. The first municipal officers were elected on April 7, 1823. Dr. William Carr Lane was chosen mayor. Thomas McKnight, James Kennerly, Philip Rocheblave, Archibald Gamble, William Savage, Robert Wash, James Loper, Henry Von Phul and James Laknan comprised the first board of aldermen.[1]

Lane was born in Fayette County, Pennsylvania, December 1, 1789, the son of a prominent citizen who in 1796 represented his district in the Pennsylvania senate. Young Lane at the age of thirteen entered Jefferson College, where he studied for several years. During 1805, he worked in the office of an elder brother who was the prothonotary or law clerk for Fayette County. This experience gave him a familiarity with political and legal matters which was of great value in his later career. In 1810, after two years residence, he was graduated with high honors from Dickinson College in Carlisle. The following year he began his study of medicine in the office of Dr. John Collins, a noted physician of Louisville, Kentucky.[2]

In 1813, Lane went with a regiment of Kentucky Volunteers to Fort Harrison on the Wabash, sixty miles north of Vincennes, where he served as post surgeon.[3]

After the war he spent the winter of 1815-1816 attending the medical course at the University of Pennsylvania in Philadelphia. In 1816, he was appointed post surgeon in the U.S. Army and served at Fort Harrison, on the upper Mississippi River, and at Bellefontaine, Missouri. He resigned from the army on May 3, 1819, and took up his residence in St. Louis.[4]

The charter incorporating St. Louis conferred on the city council the following powers:

> to make regulations to prevent the introduction of contagious diseases, to make quarantine laws for the purpose, and enforce the same within ten miles of the city, and within the jurisdiction of the state, to make regulations to secure the general health of the inhabi-

tants, to prevent and remove nuisances...[5]

The council was also given power "to provide the city with water" and "to erect pumps in the streets for the convenience of the inhabitants."[6]

Public health was a matter of deep concern to Mayor Lane. In an address delivered April 14, 1823, to the newly elected council, Mayor Lane recommended the appointment of a board of health, with ample power to search out and correct nuisances which he warned constituted a grave health problem.[7] He also suggested that steps be taken to eliminate obstructions to the natural system of drainage of the city through the sink holes and ravines emptying into the river. In the building of the city's north-south streets, the normal descent of rain water to the river frequently was blocked, creating stagnant pools.[8] Mayor Lane proposed the establishment of a public infirmary to take care of the health needs of immigrants and of the city's own working class.[9]

A controversy in the press regarding the healthfulness — or unhealthfulness — of St. Louis may have been in part responsible for the city council passing an ordinance on August 15, 1823, requiring doctors within the city to make regular reports to the mayor regarding deaths occurring among their patients. On the reports of deceased persons doctors were instructed to give the cause of death, age, sex, name and length of residence within the city.[10] Summaries of this information were provided to the press by the recently organized board of health, beginning with the week ending August 25, 1823.[11]

Concerned over the continued rumors of St. Louis's unhealthiness, the St. Louis *Missouri Republican* issued a challenge to their accuracy:[12]

The surveyor returns to St. Louis from his exposure in the woods; the fur trader from his year of abstemiousness; the miner from his bad diet at Fever River; and the boatman from the debility of a New Orleans voyage. These classes swell our bills of mortality. But notwithstanding, such is the innate salubrity of our position, that the amount of deaths in St. Louis will advantageously compare with those of any other town on the Western waters.

An ordinance was enacted by the council prohibiting the digging of graves within the city limits.[13] With a view of reducing the canine population — and thus the risk of hydrophobia — the council levied a tax of $2 annually on dogs.[14] On May 23, 1823, an ordinance was approved for the regulation of the St. Louis market through the establishment and enforcement of wholesome food standards. This law was strengthened in 1828.[15]

The tide of immigration moving through St. Louis increased in the 1820s. Many of the newcomers, as a result of the long trans-Atlantic voyage and the trip up the Mississippi River from New Orleans, reached the city depleted in health and finances. The charter of St. Louis did not give the city government specific authority to establish a hospital to meet this need.

In 1823, application was made to the Mother House of the Sisters of Charity in the United States at Emmitsburg, Maryland, to provide nurses to open a hospital in St. Louis. John Mullanphy had donated a lot for this purpose. Four sisters arrived on November 6, 1828. They commenced their work in a log house, containing two rooms and a kitchen, located on Spruce Street between Third and Fourth streets. The foundations for a three-story brick structure fronting on Spruce

Street were laid during 1831. The building, completed the following year, was the first hospital of its kind established west of the Mississippi River.[16]

The Sisters received help in their enterprise from St. Louis's Bishop Joseph Rosati who shared with the nurses membership in the order of St. Vincent de Paul.[17] Financial support was granted by the state legislature which on February 9, 1833, authorized the conduct of a lottery to raise $10,000 for the hospital's operations.[18] The Sisters did not have to wait long for patients to fill the additional space provided by their new building.

2. The Cholera Epidemic of 1832

The St. Louis *Beacon,* in an editorial entitled "Cholera" in its March 8, 1832 issue, warned of an approaching danger:[19]

> This terrible disease which has carried desolation and death over some of the most populous countries of the Old World — which, in the short space of fourteen years has extended through every climate, and prevailed at every season, being equally dreadful in its ravages in the cold of winter and the heat of summer, and which has swept off, as with the besom of destruction, more than fifty millions of the human family — this fell scourge of man, has made its appearance in the north of England . . .
>
> Without some Providential interposition, we may expect to see cholera in the United States during the present year.

On June 8, 1832, cholera appeared at Quebec, carried thither in the crowded holds of immigrant ships. During the first week of July, it was reported in New York City.

The St. Louis Board of Aldermen on July 7, 1832, in its initial reaction to the cholera threat, authorized the mayor to appoint one responsible individual in each of the three wards to oversee a campaign to remove all nuisances in his area. The undertaking involved cleaning and purifying streets and alleys, river shores, slaughterhouses, market places and toilet vaults. The ordinance provided no pay for the sanitary officers, but they could file for reimbursement of expenses.[20]

On July 15, 1832, General Winfield Scott wrote to Governor John Reynolds of Illinois informing him that cholera had broken out among U.S. Army troops being transported by water between Buffalo and Chicago. But he assured the governor that infected personnel were being confined to camp in the Chicago area.[21] This movement of troops brought the cholera closer to St. Louis.

On the evening of August 3, a citizens' meeting was held at the courthouse to determine a course of action. Edward Bates was called to the chair. The following resolutions were introduced and unanimously adopted.[22]

> Resolved, That in view of the approaching pestilence that has ravaged so large a portion of Asia and Europe, and is now invading our eastern cities and the northern frontier of our western valley, it is expedient that this meeting recommend to the inhabitants of the city of St. Louis a day of fasting, humiliation and prayer, to entreat the God of Providence to avert his righteous judgments.
>
> Resolved, That Friday, the 10th of August, be set apart, in accordance with the foregoing resolution, and that it be recommended to the churches and congregations in the city to meet on that

day in their respective places of worship, to humble themselves before God and supplicate his mercy, and the sanctification of the dreadful events of his Providence if it shall be his will to visit us.

A second mass meeting assembled at the town hall on the evening of September 10. General Bernard Pratte was appointed chairman of a committee charged with proposing to the Board of Aldermen measures to help ward off the approaching epidemic. The committee made five recommendations: (1) the division of the city into districts, not exceeding fourteen, with a sanitary officer, who was to be paid an adequate compensation, in charge of each district; (2) the prohibition of the sale within the city of watermelons, green corn, cucumbers, cabbage, and also fresh pork; (3) the revival and enforcement of quarantine laws; (4) the employment of enough scavengers and carts to remove nuisances and purify the various districts; (5) the negotiation of a loan to finance the proposed projects.[23]

The board of aldermen assigned to a sub-committee of its members the task of studying the suggestions from the citizens' meeting. The sub-committee rejected the ban on the sale of certain fresh vegetables as an infringement of individual freedom and preferred the issuance of a warning against the intemperate use of these foods during the epidemic. The sub-committee considered quarantine regulations as useless, except in the case of certain contagious diseases.[24] The city council, on January 18, 1832, had enacted legislation aimed at preventing the introduction of smallpox on ships from New Orleans.[25] It was commonly assumed, however, that cholera was an air-borne infection and thus able to evade barriers set up against it.

The sub-committee put its own ideas for dealing with the cholera epidemic into a draft ordinance which was passed by the board of aldermen on September 13. The ordinance called for the establishment of a board of health, consisting of the mayor, the health officer and the street commissioner.[26] Previous health boards had apparently become quiescent when the crisis, which called them into existence, had passed. The board of health was enjoined to lay off the city into districts, not exceeding six. To each district the mayor would appoint an agent to have charge of the work of removing nuisances and cleansing the city. The agents were clothed with authority to enter upon private property and, where nuisances were found, to direct the owner or owners to correct the condition. The agents were entitled to $2 per day pay for their services.[27]

The cholera was brought to St. Louis apparently by the steamboat *Winnebago*, which on September 7 stopped for a few minutes at the city wharf on its way to Jefferson Barracks, ten miles down river. The boat carried Black Hawk and twelve other chiefs of the Sac and Fox tribes, as well as American troops returning from the Indian conflict.[28] By September 18, cholera had broken out at Jefferson Barracks, taking the lives of a number of officers and men.[29] At about the same time, the pestilence manifested itself in St. Louis. The *St. Louis Beacon* of September 27, 1832, reported that in the previous ten days there had been several mild cases of cholera and two deaths, apparently from the same cause.[30] For the week ending October 4, there were four cases of cholera which ended fatally.[31] A board of health report, issued October 18, listed an unusually high number of deaths but did not identify the causes.[32] During the week which ended October 25, "the disease . . . raged with unprecedented violence."[33] However, the general opinion was that the pestilence was abating.[34]

The plan of the St. Louis Board of Health for reporting deaths broke down in the crisis. Two explanations exist for this failure. The immense amount of time spent by the doctors in making house calls on their sick patients may have prevented them from filing their reports. There is the possibility too that the local government may have withheld information, since publicizing the seriousness of the city's health problem could have brought business to a standstill.

On November 15, five of St. Louis's prominent physicians issued a statement informing their fellow citizens that the malignant cholera had disappeared from the city.[35]

3. The Improvement of St. Louis's Water Supply

By 1830, the population of St. Louis had reached 6,252.[36] The city limits had overrun the western boundary of the old town and pushed deep into the former commons and common fields. As the population grew, the demand for water increased. The method of hauling water from the river in barrels became unsatisfactory. Although the sinking of wells on the 1,000 foot incline from the river to "the Hill" had been frustrated by the limestone bedrock, the prairie region beyond "the Hill" yielded a plentiful supply of good water to homeowners who dug shallow wells. Water for private homes could also be secured by collecting in cisterns the run-off from the roofs.

These expedients, however, did not meet adequately the demands of large users, such as hotels, businesses, industries and the fire department. A public supply, that could be expanded as the city grew, was needed.

The board of aldermen on May 30, 1831, passed an ordinance authorizing the mayor to borrow the sum of $25,000 for the purpose of erecting waterworks.[37] The revenues from the operation of the waterworks and the land on which they were situated would be pledged as security for the repayment of the loan.

The site chosen for the reservoir was an Indian mound located at Ashley Street and Broadway,[38] about ten blocks north of Walnut Street. The pumping station, housing a steam engine, was placed at the foot of Bates Street,[39] within four or five blocks of the reservoir. The reservoir had a capacity of 400,000 gallons. Its elevation enabled it to supply by gravity flow the existing town. No treatment of the water occurred in the reservoir. Since the water was pumped out into the distribution system almost as fast as it reached the reservoir, little sedimentation could take place. Fortunately, the pumping site was north of the heavily settled areas of town, so contamination of the water supply from sewage and industrial wastes was minimal.

The board of aldermen, on June 19, 1832, passed an ordinance providing for the appointment by the mayor of a superintendent of the waterworks. The superintendent was empowered to negotiate contracts for periods not exceeding one year with persons wanting to be supplied with water. The household rate was based on the number of persons in the family. Charges for different kinds of businesses, e.g. hotels were set in accordance with their estimated water usage.[40] There were no water meters. The charges were flat rates, regardless of the amount of water actually used. The necessary hydrants and pipes for conveying water from the city mains to the place where it was to be used had to be provided at the expense of the consumer.[41]

Serious problems arose from the city's dependence upon a single reservoir. The periodic cleaning of mud from the bottom of the reservoir necessitated the shutting down of the waterworks for several days. The capacity of the reservoir had been enlarged by constructing a brick parapet atop the stone retaining walls. The danger of a breakage existed if the reservoir was filled to its maximum level.

In November 1840, a committee of the board of delegates[42] recommended that a new reservoir be built on a site about a mile west of the river-front reservoir. The site was ideal for distributing water throughout the city, being about five feet higher than the top of the existing basin on the Indian mound.[43] The board of aldermen, however, was dilatory in acting on the proposal. Besides, the city council's authority to levy a special tax for this purpose, without the approval of the general assembly, was in question.[44] In November 1843, the council asked the voters to choose between two alternative solutions to the municipal water issue: (1) build a new waterworks; (2) repair and enlarge the old one.[45] The citizens apparently chose the second alternative, for on July 6, 1844, the council voted to improve the existing works.[46]

In 1845, a wooden tank one hundred feet square by twelve feet deep was constructed on top of the old reservoir. Previously, a stone wall had been erected, surrounding the old basin. This wall carried the edges of the new wooden tank. Massive upright timbers, spaced about twelve feet apart throughout the lower basin, provided interior support.[47]

The improvement more than doubled the city's water supply. The new basin made it possible for the waterworks employees to clean one reservoir without depriving the city of water.

4. The Development of a Medical Profession

Important changes occurred in the medical profession of St. Louis in the decades immediately following the admission of Missouri as a state in 1821. The medical fraternity, which in 1821 numbered thirteen, had grown to a group of 188 by 1854.[48] Approximately seventy percent of these doctors traced their origins to the border states and the states of the Deep South.[49]

The trend during the period was toward a higher level of medical training and skill. Although most doctors had acquired a major part of their training through the preceptorial system, many were adding sufficient instruction in medical colleges to secure their diplomas. The medical school of the University of Pennsylvania was the goal of the most ambitious students. Others attended the medical departments of Transylvania University in Lexington, Kentucky, of the University of Louisville, and of Cincinnati College. A few had the advantage of graduate study and clinical observation at the famous medical schools and hospitals of London, Dublin, Edinburgh and Paris.

The St. Louis doctors were men of broad versatility and many interests. They engaged actively and successfully in politics. On the controversial issues of the day, e.g. slavery, they were found hotly defending their positions.

The leader of the profession in St. Louis was Dr. Bernard G. Farrar, whose career, beginning in 1807, had continued on an uninterrupted upward course. But he had many able peers.

Dr. William Carr Lane, after being elected St. Louis's first mayor in 1823, was reelected for five succeeding terms; he was elected also in 1838 and 1839.[50] He served in the Missouri House of Representatives during the sessions of 1826-1827, 1830-1831 and 1832-1833.[51] Beginning his career in politics as a Democrat,[52] he broke with Andrew Jackson over his populist policies and joined the Whig party.[53] A defender of the institution of slavery, he served as chairman of a meeting at the courthouse on October 27, 1835, at which a vigilance committee was appointed to oppose the spread of abolitionist propaganda.[54] Illustrating the wide range of interests in which doctors invested their surplus funds, Lane was the owner and operator of the largest gunpowder factory in the St. Louis area.[55]

Dr. Samuel Merry, who had recently arrived from Virginia, was admitted into partnership with Dr. Lane in 1821. Like his professional associate, he had a love of politics. He was a Democrat in political affiliation. Beginning in the fall of 1830, he served two terms in the Missouri Senate as a representative of St. Louis County. For a number of years, under appointment by President Andrew Jackson, he held the position of Receiver of Public Moneys for the land district of St. Louis.[56] Dr. Merry was the winner in the race for mayor in 1833 but was deprived of the office by the board of aldermen because he was holding a federal job.[57]

During the latter part of his service years, Dr. William Beaumont, a regular army surgeon, was stationed at Jefferson Barracks. About 1836, Dr. Beaumont resigned from the army and made his home in St. Louis, where he quickly built up a large and lucrative practice. In 1833 his book, *Physiology of Digestion and Experiments on the Gastric Juice,* had been published and had won him worldwide fame. The book described his observations of the digestive process in the

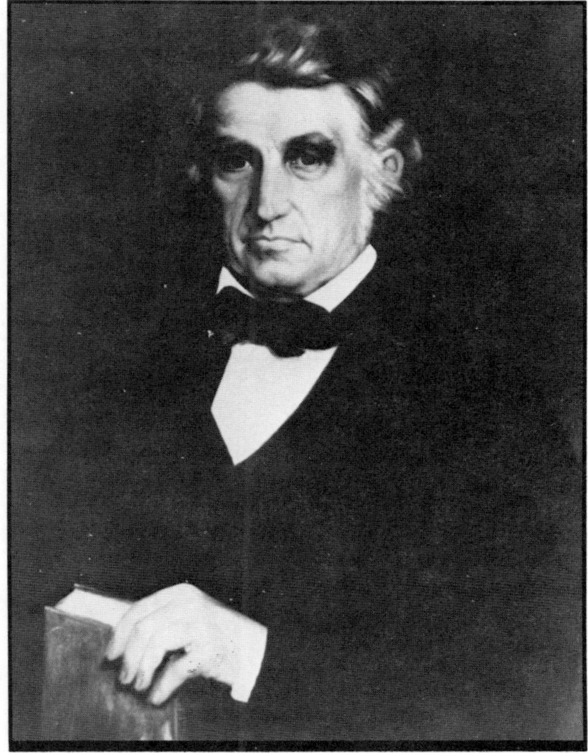

Courtesy of the State Historical Society of Missouri. Permission to use the Chester Harding portrait of Beaumont was given by the Archives, Washington University School of Medicine.
Dr. William Beaumont

stomach of Alexis St. Martin, a Canadian boatman, who suffered a gunshot wound which in healing left a peephole into the stomach's interior.[58]

With impressive credentials and connections, Dr. Joseph Nash McDowell arrived on the St. Louis scene in 1838. A nephew of Dr. Ephraim McDowell, who in 1809 had performed the first successful ovariotomy, and a brother-in-law of the famous Dr. Daniel Drake, he had taken an active part in the founding of two medical colleges and had served as professor of anatomy at Cincinnati College. His ambition was to establish in St. Louis the first medical college west of the Mississippi,[59] in which he would be the distinguished professor of surgery.

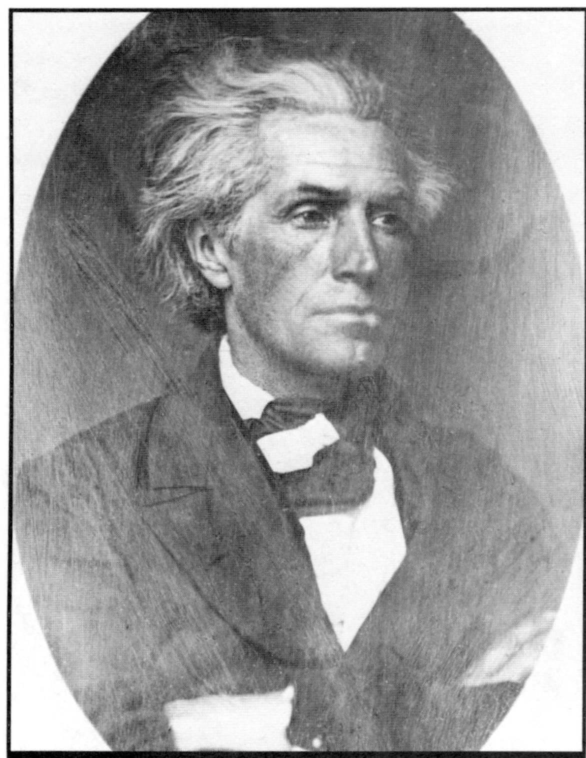

Missouri Historical Society. Dr. Joseph Nash McDowell, dag. by Fitzgibbon Por-M-103.
Dr. Joseph Nash McDowell

McDowell was a forceful speaker, utilizing the windy oratorical style of the times. He did not confine himself to medical subjects, but spoke on all the controversial issues. One of his favorite theses was that Britain was the instigator of abolitionist agitation in the United States, her purpose being to destroy the slave-based economy of the South, the cotton production of which competed in world markets with that of the East India Company.[60]

A well-educated native of Maryland, Dr. Stephen W. Adreon joined the medical profession of St. Louis in 1832. He combined a successful medical practice with service on the city council under Mayors Luther M. Kennett, Washington King and Oliver D. Filley. As pres-

ident of the board of health, Dr. Adreon contributed importantly to the development of that department. He also served as municipal health officer.[61]

Dr. John S. Moore was born in Orange County, North Carolina, in 1807. He received an excellent general education, attested by A. B. and M. A. degrees from Cumberland College, Princeton, Kentucky. He read medicine in the office of Dr. G. B. Taylor in Mansfield, Kentucky. In 1836, he received a diploma in medicine from Cincinnati Medical College, where he was a favorite pupil of Dr. Joseph N. McDowell. After a short period of practice in Pulaski, Tennessee, Moore joined Dr. McDowell in the task of establishing the first medical school in St. Louis, popularly known as "McDowell's College." He was a member of the first faculty of the college and continued to teach there until McDowell's death. He was an active member of the St. Louis Medical Society.[62]

Dr. Charles Alexander Pope, of Alabama background, entered the profession of St. Louis in 1842 with the finest medical education available in the United States and Europe. He had studied under Dr. Daniel Drake at Cincinnati Medical College, had taken his diploma from the University of Pennsylvania, and then spent several years in advanced study in medical schools in France, England and Ireland. He played a major role in the founding of the Medical Department of St. Louis University which was generally called "Pope's College."[63]

Seven years of practice in Kentucky, followed by two years of study in the best medical schools and hospitals of Europe, were cited by Dr. J. V. Prather in his advertisement in the _St. Louis Missouri Argus_ of September 4, 1835. Dr. Prather stated that he was skilled in the use of auscultation for diagnosing diseases of the heart and lungs.[64] He was proba-

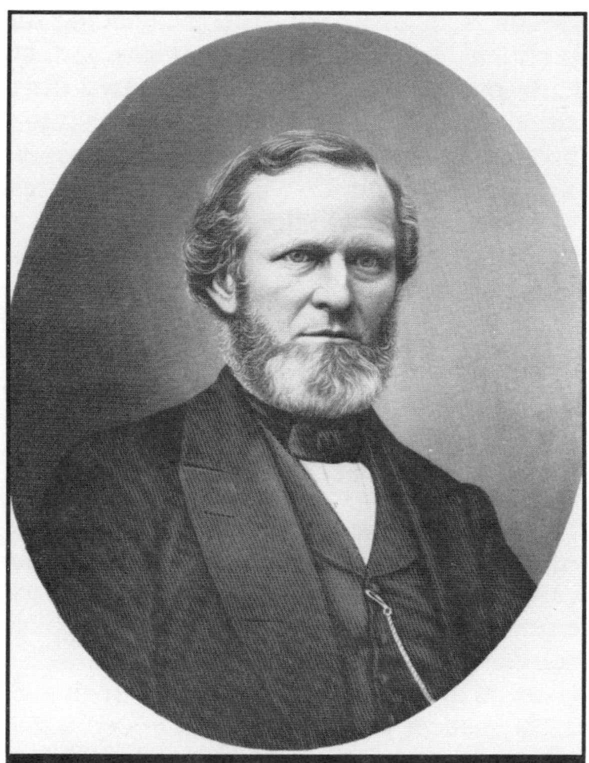

Coutresy of the State Historical Society of Missouri.
Dr. Charles A. Pope

bly the pioneer in introducing this technique, widely used in Europe, in St. Louis medical practice.

John Bates Johnson was born in Fairhaven, Massachusetts, April 26, 1817. He began his study of medicine in the office of Dr. Lyman Bartlett in 1835. Johnson graduated from Berkshire Medical College in 1840, and subsequently was honored with a medical degree from Harvard University. He served a year on the staff of the Massachusetts General Hospital where he associated with the leading physicians of Boston. He came to St. Louis in 1841.[65]

Although the large majority of doctors continued to offer their services in the whole range of practice — medicine, surgery and obstetrics — signs of specialization had begun to appear. One of the first physicians to announce a professional preference was Dr. William Van Zandt, an eye and ear specialist, who began service in St. Louis in 1835.[66] Dr. R. Simmons[67] in 1837 and Dr. F. Knox the following year started to confine their practice to diseases of women and children. Dr. Wilder, in 1841, announced that his special concern was orthopedic surgery.[68]

Women began to offer their medical services. Mrs. Cail, a practical midwife, in July 1837, announced that she had been trained in the Lying-In Institution of Dublin and had acquired ten years experience delivering babies in the United States.[69] Madame Uranie Trouette, with a diploma as an accoucheuse from the faculty of medicine in Paris in 1842, offered her medical assistance not only in midwifery but in the general field of women's diseases.[70] Women had been acting as midwives in St. Louis long before these instances, but previously had not resorted to the press to announce their availability.

As early as 1820, a small group of St. Louis doctors met regularly at the city hall to consider their common problems. However, as the number of doctors increased, the need was felt for a formal organization which would embrace not only the older, established practitioners but also the newer entrants into the local profession. On January 2, 1830, a standing committee consisting of Drs. John Woolfolk, Horace Gaither and H. L. Hoffman issued a call for a meeting of the medical society of St. Louis on Monday evening, January 4. The announced purpose of the meeting was "the cultivation of Medical Science."[71] Drs. Woolfolk and Gaither had arrived in St. Louis a few months previously. Hoffman, a druggist as well as doctor, had been in St. Louis since 1819.[72] This effort to establish a professional organization apparently failed.

A second effort, backed by the entire medical fraternity of St. Louis, numbering twenty physicians, was made in 1835. On Christmas evening of that year, the group held its first meeting at the Masonic Hall, Third and Elm streets. A committee for drafting a constitution was set up. At a second meeting at the Masonic Hall on January 7, 1836, the doctors "agreed to bind themselves by a charter which would govern their professional lives."[73] The new association, obviously hoping to become more than a mere local organization, called itself "The Medical Society of Missouri." In the choice of officers, Dr. Bernard Farrar was elected president. He appointed Dr. William Beaumont as chairman of the group's membership committee with responsibility for investigating and evaluating the qualifications of all prospective members.

In carrying out their aim to separate themselves from the widespread quackery in St. Louis, the medical society attacked two of its offensive practices — misleading advertisements and patent medicines. Cynthia De Haven Pitcock, in her article "Doctors in Controversy," in the *Missouri Historical Review* of April 1966, gives the rationale for the medical society's campaign:[74]

> Fraudulent medical practitioners customarily collected a fee for routine examination of a patient and then imposed an additional charge for a miracle tonic or pills which were kept in ready supply. These creators and peddlers of patent medicines advertised their wares as a cure for a variety of ills and prescribed them indiscriminately. The medical society ruled that both practices — advertising and the dispensing of drugs — were unethical.

This position of the society represented a considerable renunciation of privilege by the members. A number of them, including the president, Dr. Bernard Farrar, at least in their early professional days, had operated drugstores as well as practiced medicine. Most had placed advertisements in the newspapers announcing the availability of their services. The society's prohibition was aimed only at extravagant claims, as the following provision from its by-laws indicated:[75]

> No person . . . shall by publication in a newspaper or otherwise announce his pretensions to superior qualifications in the ascertainment and cure of any particular disease or diseases.

One of the first members of the society to run afoul of the advertising prohibition ironically was the chairman of its own special committee for developing improved ethical standards.

Dr. William Beaumont, in the spring of 1839, made it known that he intended taking an associate into his private practice. Several young doctors definitely were interested. Dr. Joseph Nash McDowell, on the basis of training and experience, appeared to be the logical choice. However, Beaumont rejected his petition for a partnership and selected Dr. James Sykes, a young doctor of lesser qualifications. Dr. Beaumont apparently was seeking an assistant, not a full partner.[76]

Dr. Sykes, anxious that the public be informed promptly of the new arrangement, drafted an announcement for the press which Beaumont, after a superficial examination, approved. Sykes, in his advertisement in the *St. Louis Missouri Republican* of March 19, 1839, stated that he had gained "much experience in Ophthalmic surgery" and would be able "to afford effectual relief in most of the diseases of the eye."[77] The young doctor's advertised estimate of his professional competence obviously was inflated.

For April 12, 1839, a special session of the society was arranged to consider Sykes's offense. Dr. Beaumont, who originally was only indirectly involved, chose to side with his associate in defending the advertisement.[78]

During the time between the first publication of the advertisement and the extraordinary session of April 12, the society appointed a committee to investigate the issue and make recommendations. The committee, headed by Dr. Franklin Knox, reported to the session of April 12 that they found Beaumont and Sykes acted in violation of the society's by-laws in regard to advertising. In the discussion of the committee report, conducted while Beaumont and Sykes waited outside the meeting room, Dr. Knox led the faction demanding the expulsion of the two erring doctors. The report, after a stormy debate, was tabled, and the chairman of the meeting called for another session on May 3.[79]

On the day following the April 12 meeting, Drs. Beaumont and Sykes called on Dr. Joseph N. McDowell, the society's recording secretary, and asked permission to read the minutes of the meeting. McDowell injudiciously showed them the notes he had taken during the debate, and also described the arguments in detail, recalling the speeches of each member in the closed session. Prominent among the enemies of the two accused doctors, according to McDowell, were Stephen W. Adreon and E. Y. Watson.[80]

Having learned that Adreon and Watson had spoken against them, Beaumont and Sykes cut off relations with the two doctors. The hostility between the two groups became a matter of public knowledge, and the society split into opposing camps. Finally, Sykes, who had started the controversy, took the initiative in arranging a meeting of Adreon, Watson, Beaumont and himself in Beaumont's office. McDowell was invited to attend.[81]

The result of this meeting was the repudiation and isolation of McDowell. His report to Beaumont and Sykes regarding the happenings at the closed meeting of April 12 was contradicted by Adreon and Watson.[82] It is possible that the two, in the presence of Beaumont and Sykes, toned down the critical remarks which they had made earlier in the closed session. The four doctors emerged from the meeting firmly aligned against McDowell who stood charged with falsifying the record.[83]

When, at the meeting of May 3, McDowell read the controversial minutes of the earlier meeting, he was attacked by Adreon, Beaumont and Sykes, who accused him of misrepresenting the facts. His honor impugned and, with the society apparently solidly against him, McDowell requested an extraordinary session of the society to present his side of the matter. This was scheduled for June 7.[84]

Following the fight over the minutes, the society took up a pending resolution, which censured Beaumont and Sykes for the advertising offense. The mildly worded resolution, which was passed, politely requested the two physicians to discontinue the advertisement.[85]

At the June 7 meeting, Dr. McDowell presented a written statement in the form of a resolution in which he asserted that the meeting at Dr. Beaumont's office was part of a plot to victimize and discredit him. The resolution passed with only Beaumont, Sykes, Adreon and Watson voting against it.[86]

In response to McDowell's demand for a public hearing, the society appointed an investigating committee which took testimony from the parties involved in the McDowell affair. The committee completed its investigation in early July and made its report. On July 8, after discussing the committee's findings, the society adopted the following resolution.[87]

> Resolved that it is the opinion of the Medical Society . . . that the conduct of Dr. J. N. McDowell . . . has been highly reprehensible. It is further resolved . . . that Drs. Beaumont and Sykes are . . . not guilty of any dishonorable conduct towards McDowell.

Following the adoption of the resolution, McDowell was asked to resign his office as recording secretary. As the question of his continuing membership in the society was about to be discussed, McDowell rose to his feet and made verbal resignation of his association with the society. He left the hall alone.[88]

The McDowell affair had important consequences. The public image of the medical society was tarnished. Serious flaws of character were revealed in the key figures involved in the controversy. Finally, the development of medical education in St. Louis was largely determined by the outcome of the matter.

Beaumont's triumph was only temporary. Within less than a year, Beaumont himself was to suffer public discredit and humiliation. Like events in an ancient Greek tragedy, his triumph and his humiliation were interconnected.

On November 5, 1840, one of the most famous murder trials in the city's history began in the St. Louis Criminal Court; before it ended the suspicion of malpractice had been raised against a well-known St. Louis surgeon.

The train of events leading up to the trial resembles the scenario of a Hollywood movie: a libelous attack on a respectable citizen published in the local paper; rumors of revenge reverberating in the town; a meeting at High Noon on one of the busiest streets between the newspaper publisher and the aggrieved citizen; finally a savage attack with a lead-headed cane that brought death to a person, who, until the published insult, had been a close friend of the assailant.

The setting for the tragedy was the "Log Cabin and Cider Campaign" of 1840. The major issue which had emerged was whether the country should have a new national bank to replace the one that President Andrew Jackson had destroyed. The Van Buren Democrats generally were opposed. However, in St. Louis a splinter group of pro-bank Democrats emerged. The group was headed by Dr. Thomas J. White, president; William P. Darnes, secretary; and C. C. Carroll, chairman.[89] Darnes, a native of Virginia, was a young workingman, who had made a name for himself in the Democratic organization before his defection. Through his own efforts, he had acquired a good education and gained acceptance in the polite social circles of St. Louis.

In the early summer of 1840, the St. Louis *Argus*, a Democratic paper under the new management of Andrew Jackson Davis as owner and William Gilpin, editor, began to attack the leaders of the pro-bank splinter group.[90] The attacks, in line with the gutter journalism of the time, were of a libelous nature.

On May 30, Darnes wrote a note to Davis asking if the abusive language in the *Argus* applied to him personally. He got his reply, not in a conciliatory communication from his former friend Davis, but in the following column of the *Argus*.[91]

> June 1, 1840, a fellow by the name of WPD, a common street loafer and vagabond, and fit subject for the vagrant

act had the impudence, on Saturday last to send a note by Thornton Grimsley to the proprietor of the *Argus,* Andrew J. Davis, asking from him the meaning of certain phrases of ours, which appeared in the paper that morning.

The blackguard style in which the note was couched, and the degraded character of the fellow who put his name to it as the author, rendered it necessary, of course, that it should be returned to Mr. Grimsley without a reply. None but a jackass or poltroon would think of calling for explanation of the meaning of an article, deemed offensive except by making application to its known and acknowledged author.

Darnes and Davis met about 2 P.M., June 1, in the center of Market Street in the vicinity of the National Hotel. After a few minutes conversation, during which Davis may have said something that provoked Darnes further, Darnes struck him with his hand and followed up with repeated blows upon Davis's head with his cane. Davis, bleeding profusely, was carried into the National Hotel. Dr. Thomas McMartin arrived quickly from his nearby office. Dr. Sykes was next on the scene. Since Dr. Sykes's specialty was diseases of the eye and ear, he suggested that his partner, Dr. Beaumont, be called, and this was done. Davis was removed to the Sisters' Hospital, where intensive care would be available.[92]

The preliminary examination by Drs. McMartin and Sykes revealed four major wounds, all on the left side of Davis's head. The first was upon the prominentia frontalis in the forehead area. This was a compound fracture, with the skin as well as bone broken. It was a pointed fracture, the center of the depression being lower than the margin. The second fissure was near the median line of the forehead. The skin and muscles were broken through. The third fracture was found upon the left   temple. Here the skull was shattered into a number of small pieces and was depressed upon the brain. The fourth injury was a fracture over the left ear. The muscles and skin of the ear were broken and the bones badly crushed.[93]

The initial examination indicated that Davis's sensorial functions were only slightly affected. He answered questions briefly but intelligently. When asked how he felt, he stoically said, "comfortable." The symptoms which ordinarily follow compression of the brain were not in evidence.[94]

When Dr. Beaumont arrived at the hospital, he talked with McMartin and Sykes, and then made his own survey of Davis's wounds. He concluded that an operation was immediately necessary. The fracture upon the prominentia frontalis and the one upon the left temple seemed the most dangerous since they were deeply depressed and consequently were impinging upon the brain. Using a trephine, he cut buttons of bone in the immediate vicinity of the two fractures, removed the splinters of shattered bone lying on the brain covering and elevated the depressed areas. He applied medication and bandages. For the other two fractures, he employed medication and bandages, without resorting to the use of the trephine. No attempt was made at this time to institute the customary depletion regimen of bleeding, cathartics and enemas, designed to prevent inflammation.[95]

On Thursday, June 4, Davis's condition took a turn for the worse. He exhibited a strong pulse, high fever and delirium. Dr. Sykes bled him copiously, taking thirty ounces of blood. As Davis's health continued to deteriorate, he repeatedly was bled and purged by medicine and enemas. On Friday, he suffered violent spasms and paralysis of the right side of his body. He died on Monday, one week after his beating.[96]

The trial of Darnes, in early November 1840, on manslaughter charges brought into the courtroom a number of St. Louis's leading lawyers. The case for the prosecution was presented by Peter Engle and Thomas Gantt. The defense entrusted its representation to Henry S. Geyer, Beverly Allen and Joseph B. Crockett.[97]

Geyer was a brilliant legislator and lawyer of St. Louis. As a member of the Missouri House of Representatives, he had introduced, in 1839, the Geyer Bill under the terms of which the University of Missouri was organized. He succeeded Thomas Hart Benton as U.S. Senator in 1851.[98] Geyer was the Clarence Darrow of his day, with an extraordinary ability to analyze evidence and present it to the advantage of his client.

The prosecution, after presenting witnesses to establish the facts of Darnes's assault on Davis, put on the stand Drs. McMartin, Sykes and Beaumont, who defended the medical treatment of Davis. They stressed the serious nature of Davis's wounds, particularly the two where Darnes's cane had shattered Davis's skull and depressed the bone against the surface of his brain. They agreed that the use of the trephine represented the only method of treatment offering the slightest chance of success.[99]

The defense called as its medical witnesses Drs. Thomas J. White, William Carr Lane and Franklin Knox. They testified that Beaumont and Sykes made a mistake in applying the trephine in the absence of symptoms indicating compression of the brain. The depletion program should have been instituted first, they argued. The trephine, in their judgment, was a dangerous instrument to be employed

only as a last resort. To back that point, Dr. Lane cited his own experience. Of numerous patients on whom he had used the trephine, only three or four survived.[100] The high fatality rate resulted not only from injury to the brain by the sawteeth of the trephine, but also from post-operative infections, which were rampant before the advent of antiseptic and aseptic surgery.

To what extent the defense doctors were influenced by personal considerations is impossible to determine. Dr. White was a close friend and political associate of Darnes. He and Beaumont had on occasion been involved in open rivalry in the St. Louis Medical Society.[101] Dr. Knox had an old score to settle with Beaumont and Sykes, dating back to the May 12, 1839 meeting of the medical society in connection with newspaper advertising by doctors. At that meeting, Beaumont and Sykes were admonished mildly to discontinue their notices in the paper. Dr. Knox, who also had violated the anti-advertising rule, was publicly censured. Both Beaumont and Sykes ostentatiously had joined in the vote of condemnation.[102]

Geyer, in the final argument for the defense, summarized the major points that had been raised by his side in the trial. He told of the friendship of Darnes and Davis and mentioned that Darnes, in seeking a settlement with Davis, had provided himself with a light cane — not a dangerous weapon, according to Geyer. Geyer contended that, under Missouri law, the right of self-defense was more extensive than under the English common law and included the defense of one's good name.[103]

Geyer cited the various medical authorities, mostly English, which supported the testimony of the medical witnesses for the defense. Concerned lest the international reputation of Dr. Beaumont might influence the jury in the doctor's favor, Geyer cleverly neutralized this threat. Holding in his hand a copy of Dr. Beaumont's book on digestion, he read an extract or two to demonstrate the allegedly trivial matters with which it dealt. He pointed out that Dr. Beaumont, instead of closing the wound in the stomach of Alexis St. Martin, had kept it open for years in order to carry on his observations. He added: "It was upon the same principle of curiosity that he bored a hole in Davis's head, to see what was going on in there."[104] This statement amounted to a charge that Dr. Beaumont acted on the basis of idle — if not criminal — curiosity in trephining Davis, when he might have saved his life by following the approved type of treatment. The jury found Darnes guilty of a lesser offense than that charged in the indictment.

5. A Center for Medical Education

The expulsion[105] from the local medical society did not cause Dr. Joseph N. McDowell to give up his intention to establish a medical college in St. Louis. Fortunately, his plan coincided with a cherished project of Jackson Kemper, Episcopal Missionary Bishop of the Northwest, comprising Missouri and Indiana. Aware of the difficulty of getting priests from the older states to serve in frontier parishes, he determined to establish a college which would serve as a seminary for Western youth. For the implementation of this dream, he was able to raise $20,000 in the Eastern states. A 125-acre tract, about five miles west of St. Louis, was acquired and a three-story brick edifice constructed in 1837. A charter had been secured from the legislature on January 6, 1836, specifying the broad powers and privileges of the institution, to which the lawmakers gave the name "Kemper College."[106]

The college opened in the fall of 1838, with Dr. McDowell a member of the original academic faculty. His province was the social sciences, including world history, anthropology, sociology and government.[107] In addition to his classroom duties, McDowell gave public lectures for which a fee was charged. He appeared frequently on the programs of the St. Louis Lyceum.[108] He continued, also, his practice of medicine and surgery. To establish an association with the leading doctors of St. Louis, he had joined the medical society and had taken an active role.

In the spring of 1840, plans were announced for the organization of the Medical Department of Kemper College. This department was a proprietary institution of which Dr. McDowell and his friend Dr. John S. Moore were the principal owners. The connection with Kemper College was nominal. Dr. McDowell, in April 1840, took a lease on two adjacent lots at the intersection of Ninth and Cerre streets. The location was on the south bank of Chouteau's Pond, in the general vicinity of present Union Station. He arranged for the construction of a large two-story building, with a gable roof surmounted by a small tower. The first lectures of the new institution were delivered in the fall of 1840.[109]

Since he was at odds with the local medical society, McDowell chose his faculty from outside the city. He occupied the chair of anatomy and surgery. Dr. J. W. Hall of Kentucky was chosen as professor of theory and practice of medicine. Dr. Hiram A. Prout, professor of chemistry and botany in Lagrange College, Alabama, became professor of materia medica and medical botany. Dr. Prout was a noted paleontologist; he assisted in the organization of the St. Louis Academy of Science. Dr. John S. Moore of Tennessee, a former pupil of Dr. McDowell's at Cincinnati

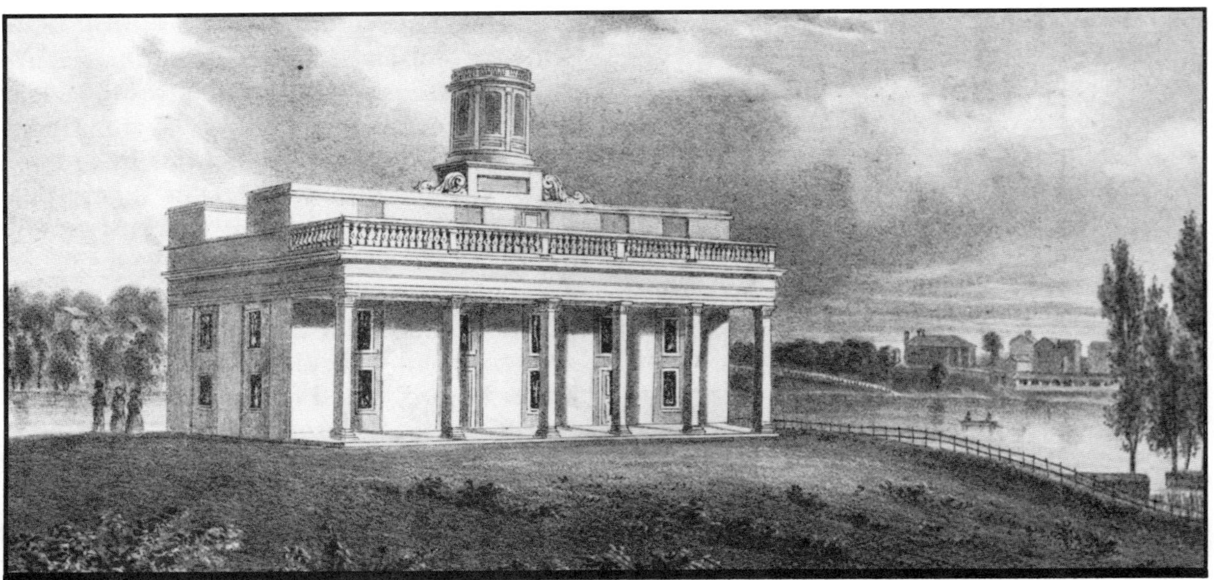

Missouri Historical Society. St. Louis Medical College, plate XII, Valley of the Mississippi, illustrated by J. C. Wild.
Kemper medical college building

Medical College, served as professor of the institutes of medicine and obstetrics. Dr. John De Wolf of the staff of the Berkshire Medical School in Vermont became professor of chemistry and pharmacy.[110]

Requirements for graduation in the Medical Department of Kemper College followed the pattern of other Middle Western institutions. No general education requirements were specified, but candidates were expected to have had three years of preliminary medical training under the preceptorial system. Students were required before receiving their M.D. degree to attend two full courses in the Medical Department of Kemper College, or one in some respectable school, with the final one in the Kemper department. Present practitioners of medicine applying for degrees must have been in reputable practice for three years, followed by attendance of one course at Kemper. The medical program was not graded into preliminary and advanced studies; the second year was substantially a repetition of the first. The regular lectures began the first Monday of November and ended on the first of March. The room for practical anatomy was open during October with free lectures provided for students who arrived early to begin their work. There was no comprehensive tuition charge for the year's training. A fee of $15 was paid to each professor by the student to gain admittance to his class.[111] The tuition fees, with certain incidental charges, were the sole compensation of the professors; they received no salary from the college. Most medical college professors also engaged in private practice.

The first commencement of the Medical Department of Kemper College took place in the Baptist Church, February 23, 1841. Three students graduated. Attendance grew from this low point. For the year 1841-1842, there were 60 students and 13 graduates; for 1842-

1843, 75 students and 19 graduates; and for 1843-1844, 100 pupils and 27 graduates.[112]

When attendance outgrew his first medical quarters, Dr. McDowell constructed a large octagonal building of gray stone, flanked by two wings. It was located at Eighth and Gratiot streets, near the first building. A spacious open area stretched from the medical building to Chouteau's Pond.

McDowell proceeded to transform his college into a fortress. He bought 1,400 condemned muskets from the U.S. Government and trained his students in their use.[113] There was some insurance value in this precaution. No legislation had been enacted in Missouri to provide medical schools with cadavers for their anatomical studies. So bodies had to be secured by surreptitious means, including grave robbing. This could easily lead to a riot and an attack on the college.

Other motives sprang from the strange, complex personality of McDowell. He had a strong love for military showmanship. On national holidays, wearing a three-cornered hat of the Continental Army with a large cavalry sabre strapped to his waist, he led his students in a parade on the nearby open area. This ended with the firing of a home-made cannon.[114] In his jingoistic reveries, he imagined himself invading and capturing a province of Mexican territory as leader of a filibustering band made up of his medical students.[115] He actually did apply for and receive a commission as colonel in the revolutionary army of Texas, but saw no action.

The fortress style of his building fitted in with his persecution complex and with his manifold fears and hostilities. His expulsion from the medical society was a traumatic experience, which his subsequent readmission in 1843 probably did not erase from memory. He had a strong antipathy to the Roman Church, of which he was constantly reminded by the presence of the Christian Brothers' Academy next door to his own medical building on Eighth Street. The opening of a rival medical school under the auspices of St. Louis University strengthened that feeling.[116] He hated abolitionism — and all the other isms of his day. In politics he was a Know-Nothing, opposed to unrestricted foreign immigration.

In July 1841, arrangements were made for Kemper Medical Department professors to deliver clinical lectures at the Sisters' Hospital.[117] This valuable bedside experience would supplement in an important way the students' classroom instruction.

On April 3, 1843, Dr. McDowell announced the opening at the college building of a public dispensary and a private infirmary and extended to the citizenry an invitation to take advantage of these new facilities:[118]

> The citizens of St. Louis and the South and West, are informed that the various operations in surgery, not excluding any part, will be performed on the poor from any portion of the world, free of charge. Those from a distance who are unable to pay for surgical attendance, will be expected to board themselves in the city, or in the Infirmary as may be thought best, and every attention will be given them as would be given the rich. Persons residing in the city, can have operations performed, and medicine given them if unable to pay, and their word is all that is required to demand the services proposed.

While Dr. McDowell was getting his medical school established, a second St. Louis medical college, organized five years earlier, was still in a state of suspended activity. In September 1836, the president of St. Louis

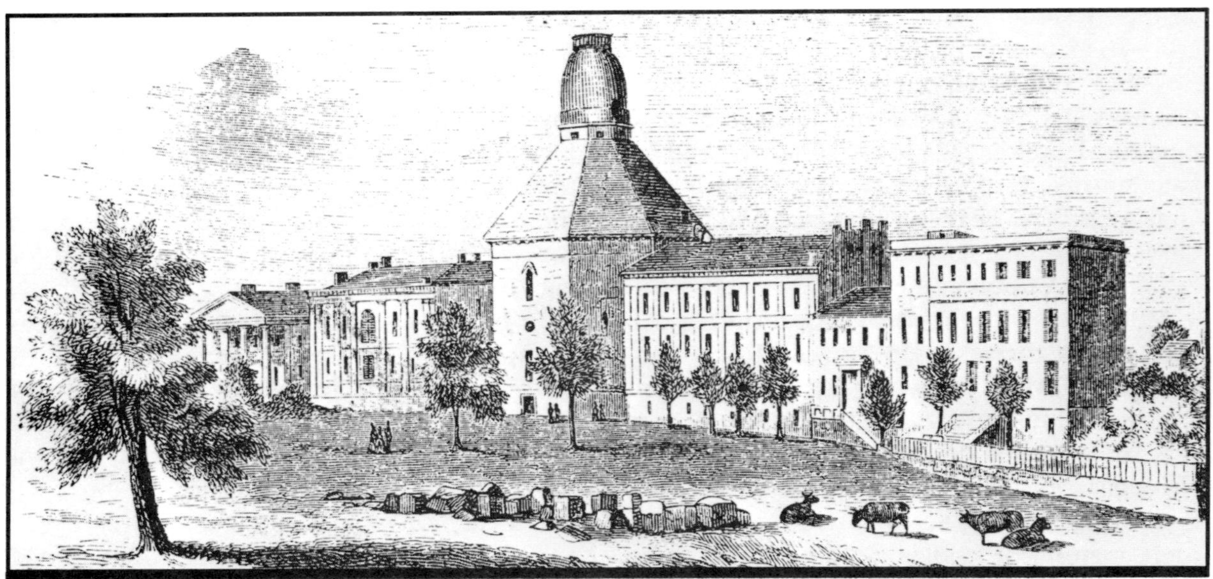

Missouri Medical College (McDowell's College). Courtesy of the State Historical Society of Missouri.

University had sent a letter to the medical society asking its cooperation in the institution of a department at the university.[119] The suggestion was received favorably. The university named a nine-member board of trustees as follows: Dr. Bernard G. Farrar; Dr. H. L. Hoffman; Colonel John O'Fallon; Colonel J. W. Johnson; the Reverend William G. Eliot; the Reverend T. P. Green; General William H. Ashley; M. P. LeDuc; and William Renshaw.[120] The board was representative of major religious and professional groups in St. Louis and contained men of distinction. Dr. Farrar presided over the St. Louis medical fraternity. Colonel John O'Fallon was a generous benefactor of civic causes. The Reverend William G. Eliot later founded Washington University. General Ashley pioneered the development of the Rocky Mountain fur trade.

The medical society appointed the following faculty: Dr. Charles J. Carpenter, professor of anatomy and physiology; Dr. William Beaumont, professor of surgery; Dr. Henry King, professor of chemistry; Dr. Edmund H. McCabe, professor of materia medica; Dr. Hardage Lane, professor of obstetrics and diseases of women and children; Dr. Joseph Johnson, professor of theory and practice and medical jurisprudence.[121]

Before further steps could be taken the Panic of 1837 prostrated the national economy. The financial crisis lasted for five years and effectively discouraged public and private enterprise.

In October 1841, the management of St. Louis University resumed the planning for a medical department. They appointed a board of trustees from the various religious denominations, Protestant and Catholic. Drs. Joseph Wells Hall, Hiram Augustus Prout, James Vance Prather, Daniel Brainard and Moses L. Linton were chosen as members of the school's professional staff. The first lectures

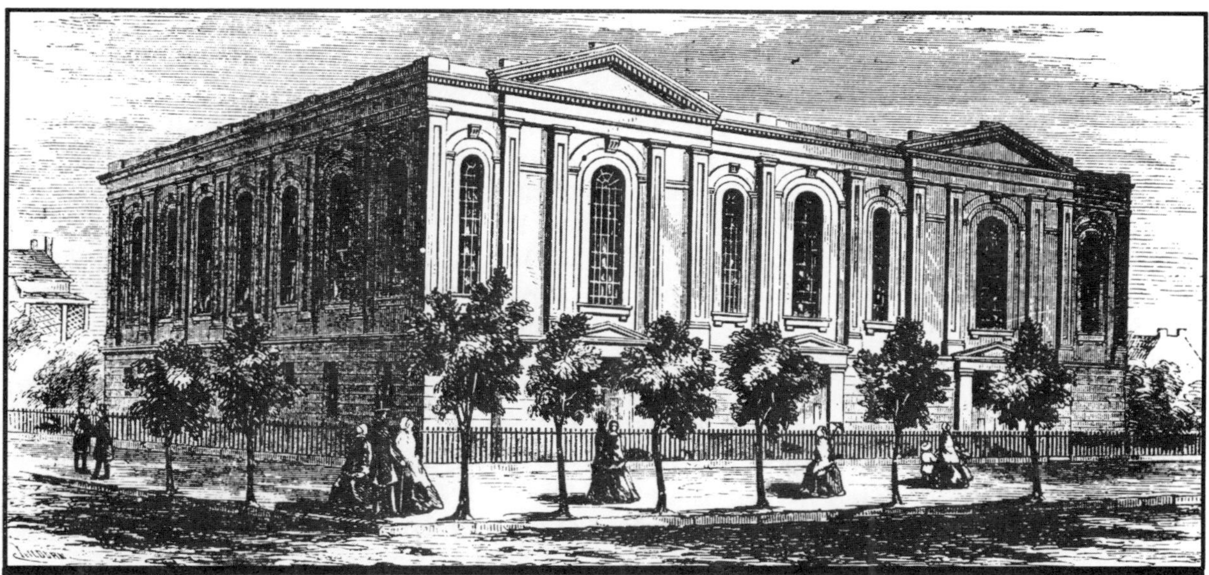

St. Louis Medical College (Pope's College). Courtesy of the State Historical Society of Missouri.

were delivered in the fall of 1842, in a small house on Washington Avenue, near Tenth Street. The house belonged to Dr. Prather, who had been named dean of the college.[122]

The emergence of a second medical college in St. Louis was not universally welcomed. Dr. McDowell angrily railed against the breaching of his monopoly of medical education. His ire increased when the new college hired two of his best professors — Drs. Hall and Prout. The St. Louis *Missouri Republican* considered the action of St. Louis University ill-advised, since St. Louis could not adequately support more than one medical school. The paper indicated that it would continue to back the Kemper College Medical Department.[123] The ideal solution to the medical school issue, according to the St. Louis *Missouri Republican,* would have been a medical college organized as part of the state's educational system and affiliated with the university established at Columbia. Such a

school would have a better chance of securing needed financial assistance.[124]

At the end of the first term, Drs. Prout and Brainard resigned. Dr. Brainard returned to Chicago where he was instrumental in founding the Rush Medical Center of the University of Chicago. Drs. Abram Litton of Nashville, Tennessee, Joseph Granville Norwood of Madison, Iowa, and Charles Alexander Pope joined the faculty ranks in the fall of 1843.[125]

On February 25, 1844, hundreds of rioters, incited by a report of the improper disposal of the remains of dissected bodies[126] and by rumors of grave robbing by faculty and students of the Medical Department of St. Louis University,[127] invaded the medical building and destroyed a valuable scientific museum and its exhibits. The board of aldermen in July 1844, rejected a petition to have the Medical Department of St. Louis University declared a public nuisance and closed down. The board did, however, set up a program of periodic inspection of the Medical Department's anatomical division.[128]

Dr. Prather was followed as dean by Dr. Moses L. Linton and Dr. Charles A. Pope. In 1846, Dr. Pope married Caroline O'Fallon, daughter of Colonel John O'Fallon. As a contribution to the advancement of the career of his son-in-law, Colonel O'Fallon built, at Seventh and Spruce streets, a handsome medical building with two lecture rooms, two anatomical quarters and other accommodations.[129] The year of his marriage Dr. Pope became dean, a position he held for almost two decades. The length and distinction of his service caused his school to be known generally as "Pope's College." Dr. Pope's work was recognized nationally by his being elected president of the American Medical Association in 1854.[130]

The tie of the Medical Department to St. Louis University, a Jesuit institution, came under increasing criticism. The tide of Know-Nothingism was sweeping the country, with the Catholic Church and its institutions a major object of attack. In St. Louis, Dr. McDowell was a leader of the anti-foreigner movement.[131]

Dr. Moses Linton, in his lecture introducing the fall term of 1845, attempted to clear away the misinformation regarding the relationship of the Medical Department to St. Louis University. He categorically denied that the medical school was under the influence and control of the Jesuits and asserted further that

> no one has any power over the medical department of the St. Louis University, but the Faculty and Board of Trustees, and that there is but one Catholic in the Faculty, and that he was not known to be such when he was invited to St. Louis.[132]

He pointed out that the medical institution had been built up by the individual efforts of its professors who were alone responsible for the school building with its apparatus, library and museum.[133]

Convinced that the association with St. Louis University brought no material benefits to the medical college, but did create serious public relations problems, the medical faculty in 1848 asked the trustees of St. Louis University to allow the college to separate from the parent institution. The request was denied.[134]

The connection between McDowell's College and Kemper College was severed by the financial failure of the latter institution. In 1847 McDowell's College became the Medical Department of the University of Missouri at Columbia. This again was only a nominal relationship. The Medical Department received no funding from the university. As evidence of the tie, the university president attended commencement exercises of the Medical Department and occasionally delivered the graduation address. The department from this time was commonly called the Missouri Medical College.[135]

The faculty of the Missouri Medical College in 1847-1848 consisted of the following teachers: Dr. Joseph N. McDowell, anatomy; Dr. John S. Moore, practice of medicine; Dr. Richard Barrett, physiology and materia medica; Dr. Thomas Barbour, obstetrics and diseases of women and children; Dr. John B. Johnson, pathology and clinical medicine; and Dr. Edward H. Leffingwell, chemistry and pharmacy.[136]

6. St. Louis as a Hospital Center

St. Louis's role as a hospital center was a natural consequence of its geographical position and its commercial development. The city was located at the point where the old National Road, present Interstate 70, crossed the Mississippi River. Before the development of railroads, this was the main land route for millions of westward-moving Americans. The trip from the Eastern states to St. Louis was a long and arduous one in the 1840s and 1850s and sickness frequently occurred. Since the towns along the highway in Illinois were small, persons needing medical and hospital care often waited until they got to St. Louis to seek it.

St. Louis was the major port in the central part of the country on the Mississippi-Missouri rivers system. A large portion of the German and Irish immigration of the pre-Civil War period came through New Orleans rather than New York. After spending weeks in the cramped quarters of sailing vessels with limited food and water, they transferred almost immediately in New Orleans to the decks of river boats for the trip to St. Louis and points north and west. Thousands arrived in St. Louis suffering from various epidemic diseases.

As the busiest river port on the central network, St. Louis was the home of many of the men who operated the steamboats, barges and flatboats. The craft usually were unscreened and the crews exposed to the malaria-spreading mosquito. Sickness was particularly high among the crews of flatboats with an estimated forty percent fatality during a single trip downriver to New Orleans.[137]

The early St. Louis hospitals were houses of refuge in case of sickness or other emergencies, for transient strangers and for the city's own indigent citizens. Families in comfortable circumstances did not ordinarily patronize hospitals. They were able to pay doctors to make house calls. Nursing care was provided by family members and by servants.

Since the Sisters of Charity had established in 1828 a small hospital, later considerably enlarged, the city council inaugurated the practice of sending sick persons, for whom it was responsible, to this private institution. The hospital accepted patients suffering from mental as well as other kinds of diseases. The city paid thirty-one and one quarter cents per day for each of its patients sent to the hospital in return for the medicine, board and nursing care provided by the institution.[138] The city health officer was responsible for medical attendance.

From time to time the city conducted studies to find out who was using the hospital service, the place of origin of the patients, the type of ailment or disability, the length of stay and the cost to the government. Of 659 persons sent to the hospital at city expense from April 30, 1844 to April 30, 1845, 467 were foreign-born, while 192 were born in the United States. Of the foreign-born, 200 were from Ireland and 155 from Germany. Only twelve out of the 192 patients born in the United States were natives of Missouri.[139] These figures indicated that a large portion of the city patients were newly arrived immigrants and citizens of other states, brought to St. Louis for the specific purpose of entering the hospital.[140] The studies showed also that a considerable fraction of the patient load consisted of blind, deranged, aged, orphaned, crippled and unemployed persons who could be better taken care of in an almshouse or workhouse.[141]

As the annual costs of sending patients to the Sisters' Hospital mounted, the city government conducted preliminary investigations which suggested that it might save money by building and operating its own hospital. On November 1, 1843, an ordinance was approved setting aside a lot, described as the west half of block no. 3 of the city commons, as a future hospital site.[142] The tract comprised about twenty-eight acres situated at the junction of Park and St. Ange avenues and Linn Street. It was on the western limits of the city on high ground above the smoke of factories and the fogs emanating in summer from the river and Chouteau's Pond. Ample springs of excellent water gushed on the hospital grounds.[143]

Before taking the final step of getting involved in hospital administration, the city council proposed that the Sisters of Charity lower their rates. For 1844, the city had paid $18,000. The Lady Superior of the order rejected the suggested new rates as inadequate to cover the services rendered.[144]

In early July 1845 the city council appropriated $5,000 for beginning the construction of a municipal hospital.[145] The original plan called for a three-story building, 213 feet long, 50 feet wide, flanked by two wings. Because of a shortage of funds, only one half of the planned structure was built during 1845-1846. The hospital opened on August 20, 1846, when ninety-one patients were received. Attendance averaged ninety-six persons per day. The overall cost of the completed half of the building was $20,586.37. As of early November 1846, the hospital board of managers estimated that the city was saving $3,764.42 annually by operating its own hospital. The new facility lacked accommodations for insane patients.[146] Thirteen were left at the Sisters' Hospital,[147] where they were housed in the basement of the east wing.[148]

In March 1846 the hospital committee of the city council approved a plan for the organization and government of the City Hospital which made the salaried resident physician the key to the treatment program. This office called for a person of recognized professional competence and wide experience in the preparation of drugs, the diagnosis and treatment of diseases and the conduct of emergency operations. He was to be assisted and supervised by a board of four attending physicians, each of which would be on duty for a three-months period. The attending physicians would not be compensated. The resident and attending physicians would, in turn, be supervised by a panel of nonremunerated consulting physicians.[149]

The board of aldermen, in May 1847, confirmed for appointment the following hospital staff officers: Dr. D. O. Glascock, residing physician; Dr. M. M. Pallen, attending physician for July, August and September 1847; Dr. C. A. Pope, attending physician for October, November and December 1847; Dr. J. B. Johnson, attending physician for January, February and March 1848; Dr. Thomas P. Barbour, attending physician for April, May and June 1848; Drs. M. L. Linton, William M. McPheeters, George Engelmann and John S. Moore, consulting physicians; Susan Wyman, matron; Nehemiah Wyman, steward.[150]

An address on "National Hospitals in the West," delivered by Dr. Daniel Drake on January 6, 1835, at the Medical Convention of Ohio in Columbus, initiated a movement which eventually brought St. Louis a second public hospital. Dr. Drake pointed out that the volume of inland commerce on the Mississippi-Missouri system and the Great Lakes was equal to two-thirds of the nation's oceanic trade. This interior traffic employed approximately 43,000 boatmen.[151]

While the maritime workers were provided medical and hospital care, the boatmen on the inland waters lacked this protection.[152] The service on the interior waterways, particularly the Mississippi River, was especially hazardous because of the danger from malaria and yellow fever. The boatmen in many instances did not meet the residence requirement entitling them to medical benefits in their home ports.[153] Besides, the boatmen often fell sick far from their home stations. A system of hospitals in key cities on the inland rivers and the Great Lakes was needed so that sick boatmen would never be more than several days away from medical attention.[154] Since the lake and river traffic was part of interstate commerce, a national, rather than a state system of hospitals, was constitutionally justified.

Copies of Dr. Drake's address were sent to the president of the United States and members of Congress. On March 3, 1837, Congress approved legislation providing for the selection and purchase of suitable sites for marine hospitals on the Ohio and Mississippi rivers and the shores of Lake Erie.[155] In August 1837, it was reported that a board of surgeons of the United States Army had selected St. Louis as a hospital site.[156] However, it was not until 1858 that a marine hospital actually opened in St. Louis. A dispute among local doctors regarding the best location for the institution was a major factor in causing the long delay.[157]

In 1848, a group of St. Louis doctors opened the "Hotel for Invalids," a private hospital. They leased and remodeled the Paul House, a former hostelry, at the corner of Second and Walnut streets. St. Louis had a need for such an institution. The City Hospital and the Sisters' Hospital, being charitable societies, could not offer the privacy and personal attention of high quality medical care. The services of the private hospital particularly were designed for the class of patients who otherwise would have to arrange for medical and nursing attention in their hotel or boardinghouse rooms.[158]

The rates were determined by the type of room occupied. The charge for a private room was $4 per day. Accommodation in a general ward was $2 daily. The room charge covered everything — nursing care, medical treatment, drugs, board and laundry charges.

Drs. J. H. Johnson and E. S. Frazier were the attending physicians and surgeons. Drs. R. F. Barrett and J. S. Moore acted as consulting physicians and surgeons. The staff were able to call on the entire faculty of the Missouri Medical College for consultation in critical cases.[159]

Drs. James Sykes, H. Augustus Prout and H. Van Studdiford had opened an eye infirmary in November 1841 at their offices on Main Street. They offered to provide operations and medicines for nonpaying, as well as paying patients.[160]

7. *Public Health Legislation*

On September 2, 1843, the city council approved a comprehensive health ordinance that consolidated prior laws and covered new subjects. The ordinance was a model of organization and clarity. A. B. Chambers, the editor of the St. Louis *Missouri Republican*, played a major role in the drafting of the document.[161] Chambers, as his frequent editorials indicated, had a sound knowledge of public health issues. To aid him in the task, he took advantage of the administrative experience and the current health ordinances of the cities of Boston, New York, Philadelphia and New Orleans.[162]

The ordinance established a board of health consisting of the health officer and one member of the board of aldermen from each ward.[163] The board, by its composition, was a political rather than a strictly professional body. It is noticeable that the mayor was not included.

The general powers and duties of the board of health were expressed in the following sections of the ordinance:[164]

Section 4. The Board of Health shall have a general supervision over the

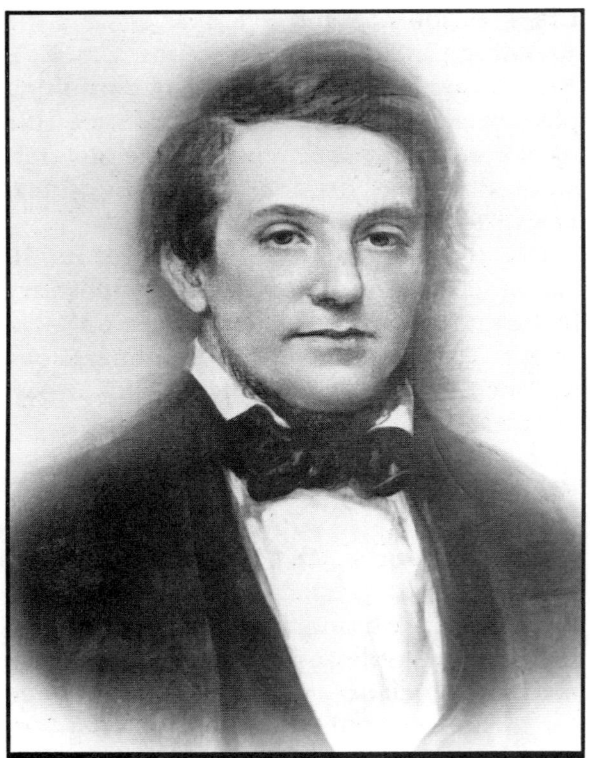

Missouri Historical Society, A. B. Chambers, Por-C-35.
A.B. Chambers

Health of the city, the cleanliness of the streets, alleys, avenues, market places, public squares, lots, yards, buildings, and enclosures, of every description; the small pox Hospital; and persons sent to any Hospital at the expense of the city.

Section 5. The Board of Health shall have power to elect a President; to enforce all ordinances concerning or relating to quarantine, the removal of filth, the removal or suppression of nuisances; the removal or safe keeping of persons infected with contagious diseases; to examine and cause to be entered and shall have examined, in the day time, all houses, cellars, enclosures and all other places; and all other powers necessary to carry the foregoing into execution.

The several street inspectors, with their staffs of daytime and nighttime scavengers, served as officers of the board in keeping the city clean and sanitary.[165]

The ordinance provided that the mayor should select the health officer alternately from the faculties of the medical departments of Kemper College and St. Louis University. His duties were to visit regularly all parts of the city and report cases of nuisances or contagious disease; to vaccinate, free of charge, all persons who had not been vaccinated; to attend the persons sent, at city expense, to the Sisters' Hospital, and to treat the inmates of the Small Pox Hospital, the city workhouse and the city prison; to examine boats coming into ports with possible cases of smallpox and other contagious disease, and assist in enforcing quarantine regulations.[166]

Admission to the Sisters' Hospital, at public expense, was limited to persons who had resided in the city for at least six months and had no means of support. However, the city register was authorized to waive this residence requirement in cases of extreme sickness or necessity.[167]

The ordinance specified that students of both medical colleges should be admitted to the city wards of the Sisters' Hospital during the college sessions, and also to the clinical lectures delivered by the professors of either college.[168] This provision put an end to the rivalry that had existed for several years between the two schools over the privilege of taking students to the Sisters' Hospital and of delivering clinical lectures. The city patients at the hospital were attended by the health officer. Each medical school was interested in having one of its faculty members appointed health officer, so that he could obtain the monopoly of conducting clinical lectures for his students. So determined was Dr. Joseph N. McDowell to win this advantage that he, after much lobbying, persuaded the city council to reduce the health officer's salary from $700 annually to a token payment of $1. This rendered it impossible for any doctor other than a medical school professor to hold the job. Since the office involved visiting not only the hospital patients, but also the sick at the Small Pox Hospital, the city prison and the workhouse, even a medical faculty member took the municipal job at considerable personal sacrifice.[169] Both Dr. McDowell from the Kemper Medical Department and Dr. J. V. Prather from the Medical Department of St. Louis University quickly tired of working for nothing.

A further provision of the act made it unlawful for the sexton of a cemetery within the city to inter any person without a certificate from the attending physician giving complete mortality information.[170]

In a meeting of the board of aldermen, June 6, 1845, the chairman of the committee on hospital spoke in favor of restoring a moderate salary as a means of securing better service from the health officer. He also advocated the passage of an ordinance prohibiting the city register from admitting to the hospital persons who had resided in the county more than a year. A recent act of the general assembly had made it the responsibility of the county courts to support poor and sick persons who were long-time residents. For years, St. Louis, a subdivision of the county had assumed this obligation.[171] Protracted negotiation was required to induce St. Louis County to take over this burden.[172]

The 1843 ordinance provided for the periodic cleaning of privy vaults by a crew of night scavengers. The carts containing human wastes were driven to the river bank and the contents tilted into the stream. The excrement washed ashore in the southern part of the city and caused frequent complaints by citizens and politicians from that area. In June 1845, arrangements were made to acquire a scavenger boat and to outfit it with the proper equipment for waste disposal service. The board of health was assigned general responsibility for the craft and its operation.[173] The craft, when put into commission, would transport its cargo well below the southern limits of the city before dumping it overboard.

For two public health problems, the city council failed to provide quick solutions. Following a heavy rain, a half-mile square area in northwest St. Louis, with its center at Seventh and Wash streets, was inundated. Water from spring rains remained throughout the summer, becoming stagnant and full of rubbish and filth. A cheap plan to drain the district through opening of sink holes had failed to provide relief. Henry Kayser, city engineer, at a meeting of the board of delegates on June 10, 1844, presented a detailed plan for constructing a storm sewer from Seventh and Wash streets to the river.[174] No action was taken. Rather unfairly, the continuing public nuisance became popularly known as "Kayser's Lake."

The second problem was posed by Chouteau's Pond. Once a wholesome and attractive spring-fed lake, a popular resort for boating and fishing, the lake had become contaminated by industrial wastes from plants lining its banks. In summer when the lake level dropped, the scanty water and exposed shores exuded foul odors and, it was feared, noxious miasmata. In January 1848, the board of health requested the city council to appoint a committee to inquire of the owners their price for selling the pond. If the owners would not sell to the city, the committee was instructed to ascertain on what terms they would take down their mill dam and drain the area.[175] The response of the proprietors was negative.

8. The State of Medical Science

Medical practice in St. Louis during the period 1821-1848 was dominated by the theory of Benjamin Rush that all diseases are caused by disorder or tension in the capillaries.[176] This condition called for purging and copious bleeding, followed by the administration of stimulants. The Rush system came under increasing criticism. But because of the absence of a satisfactory alternative, most doctors were still bleeding and purging in the 1840s and even 1850s.[177] This practice at least met the demand of the patient that the doctor do something for him. It relieved the doctor of the necessity of admitting that in most cases his medical science was ineffective or counterproductive.[178] However, in the leading medical centers of the Eastern states and of Europe, this reliance on "heroic" medicine was being abandoned, and more emphasis in treatment was placed on the natural defensive and curative powers of the human body.[179]

Surgery also was at a primitive stage. The early doctors advertised that they practiced surgery as well as medicine, although their training and experience in performing operations was extremely limited. They were saved from causing more havoc than they did by the reluctance of patients to submit to the surgeon's knife. Since there were no effective pain killers, surgery was a devastating experience.

Surgery in the main was limited to amputations and the adjustment of fractures and dislocations.[180] Because of the danger of infec-

tions, there was a standing rule that the surgeon should not invade the major body cavities. Dr. Ephraim McDowell in Kentucky in 1809 successfully violated this rule with his pioneer ovariotomy.

The following items from a fee bill adopted on November 23, 1829, by thirteen St. Louis physicians, illustrates the types of surgical operations they were called on to perform: Natural labors, $8 to $20; preternatural, difficult labors, $30 to $40; amputating fingers, toes and other small members, $10; amputating arm, leg or thigh, $50; reducing luxation of the lower jaw, $5; reducing luxation of the wrist, $5; reducing luxation of the elbow joint, $25; reducing luxation of the shoulder joint; $20; reducing luxation of the ankle, $20; reducing luxation of the knee, $20; reducing luxation of the hip, $50; reducing a simple fracture of the arm or leg, $25; reducing a simple fracture of the thigh, $40; reducing a simple fracture of the clavicle, $20; reducing a simple fracture of the patella, $20; operating with trephine, $50; elevating the skull when the trephine is not used, $5 to $70; introducing catheter, $5; extracting tooth, $1; cupping, $1; bleeding, $1; opening abscess, $1 to $2; amputating corpus or torsus, $60; amputating the breast, $50; extracting cataract, $50; couching cataract, $50; removing polypus from uterus, $30 to $70; removing polypus from naves, $10 to $20; extirpating testicle, $30; tracheotomy, $25; operation of paraphimosis, $5; operation of strangulated hernia, $60; reducing strangulated hernia by taxis, $10; operation for hydrocele, $20 to $50; lithotomy, $100 to $200.[181]

Information is lacking regarding the frequency and success with which these operations were performed by St. Louis physicians. Doctors were just beginning to collect and study clinical statistics.[182] Dr. Joseph N. McDowell of the Medical Department of

Kemper College in January 1841 surgically removed the cancerous breast of a female patient;[183] in October of that year, he extracted stones from the bladder of a second sufferer.[184] The fact that these operations were reported in some detail in the press suggested that they were rare rather than routine accomplishments. Dr. McDowell was recognized as the city's most successful surgeon.[185]

In 1844, the executors of the estate of Mary Dugan instituted a malpractice suit in the St. Louis Circuit Court against Drs. William Beaumont and Stephen Adreon, in which Drs. Franklin Knox, Hardage Lane, William Carr Lane, Charles Pope, Thomas Reyburn and James Sykes testified against Beaumont and his associate.[186] The threat of such suits must have exercised some restraint on experienced — as well as inexperienced — surgeons.

9. Sectarian Medical Systems

The reliance of the regular or allopathic doctors upon bleeding and the use of massive dosage of calomel and other metallic drugs prompted the rise of rival systems with gentler methods of treatment. The most important of these was homeopathy, a school founded by Samuel Christian Frederick Hahnemann, who in 1796 had revived the Paracelsian doctrine of *similia similibus curantur.* Hahnemann taught that "diseases or symptoms of diseases are curable by drugs which produce pathologic effects on the body similar to those produced by the disease." He further propounded that "the dynamic effect of drugs is heightened by giving them in infinitesimally small doses."[187]

Homeopathic medicine was introduced in St. Louis by Dr. J. G. Rosenstien who, in April 1842, opened an office at the Planters' House.[188]

A second medical sect with widespread popular support was the botanic system, founded in 1806 by Samuel Thomson, a New Hampshire farmer. His mode of treatment was based upon commonly available plants and upon steam baths. Thomson sold rights to practice his patented system at a price of $20 for laymen and $500 for physicians.[189]

The first of these botanic doctors in St. Louis was C. Rice who, in February 1833, established his practice at Third and Market streets. A month or so later Rice became involved in a controversy in the columns of the St. Louis *Free Press* with his former partner Dr. J. L. Craft. Dr. Rice charged that after Dr. Craft had purchased the right to practice the Thomsonian system, he financed Craft's move to St. Louis and took him into partnership. Rice alleged that upon the dissolution of the association, Craft had gotten an improperly large share of the firm's assets.[190]

The contest between the two quarreling practitioners ended with Dr. Craft receiving official indorsement as agent of the Thomsonian Botanical System of Medical Practice in St. Louis.[191] In an advertisement in the St. Louis *Free Press* of April 11, 1833, Dr. Craft announced that he had on hand a full assortment of "Doctor" Thomson's medicines also sixty sets of Thomson's book on medical practice, entitled *New Guide to Health.* He declared that he used no mercury, nitre or antimony. To aid in diagnosis, he required a vial of urine from new patients.[192]

10. Problems of Disease Classification and Identification

Municipal legislation dating back to 1823 required St. Louis doctors to provide information, including cause of death for patients who died under their care.[193] The lack of a standard system of classification of diseases made it necessary for each doctor to devise his own system. It was common practice among physicians to classify diseases, except for the easily-recognizable affections, by their most prominent symptoms, e.g. fever, inflammation, convulsions and debility.[194] Some of the common diseases had multiple names. Malaria fever was referred to under the following pseudonyms: autumnal, bilious, intermittent, remittent, congestive, miasmatic, marsh, malignant, chill-fever, ague, fever and ague, and *the Fever.*[195]

Another problems was that of disease identification. In the 1820s and the 1830s medical science, especially in France,[196] was beginning to establish for each disease entity a complete picture, including clinical symptoms, autopsy findings, and ultimately the isolation of the causal germ or virus. American medical practice, however, still lagged several decades behind European progress and continued to rely on clinical observations for the identification of diseases. This was an imprecise method for differentiating between closely related infections.

The St. Louis Board of Health grouped its mortality listing by the cemeteries in which interment occurred. The report of August 14-20, 1840, from which details of sex, race and age have been omitted, shows some of the disease categories which were employed. *St. Louis Cemetery:* dentition, whooping cough; drowning; congestive fever; summer complaint; unknown; gastroenteritis; asthma; bilious fever; dysentery. *Methodist Cemetery:* typhoid fever; inflammation of bowels; bilious fever; brain fever; congestive fever; bloody flux; convulsions. *Presbyterian Cemetery:* dysenteria biliosa; bowel complaint; spasms and cramp; congestive fever; fever; inflammation of the brain.[197]

No attempt was made by the early boards of health to organize the disease statistics into a permanent record. It was not until 1850 that annual summaries were prepared at first only for typhoid fever, smallpox, consumption and cholera.[198] Health reports earlier than 1850 were probably destroyed in the 1849 St. Louis fire.

11. Medical Journals

Almost contemporaneous with the organization of St. Louis's two medical schools was the establishment in 1843 of its first medical publication — the *St. Louis Medical and Surgical Journal.* Dr. M. L. Linton was the first editor. Born in Nelson County, Kentucky, in 1808, he secured his higher education at Transylvania College. Much of his professional training was acquired in Europe at a time when important advances were being made in medical science. While abroad he became acquainted with Dr. Charles A. Pope who later invited him to take the chair of theory and practice of medicine in the Medical Department of St. Louis University. Linton wrote a book entitled *Outlines of Pathology* which was widely used as a text.[199]

A mutually beneficial relationship was created between the medical schools and the new journal. The schools attracted to St. Louis distinguished physicians, who contributed articles for its columns. The opportunity for publication encouraged the faculty members — and also other St. Louis doctors — to conduct medical experiment and research. Through its system of exchanges with foreign scientific publications, the journal informed doctors and students of advances in medicine and surgery in major European centers. Thus, the journal contributed to the tradition of close cooperation between American and continental medicine which existed when St. Louis was part of the French colonial empire and its early physicians were French-trained.

In May 1845, the *Missouri Medical and Surgical Journal* was started under the editorship of Dr. R. F. Stevens with the medical faculty of Kemper College as associates. In September 1848, this journal merged into the *St. Louis Medical and Surgical Journal.*

12. State Non-Intervention in Medical Matters

The initial attitude of the state of Missouri toward medical practice was one of non-intervention. The lawmakers assumed that the purchaser of medical services would have the wisdom to distinguish between reliable and quack doctors and that competition between practitioners would keep the cost of treatment reasonable.

To fill the vacuum caused by governmental inactivity, the St. Louis Medical Society set its own seal of approval upon physicians it considered qualified and responsible. But its judgments were sometimes distorted by personal controversies and animosities, as in the case of Dr. James N. McDowell in July 1839.[200] Later St. Louis's two medical schools, through the authority to grant diplomas, became local accrediting agencies.

Although the state did not say who should practice medicine in Missouri, it did place some restrictions on how the profession should be conducted. A physician who, while intoxicated, unintentionally caused the death of a patient by his treatment, was declared guilty of manslaughter in the third degree.[201] Further, any doctor who procured an abortion, unless necessary to save the life of the mother, risked being found guilty of a misdemeanor, punishable by imprisonment not exceeding one year or a $500 maximum fine.[202]

Prompted by the incident which had occurred at the Department of Medicine at St. Louis University in February 1844, the general assembly enacted a law making grave robbing for anatomical experimentation a misdemeanor, drawing a maximum punishment of one year in jail or a $500 fine, or both.[203]

Not all legislation regarding medical practice passed by the general assembly was punitive. Doctors, along with clergymen and lawyers, were exempted from jury duty.[204] Legislation was passed establishing the confidentiality of information gained by a doctor or surgeon through his professional relationship with a patient.[205]

For one class of citizens — the insane — the presumption that they had the ability to make wise decisions regarding their health and welfare could not be made. Legislation enacted on March 3, 1835, gave the county courts responsibility for these incompetents. Upon receiving a written charge by one or more persons that a certain citizen was of unsound mind, the court was authorized to set a date to investigate the allegation. The same adversary relationship that prevailed in a criminal trial was followed. The accused person was brought to court by the sheriff, the charge of being insane was read, and he was asked how he pleaded, "Guilty" or "Not guilty." A jury decided the case. No arrangement was made to provide legal counsel for the accused. There was no requirement that charges be substantiated by medical or psychiatric testimony. If a person was found insane, the county court appointed a guardian to look after him and his property. In the case of an insane person who was indigent, a guardian or some other homeowner was paid a small allowance to furnish board, lodging and necessary care. This was the procedure in Boone and possibly other counties.[206]

The major purpose of the law was to establish procedures for caring for persons incapable of managing their own affairs, particularly their estates. Existing means — the jury trial to establish the fact of insanity and the institution of guardianship — were employed in the implementation of the law. Protection of society against violently and criminally insane persons was a secondary aim of the act.[207]

In St. Louis, where for a number of years the municipal authorities were unaware that the county court was responsible for the care and treatment of insane persons, a different procedure was followed. Both the mayor and the city register had the power, after a preliminary investigation, to send sick persons, including those suffering from mental illness, to the Sisters' Hospital. The mentally deranged thus provided for were mostly homeless and indigent newcomers to St. Louis who would not likely raise the objection that their legal rights were violated by the summary procedure. The certificate by the mayor or register was merely an authorization for the hospital, at the city's expense, to admit the patient, not an order for his confinement.[208]

Chapter II
Foundations of Health Services in St. Louis, 1821-1848.

1 St. Louis *Missouri Republican*, April 9, 1823, p. 2:4.
2 Frederick L. Billon, *Annals of St. Louis in Its Territorial Days from 1804 to 1821* (St. Louis, Printed for the Author, 1888, pp. 336-337.
3 *Ibid.*, p. 337.
4 *Idem.*
5 *Laws of a Public and General Nature of the District of Louisiana of the Territory of Missouri, and of the State of Missouri up to the Year 1824* (Jefferson City, W. Lusk and Son, 1842, p. 969.
6 *Ibid.*, p. 970.
7 St. Louis *Missouri Republican*, April 23, 1823, p. 3:3-4. Dr. Lane and many doctors of his day believed that diseases were caused by miasmata or clouds of infectious particles arising from decaying vegetation, swamps, etc. In cities, stagnant waters, garbage, human wastes and other refuse, acted on by the hot sun, were thought to produce miasmatic emanations.
8 *Idem.*
9 *Idem.*
10 St. Louis *Missouri Republican*, Aug. 20, 1823, p. 2:5.
11 *Ibid.*, Aug. 27, 1823, p. 3:5.
12 *Ibid.*, Aug. 26, 1828, p. 2:4.
13 *Ibid.*, May 21, 1823, p. 3:1.
14 *Ibid.*, May 21, 1823, p. 3:2.
15 *Ibid.*, Oct. 7, 1828, p. 3:1.
16 William Hyde and Howard L. Conard, *Encyclopedia of the History of St. Louis.* Vol. II (New York, The Southern History Co., 1899, p. 1051.
17 Louis Houck, *A History of Missouri.* Vol. II (Chicago, R. R. Donnelly and Sons, Co., 1908) p. 326.
18 *Laws of a Public and General Nature of the State of Missouri Passed Between the Years 1824 and 1936, not Publshed in the Digest of 1825 nor in the Digest of 1835.* Vol. II (Jefferson City, W. Lusk and Son, 1842) pp. 374-375.
19 St. Louis *Beacon,* Mar. 8, 1832, p. 2:4.
20 *Ibid.,* July 12, 1832, p. 3:2.
21 *Ibid.,* Aug. 2, 1832, p. 3:3.
22 *Ibid.,* Aug. 9, 1832, p. 2:1.
23 *Ibid.,* Sept. 20, 1832, p. 2:2.
24 *Ibid.,* Sept. 20, 1832, p. 2:2-3.
25 *Ibid.,* Jan. 19, 1832, p. 2:5.
26 *Ibid.,* Sept, 20, 1832, p. 2:3.
27 *Idem.*
28 *Ibid.,* Sept. 13, 1832, p. 2:5.
29 *Ibid.,* Sept, 27, 1832, p. 3:1.
30 *Idem.*
31 *Ibid.,* Oct. 4, 1832, p. 2:4.
32 *Ibid.,* Oct. 18, 1832, p. 3:2.
33 *Ibid.,* Oct. 25, 1832, p. 2:5.
34 *Idem.*
35 *Ibid.,* Nov. 15, 1832, p. 3:1.
36 Cynthia De Haven Pitcock, "Doctors in Controversy, An Ethical Dispute Between Joseph Nash McDowell and William Beaumont," *Missouri Historical Review,* Vol. LX, No. 3 (April 1966) , p. 337, footnote 3.
37 St. Louis *Beacon.* June 16, 1831, p. 3:3. The waterworks originated in 1829 in a partnership of John C.Wilson and Abraham Fox to build and operate a plant to supply

"clarified" water to the city for a term of 25 years. Despite generous franchise terms and a promised bonus of $3,000 upon completion of the works, the contractors were unable to raise sufficient capital to carry out the plan. The city eventually purchased the interests of Wilson and Fox and became the sole owner of the works. The first water was delivered in the fall of 1831 or the summer of 1832, William Hyde and Howard L. Conard, *Encyclopedia of the History of St. Louis*. Vol. IV (New York, the Southern History Co., 1899), p. 2469.

38 Walter B. Stevens, *Water Purification at St. Louis* (St. Louis, n. p., 1911), p. 29.

39 William Carr Lane, *Water for the City of St. Louis* (St. Louis, n. p. 1860), p. 2.

40 St. Louis *Beacon*, June 28, 1832, p. 3:3.

41 *Idem.*

42 By 1840, a bicameral legislature, consisting of the board of delegates and the board of aldermen, had replaced the original board of aldermen.

43 St. Louis *Missouri Republican*, Nov. 28, 1840, p. 3:6-7.

44 *Ibid*, Feb. 21, 1843, p. 3:1.

45 *Ibid*, Nov. 24, 1843, p. 4:2.

46 *Ibid*, July 10, 1844, p. 4:3.

47 *Ibid*, May 3, 1845, p. 2:1.

48 *The St. Louis Directory for the Years 1854-1855.* (St. Louis, Chambers and Knapp, 1854), pp. 234-235.

49 These figures are for Missouri as a whole, but would appear to be true also for St. Louis considered separately. Roland Lanser, "The Pioneer Physician in Missouri", *Missouri Historial Review*, Vol. XLIV, No. 1 (Oct. 1949), p. 32.

50 Billon, *Annals of St. Louis in its Territorial Days*, p. 337.

51 Lanser, "The Pioneer Physician in Missouri," p. 45.

52 St. Louis *Missouri Republican*, May 10, 1824, p. 2: 3-4.

53 Lanser, "The Pioneer Physician in Missouri," p. 45.

54 St. Louis *Argus*, Oct. 30, 1835, p. 3:4.

55 *Ibid*, April 15, 1836, p. 3:3. Dr. Lane was a former Army officer, who retained his interest in military affairs. In February 1822, he had been appointed quartermaster general of the state of Missouri.

56 Billon, *Annals of St. Louis in the Territorial Days*, p. 328.

57 St. Louis *Free Press*, July 11, 1833, p. 2:5.

58 Pitcock, "Doctors in Controversy," p. 339.

59 *Ibid*, p. 341.

60 St. Louis *Missouri Republican*, Jan. 29, 1842, p. 2:1.

61 Walter B. Stevens, *St. Louis: The Fourth City 1764-1909.* Vol I. (St. Louis, The S. J. Clarke Publishing Co., 1909), p. 588.

62 R. J. Terry, "The Origins of the Missouri Medical College" (St. Louis, 1918. Reprint from the *Washington University Medical Alumni Quarterly*, April 1938), p. 136.

63 Stevens, *St. Louis: The Fourth City*, Vol. I, p. 598.

64 St. Louis *Missouri Argus*, Sept. 4, 1835, p. 3:3.

65 Max A. Goldstein, ed., *One Hundred Years of Medicine and Surgery in Missouri* (St. Louis, St. Louis Star Publisher, 1900), pp. 277-278.

66 St. Louis *Farmers and Mechanics Advocate*, Feb. 7, 1835, p. 3:6.

67 St. Louis *Missouri Republican*, June 29, 1837, p. 2:4.

68 *Ibid*, April 1, 1841, p. 3:2.

69 *Ibid*, July 7, 1837, p. 3:5.

70 *Ibid*, Dec. 22, 1842, p. 2:5.

71 St. Louis *Beacon*, Jan. 2, 1830, p. 3:2.

72 *Ibid*, Aug. 15, 1829, p. 3:3; *ibid*, Nov. 7, 1829, p. 3:2; St. Louis *Missouri Gazette*, April 21, 1819, p. 3:4.

73 Pitcock, *opus cit.*, pp. 338-339. The society held a special meeting on June 9, 1837, for the purpose of receiving the act of incorporation granted by the legislature of Missouri. St. Louis *Missouri Republican*, June 5, 1837, p. 2:4.

74 Pitcock, *opus cit.*, p. 340.

75 *Idem.*

76 *Ibid*, p. 341.

77 *Ibid*, pp. 341-342.

78 *Ibid*, p. 342.

79 *Ibid*, p. 343.

80 *Idem.*

81 *Ibid*, pp. 343-344.

82 *Ibid*, p. 344.

83 *Idem.*

84 *Ibid*, pp. 344-346.

85 *Ibid*, p. 346.

86 *Ibid*, p. 347.

87 *Idem.*

88 *Idem.*

89 Cynthia De Haven Pitcock, "Involvement of William Beaumont, M.D., in a Medical Legal Controversy: The Darnes-Davis Case, 1840," *Missouri Historical Review*, Vol. LVIV, No. 1 (Oct. 1964), p. 34.

90 *Idem.*

91 *Ibid*, pp. 35-36

92 *Ibid*, pp. 37-38.

93 Thomas S. Nelson, ed., *Full and Accurate Report on the Trial of William P. Darnes, on an Indictment Found by the Grand Jury of the County of St. Louis, at the September Term, 1840, of the Criminal Court of Said County, on a Charge of Manslaughter in the Third Degree for the Death of Andrew J. Davis, in the City of St. Louis on the first of June, 1840.* (Boston, Clarendon Harris, 1841, pp. 31-35. This is the testimony of Dr. Thomas McMartin at the Darnes trial.

94. *Idem.*

95 *Ibid*, pp. 55-59.

96 *Ibid*, p. 36

97 Ibid., p. 10.

98 Hyde and Conard, *Encyclopedia of the History of St. Louis.* Vol. II, p. 893.

99 Nelson, *opus cit.*, pp. 31-39, 55-59.

100 *Ibid*, pp. 75-81.

101 Pitcock, "The Darnes-Davis Case, 1840," p. 42.

102 Pitcock, "Doctors in Controversy,"p. 346.

103 Nelson, *opus cit.*, pp. 131-147.

104 Pitcock, "The Darnes-Davis Case, 1840," p. 44.

105 Dr. McDowell was readmitted to the medical society, which at its annual meeting on January 6, 1843, appointed him as examiner on physiology on its examining board. St. Louis *Missouri Republican*. Jan. 13, 1843, p. 2:7.

106 Terry, *opus cit.*, pp. 126-127.

107 Stevens, *St. Louis: The Fourth City*, Vol. I, p. 592.

108 St. Louis *Missouri Republican*, Oct. 26, 1840, p. 3:3.

109 Terry, *opus cit.*, pp. 132, 137.

110 *Ibid*, pp. 135-137.

111 *Ibid*, pp. 137-138.

112 *Ibid*, pp. 138-139.

113 Stevens, *St. Louis: The Fourth City.* Vol. I, p. 597.

114 *Ibid.,* pp. 592-593.

115 *Ibid.,* p. 597.

116 *Idem.*

117 St. Louis *Missouri Republican,* July 14, 1841, p. 2:2.

118 *Ibid,* April 3, 1843, p. 1:4.

119 William B. Faherty, *Dream by the River: Two Centuries of St. Louis Catholicism 1776-1967* (St. Louis, Piraeus Publishers, 1973), p. 50.

120 St. Louis *Missouri Argus,* Oct. 7, 1836, p. 3:4.

121 *Idem.*

122 William Frederick Norwood, *Medical Education in the United States Before the Civil War* (Philadelphia, University of Pennsylvania Press, 1844), p. 356.

123 St. Louis *Missouri Republican,* Nov. 2, 1841, p. 2:1.

124 *Ibid,* April 24, 1840, p. 2:3.

125 Norwood, *opus cit.,* p. 356, footnote 14.

126 St. Louis *Democrat,* Feb. 26, 1844, p. 2:1.

127 St. Louis *Missouri Republican,* Feb. 27, 1844, p. 2:1.

128 *Ibid.,* July 6, 1844, p. 4:1.

129 Stevens, *St. Louis: The Fourth City,* Vol. I, p. 598.

130 *Idem.*

131 Faherty, *opus cit.,* p. 76.

132 St. Louis *Missouri Republican,* Dec. 15, 1845, p. 2:4.

133 Idem.

134 Fahrerty, *opus cit.,* p. 76.

135 *Ibid.,* p. 354.

136 *Ibid.,* p. 355.

137 This estimate was made by Dr. Daniel Drake in an address on "National Hospitals in the West," given at the Medical Convention of Ohio, Columbus, Jan. 6, 1835. St. Louis *Farmers and Mechanics Advocate,* Mar. 28, 1835, p. 2:1.

138 St. Louis *Missouri Republican,* Sept. 6, 1843, p. 4:4.

139 *Ibid.,* June 11, 1845, p. 2:4.

140 *Ibid.,* Dec. 10, 1840, p. 4:2.

141 *Ibid.,* Nov. 7, 1840, p. 4:1.

142 *Ibid.,* Nov. 4, 1843, p. 2:4.

143 *Ibid.,* Nov. 9, 1846, p. 3:1; *Ibid,* Oct. 30, 1843, p. 4:1.

144 *Ibid.,* July 7, 1845, p. 4:1.

145 *Ibid.,* July 12, 1845, p. 2:1.

146 *Ibid.,* Nov. 9, 1846, p. 3:1.

147 *Idem.*

148 *Ibid.,* Oct. 30, 1843, p. 4:1.

149 *Ibid.,* Mar. 5, 1846, p. 2:3.

150 *Ibid.,* May 18, 1847, p. 3:3.

151 St. Louis *Farmers' and Mechanics' Advocate,* Mar. 28, 1835, p. 2:2.

152 *Idem.*

153 St. Louis *Missouri Republican,* Sept. 1, 1843, p. 1:1.

154 St. Louis *Farmers' and Mechanics' Advocate,* Mar. 28, 1835, p. 2:2.

155 St. Louis *Missouri Republican,* May 24, 1837, p.2:1.

156 *Ibid.,* Aug. 16, 1837, p. 2:1.

157 Hyde and Conard, *Encyclopedia of the History of St. Louis,* Vol. II, p. 1053; St. Louis *Missouri Republican,* Apr. 21, 1846, p. 2:1.

158 St. Louis *Missouri Republican,* Jan. 8, 1848, p. 2:1.

159 *Idem.*

160 *Ibid.,* Nov. 12, 1841, p. 2:5.

161 *Ibid.,* Sept. 21, 1843, p. 2:1.

162 *Idem.*

163 *Ibid.,* Sept. 6, 1843, p. 4:1.

164 *Idem.*

165 *Ibid.,* p. 4:1-4.

166 *Ibid.,* p. 4:3-4.

167 *Ibid.,* p. 4:4.

168 Idem.

169 *Ibid,* Dec. 19, 1844, p. 3:1.

170 *Ibid,* Sept. 6, 1843, p. 4:5.

171 *Ibid,* June 13, 1845, p. 4:2.

172 *Ibid,* Dec. 7, 1847, p. 4:2.

173 *Ibid,* June 3, 1845, p. 4:1.

174 *Ibid,* June 14, 1844, p. 3:1-3.

175 *Ibid,* Jan. 17, 1848, p. 4:1-2.

176 Richard Harrison Shryock, *Medicine and Society in America 1660-1860* (New York, New York University Press, 1960), ppp. 69-70.

177 *Ibid,* p. 144.

178 *Ibid,* p. 148.

179 *Ibid,* pp. 131-132.

180 *Ibid,* p. 59.

181 Goldstein, *opus cit.,* pp. 52-53.

182 Shyrock, *opus cit.,* p. 130.

183 St. Louis *Missouri Republican,* Jan. 22, 1841, p. 2:5.

184 *Ibid,* Oct. 29, 1841, p. 2:1.

185 Goldstein, *opus cit.,* p. 49.

186 Pitcock, "Doctors in Controversy," p. 348, footnote 27.

187 Norwood, *opus cit.,* p. 416.

188 St. Louis *Missouri Republican,* Apr. 18, 1842, p. 2:6.

189 Norwood, *opus cit.,* p. 418.

190 St. Louis *Missouri Republican,* Feb. 21, 1833, p. 4:3; *ibid,* Mar. 28, 1833, p. 3:5.

191 *Ibid,* Apr. 6, 1833, p. 3:2.

192 Ibid, Apr. 11, 1833, p. 4:5.

193 St. Louis *Missouri Republican,* Aug. 20, 1823, p. 2:5.

194 William Travis Howard, Jr., M.D., *Public Health Administration and the Natural History of Disease in Baltimore, Maryland 1797-1920* (Washington, D.C., Carnegie Institution of Washington, 1924, p. 192.

195 Eldon G. Chuinard, *Only One Man Died: The Medical Aspects of the Lewis and Clark Expedition* (Glendale, California, The Arthur H. Clark Co., 1979), p. 175, footnote 19.

196 Shryock, *opus cit.,* p. 124.

197 St. Louis *Missouri Republican,* Aug. 25, 1840, p. 2:5.

198 Goldstein, *opus cit.,* p. 84.

199 *Ibid,* pp. 95-96.

200 Supra, pp. 20-22.

201 *Revised Statutes of the State of Missouri 1834-1835.* 1st edition. (St. Louis, Argus office, 1835), p. 169.

202 *Revised Statutes of the State of Missouri 1844-1845* (St. Louis, Chambers and Knapp. 1845), p. 183.

203 *Ibid,* p. 210.

204 *Ibid,* p. 326.

205 *Ibid,* p. 573.

206 *Revised Statutes of the State of Missouri, 1834-1835,* pp. 323-327; Boone County, *County Court Record, 1832-1834,* meeting of June 16, 1834; Boone County, *County Court Record,* Book G, p. 354.

207 *The Revised Statutes of the State of Missouri, Revised and Digested by the Eighth Assembly During the Years 1834 and 1835* (St. Louis, Argus Office, 1835), pp. 323-327.

208 St. Louis *Missouri Republican,* Dec. 10, 1840, p. 4:2.

Chapter 3

St. Louis: Gateway to the West, 1849-1861

1. St. Louis in the 1840s

ST. LOUIS EXPERIENCED phenomenal commercial and industrial expansion during the 1840s. In a memorial of October 29, 1845, presented to the Senate and House of Representatives of the United States, requesting an appropriation of $75,000 to finish the work of improving the St. Louis harbor, the city council stated that:[1]

> St. Louis is a port of entry, and is from her central location the great emporium of the trade of the Mississippi Valley, the magnitude of which it is difficult to estimate for want of full statistics, but which may be considered as fully equal to the entire foreign trade of the United States; our registered steamboat tonnage owned here is over 20,000 tons, to say nothing of as much more tonnage furnished from New Orleans, Louisville, Cincinnati and Pittsburgh for the necessities of our trade, making ours next to New Orleans the greatest steamboat port in the United States.

By 1849, a total of 130 steamboats with a tonnage of 30,595 were owned in St. Louis. During that year, 265 steamboats, totaling 62,137 tons, visited the St. Louis port.[2] The agricultural and industrial products of the areas drained by the Missouri, Upper Mississippi and Ohio rivers were channeled through St. Louis and, in many cases, transshipped there for the continuing trip to New Orleans. From the Missouri and Upper Mississippi came furs, hides, lumber, hemp, ores, grain and meat products; by way of the Ohio system arrived metal products, machinery, merchandise, drugs, tobacco and whisky. At times, twenty or more steamboats were tied up at the St. Louis docks, loading and unloading passengers and cargo.

To its well-established commercial activities, St. Louis in the 1840s added manufactories of furniture, stoves, agricultural implements, leather goods, bricks, tobacco, flour, sugar, beer and whisky, packing house products and soap.[3]

The commercial and industrial growth of St. Louis attracted new residents. The population, which stood at 6,694 in 1830, increased to 16, 469 in 1840. By 1850, it had grown to approximately 77,716.[4] Part of this increase came from the westward movement of Americans from the older states. This was facilitated by the completion of the National Road to St. Louis.

During the 1840s, St. Louis received a large influx of immigration from Ireland and Germany. Agricultural distress prompted the Irish emigration. The potato crop which provided the main item of the diet of the small farmers, failed disastrously in 1845, 1846 and 1848. Other factors contributed to the ruin of the Irish peasantry. The repeal of the British corn laws in 1846, creating free trade in agricultural products, deprived Irish wheat of a favored market in England.[5] The division of land among the male heirs reduced the smaller farms to an uneconomic size. Finally, the extension of the English poor laws to Ireland in 1847 made it financially advantageous for the landlords to evict the impoverished tenants from their estates in order to avoid paying taxes for their support.[6] Some landlords helped finance the overseas migration of their displaced tenants.

Disappointing potato crops as well as overpopulation in the rural areas were factors in the German emigration. Gottfried Duden, in a book widely publicized in Germany, painted an idyllic picture of Missouri farm life, which initiated the exodus to Missouri. The failure of the Frankfurt Assembly of 1848-1849 to establish a unified and representative government for the German states caused thousands of the members of the commercial and professional classes, many of whom had been active in the political uprisings in their various states, to seek a new homeland.[7]

The western boundary of St. Louis, which had been established along Eighteenth Street in 1841, was moved in 1853 to a line just beyond Grand Avenue.[8] As the residential district moved westward, and southward along Carondelet Avenue and northerly by way of Bellefontaine Road, the original town from the river to Third Street was relinquished to warehouses, business establishments and professional offices.

St. Louis in the 1840s lacked many essential utilities and amenities. There were no storm or sanitary sewers. The blocking of the city's natural drainage system of ravines and sinkholes caused pools of stagnant water to accumulate in various areas.

The streets and alleys were in a filthy condition, except during epidemics when a concerted effort was made to cleanse them. The 1840s were a decade of rapid population growth. Many unimproved streets were opened up and much jerry-built housing erected to take care of the flood of immigrants. The board of health, composed of the health officer and one member of the board of aldermen from each ward, was charged with the task of keeping the city clean. They delegated the job to ward street inspectors who were responsible for making contracts with individual day and night scavengers.[9] The system did not work. There was no supervision of the performance of the scavengers; and sufficient money was not appropriated for hiring an adequate number. The problem of keeping the city in a healthful condition was not solved until a system of sanitary sewers was built and until the job of supervision was transferred to a board of public works rather than left in the hands of the infrequently meeting board of health.

The city's water supply was taken directly from the Mississippi River at the foot of Bates Street and pumped into the double-deck reservoir nearby. It was drawn out into the distribution system almost immediately. The water was unfiltered and untreated with chemicals. The rapid course through the reservoir left little time for sedimentation. The city waterworks furnished an inadequate quantity, as well as an unsatisfactory quality of water and even that was often unavailable because of plant accidents. The water was distributed to public hydrants in the streets and also to private hydrants in the yards of citizens willing to pay for the service. Many citizens had their private wells.

The town relied on volunteer companies for fire protection. The companies were semi-private clubs, with their fire stations, colorful uniforms and service traditions. The city helped to buy their equipment. A melee between rival companies in July 1857 was responsible for a movement to replace the volunteers with a paid fire department.[10]

Streets were improved by macadamizing rather than by paving. The constant traffic over the crushed limestone raised clouds of dust which the local physicians blamed for the high rate of pulmonary complaints, eye disease and general discomfort.[11]

There were no zoning regulations. Small dairies, slaughterhouses, breweries, foundries, tanneries and other industries with their noise, smoke and offensive odors made life unpleasant for neighboring   citizens.

Although one-tenth of the proceeds from the sale of the commons in 1835, was set aside for public schools, the city was slow in establishing an adequate system. In November 1840, the Reverend W. G. Eliot, in the introductory lecture of the lyceum series, stated that out of an estimated 3,000 children in St. Louis of school age, only 200 were enrolled in the city's two common schools. Church schools and private academies enrolled possibly 700-800 more. But Eliot was of the opinion that 2,000 of the local children were receiving no formal instruction. He regretted the general lack of interest of St. Louisans in intellectual and cultural matters.[12]

2. The 1849 Cholera Epidemic

The United States enjoyed a long respite following the cholera epidemic of 1832-1833. This came to an end on December 1, 1848, when the packet ship, *New York*, out of Havre arrived at New York harbor with seven of her steerage passengers dead and many others ill with the unmistakable symptoms of cholera. The dread disease, following its usual course, had from its homeland in India swept through Asia, the Middle East and Europe. In the fall of 1848 it was in England and France, poised to make its passage across the Atlantic.[13]

On September 14, 1848, Dr. Thomas Barbour of the faculty of Missouri Medical College reported in the St. Louis *Missouri Republican* that he had diagnosed and treated in St. Louis an isolated case of Asiatic cholera.[14] This claim was disputed the next day in the columns of the *Missouri Republican* by a correspondent signing himself "Medicus," who asserted that Dr. Barbour's case was one of common summer cholera which was not epidemic, and that Dr. Barbour was a publicity-seeking alarmist.[15]

In an editorial in its issue of December 21, 1848 the St. Louis *Missouri Republican* warned citizens to prepare for the inevitable visit of cholera to their city:[16]

> In all the Eastern cities, measures are already in progress, to prepare for the visitation of the cholera. Complaints are loudly made in the newspapers of the filthy condition of the several cities, and efforts to improve them strongly recommended. Something of this kind should be done in St. Louis. The general condition of the city and of every street in it, is as favorable for the spread of the disease as can possibly be imagined. Everywhere, arising to some extent, from the prevalence of wet weather and the negligence of the city scavengers, causes of complaint exist, and if our citizens desire to escape the ravages of this scourge they should at once attempt some reform in this particular.

All the writers upon the cholera urge a proper attention to cleanliness, throughout the town, as most likely to lessen its ravages. It is not now too soon to begin this work. Its existence at New York is pretty well established, and an arrival at New Orleans, from Havre, of an emigrant ship, on board of which was a large number of passengers sick, gives reasons to fear that it may soon break out there. The papers do not make mention of the disease as being cholera, though it is not improbable, from the fact that the cholera was brought to New York by a vessel from Havre, leaving about the same time as the vessel which has arrived at New Orleans. At all events, two or three months may be sufficient for it to reach St. Louis in its course from New York, and we cannot expect entirely to escape, though much may be done to mitigate its severity.

Less than a week after this warning, the steamer *Alton* arrived in St. Louis from New Orleans with a number of German emigrants aboard. On the voyage upriver a woman and five children had died, presumably of cholera, though the ship's officers said that dysentery was the cause of the deaths. When the ship docked, only one passenger was sick and he was retained on board until he recovered. The other passengers dispersed through the city, possibly carrying the germs of cholera with them.[17]

A month later the steamer *Andrew Fulton* from New Orleans docked at the harbor. Several passengers, including the pilot, developed cholera on the trip. The pilot died.[18]

By May 1849, the cholera which up to this time had been confined mostly to deck passengers on boats from New Orleans, appears to have firmly established itself within the city of St. Louis. The weekly mortality report published May 2 showed 141 deaths of which 41 were from cholera.[19] The problem of coping with the local epidemic was complicated by the arrival in St. Louis of thousands of emigrants — German and Irish refugees and Mormons from England en route to Utah. Crowds of gold seekers headed for California also were on hand.

For the hundreds of Irish who arrived in St. Louis, the steamboat trip up the Mississippi River was merely the last leg of a long and hazardous journey. Driven from their small fields by successive failures of the potato crop and by major changes in the economics of British agriculture, they had made their way carrying their scanty possessions to an Irish Channel port from which they crossed over to Liverpool. In Liverpool, they resided in cheap housing until they could make arrangements with ship brokers for passage across the Atlantic. Packed in the steerage of British or American sailing vessels, their condition was only slightly better than that in which blacks were transported earlier in the slave trade.[20]

Emigrants were carried below deck in the area which on many trips provided space for wheat, lumber, cotton or iron products. No portholes for ventilation existed; openings to the fresh air would have admitted sea water. It was common practice to berth four persons in space six feet square. Toilet facilities were often located on deck and inaccessible in bad weather. No cooked food was furnished the emigrants. They were entitled to receive a weekly ration, mostly dry food which they had to cook themselves. Often the passengers were cheated regarding the quantity as well as quality of the provisions. Since many boats had only one range for 100 persons, getting to use the stove was almost impossible. Water was strictly rationed and was often salty or spoiled. A ship's surgeon, if carried, usually was poorly trained. The ship's captain and mates maintained discipline with an iron hand. Complaints were ignored or rewarded with beatings of the complainants.[21]

After spending five or six weeks in the hold of a vessel where they suffered constantly from seasickness, malnutrition, foul air, dehydration, loss of sleep, and inability to wash or change their clothing, the emigrants were put ashore in New Orleans.[22] For a few hours many indulged, often excessively, in the consumption of types of food and drink especially fresh fruit which they had long been denied. Then once more, under the direction of ship brokers, they were herded, without any quarantine check, aboard river boats for the trip to St. Louis. On the trans-Atlantic voyage they were steerage passengers; for the 7-8 day river trip they were quartered on deck. There were no laws of the United States guaranteeing them even minimum allowances of space, food, water or medical attention. Being deck passengers they received plenty of fresh air. Protection from the summer sun, they had to arrange for themselves. They were responsible for their own meals. There were no ranges for cooking. Water was a problem. Some boats had pumps for elevating the river water to the deck; otherwise the passenger had to lower a bucket over the rail and draw up his supply. More than one passenger was pulled overboard and lost through dropping his bucket into the river while the boat was in motion.[23]

The experience of German emigrants of the farmer class paralleled that of the Irish peasants. Havre, France, was the popular port of embarkation for the Germans. Packet boats sailed from Havre to New Orleans to take on cargoes of cotton for the French mills. Since the United States imported little from France,

they would have sailed on the outward voyage practically empty had it not been for the hordes of emigrants seeking passage. Since most of the Germans hoped to buy farmland in the Middle West, New Orleans rather than New York was the logical place to leave ship. From New Orleans, they took river transportation to a wide variety of destinations.[24]

The third major group of emigrants were the Mormons, who called themselves the Poor Man's Church. During the 1840s and 1850s, they actively gathered converts in Great Britain. But it was not their aim to establish a strong church there. Instead, the converts were organized into companies under the charge of a president and six committeemen and dispatched to Liverpool. Here, they chartered their own ships for the trip to New Orleans. In 1849, 2,500 Mormons emigrated. In New Orleans, they took passage for St. Louis where they arranged transportation to Council Bluffs, Iowa.[25] On the steamboat *Mary*, bound from St. Louis to Council Bluffs in early May 1849, cholera broke out among Mormon deck passengers, with a heavy loss of lives. Wagon trains were organized in Council Bluffs for the final overland trip to Salt Lake City, Utah.[26]

In the spring of 1849, thousands of gold seekers arrived in St. Louis on the way to California where gold had been discovered in the tributaries of the Sacramento River a year previously. Some came from neighboring states by wagon trains. Others from the Eastern states and Europe traveled by boat to St. Louis and outfitted there. The city, with its long experience in organizing exploring and fur trading expeditions, had the wagons, saddlery, livestock, clothing, guns and food the prospectors would need. The adventurers probably camped on the western edge of town as they assembled their outfits. Later they moved to Independence, Westport,

Weston and St. Joseph to await the emergence of grass on the western plains needed to sustain their stock. The camp sites of the Forty-Niners, both in the state and on the long trail to California, were fertile breeding places for cholera.[27]

As summer approached, the death toll in St. Louis from cholera mounted. For the week ending May 13, the number of deaths for all causes was 273 of which 181 were from cholera.[28] During May 11-12, some 1,200 emigrants, just from Europe, had landed at the St. Louis wharf, bringing sickness, disease and death. They were not required to undergo any medical inspection before they scattered to the homes of friends or relatives or to cheap lodging in the city. The "Gateway to the West" was wide open to disease as well as to immigrants.[29]

Finally roused to action, the council hired hundreds of workers to clean the streets and alleys, and dispose of the accumulated filth and refuse.[30] It placed $10,000 at the disposal of the board of health to be used in protecting the health of the city.[31]

A report by "An Eye Witness" indicated that these piecemeal actions by the council were producing no relief at the grass roots level where hundreds were dying from the pestilence:[32]

Beyond the effort to keep the streets in a somewhat better condition than usual, literally nothing has been done and the scenes presented in some portions of our city beggars [sic] description. I will notice one occurrence of an hour since, and ask any and all of my fellow-citizens shall this state of affairs continue and we look on with supine indifference? Would the inhabitants of any other city in the civilized world suffer such scenes to pass around them, and no effort be made to ameliorate the wretched condition of their destitute fellow-creatures? I was told that on Ninth St., between St. Charles and Washington Avenue, a child had died alone and unattended; and incredulous of so horrid an occurrence in a populous neighborhood, I entered the house. In a lower room was a girl of about ten years of age, trying to soothe an infant of some four weeks old — the father and mother having gone to the hospital an hour before. In the upper story, on a bedstead covered with an old blanket, lay the corpse of a girl of about twelve or fourteen who had evidently died in the act of quenching thirst with a piece of orange, still grasped in the dead hand. Beside the corpse stood a Sister of Charity who had just heard of the death and came in the fulfillment of her beautiful mission, after having accomplished the loathsome task of laying out corpse after corpse since the pestilence had broken out with such violence in the fated neighborhood. I found that the whole block bounded by Washington Avenue, St. Charles, Ninth and Eighth streets was a perfect lazar house. Three, four and five dead bodies lying in one house at the same time. Many are anxious to get to the hospital, but poverty is added to their other miseries, and no conveyance being provided by the city they are forced to die in the pestilential atmosphere around them, thus adding fuel to the fire.

A. B. Chambers, the editor of the St. Louis *Missouri Republican,* played a role in mobilizing opinion for effective and concerted action. In the issue of June 24, he commented:[33]

One of the strangest features of the times, in the midst of this desolation, is the apathy and apparent indifference which pervades the public. It cannot be charged upon one class of society more than another. Nearly every individual seems to be alive to the importance of action, immediate and efficient, but who shall lead, who shall take the first step is the point of difficulty. As if frightened at the common calamity, all stand still, waiting the action of others, and nothing is done.

The apathy and indifference of the community seems to find consolation, and even justification, in another source, the inaction of the City Authorities. Surely no city can point to greater inactivity than is presented by the Municipal Authorities of St. Louis. We have a Mayor, a Council and a Board of Health, with the City Treasury at their command, with numerous functionaries subject to their order and ample power to increase their agents to any extent which the necessity may require, and yet, what have they done? True, we have had two or three Proclamations, and the recommendation of a few sanatory observances, but have they been enforced? Have the Council, by the passage of ordinances, and by an increase of officers caused these recommendations to be observed? Have the Board of Health, which meet three times a week, enforced obedience to their requirements? In a word, what has been done, that can be pointed to as an efficient monument of the precaution, energy and attention of the City Authorities, for the health of the people.

In response to a call signed by a number of prominent citizens, a mass meeting convened at the courthouse at 7:30 P.M. Monday, June 25, to consider the public health emergency and to make recommendations for dealing with it. Edward Bates was called to the chair. A comprehensive set of proposals was drawn up and speedily adopted. The appointment of a special inspector for each inhabited block, with responsibility for cleansing and disinfecting his area, was urged. The block inspectors would have the authority to move families from crowded, unhealthy tenements to wholesome quarters.[34]

A committee of inspectors, consisting of five members, was recommended for each ward. It would provide hospital rooms, appoint doctors to staff the emergency hospitals, supervise the block inspectors and keep records of expenses incurred. Penalties were prescribed for failure to comply with orders of the health officials or for failure of officials to perform their duties. A committee was appointed to consult with the city authorities regarding the institution of a quarantine and to assist in carrying out the quarantine when established. This committee was instructed to convey the recommendations of the mass meeting, in the form of an ordinance, to the mayor and city council. If the constituted municipal authorities were unable or unwilling to implement the proposals of the citizens' meeting, they would be asked to resign and turn back their responsibilities and powers to the people.[35]

The citizens' committee met with Mayor James G. Barry at the town hall the next morning. The mayor pledged his full cooperation in carrying out the recommendations of the committee. The two legislative boards had adjourned until Wednesday evening, June 27. The mayor summoned them to a special meeting that afternoon (June 26) at 4 P.M.[36]

The board of aldermen and the mayor met with the citizens' group at the appointed hour. The delegates were absent, their board having failed to raise a quorum of members. Alderman George Maguire, in a surprise move, introduced a substitute for the citizens' ordinance, which after discussion and slight amendment was passed by a vote of 8 to 1. The substituted ordinance, in order to carry out the proposals of the public meeting, established a committee of public health, consisting of T. T. Gantt, R. S. Blennerhassett, A. B. Chambers, Isaac A. Hedges, James Clemens, Jr., J. M. Field, George Collier, L. M. Kennett, Trusten Polk, Lewis Bach, Thomas Gray and William G. Clarke. This was the same committee, consisting of two representatives from each of the city's six wards, which had drafted the recommendations of the mass meeting.[37]

The committee of public health was given power to appoint such officials and agents as it deemed necessary to carry out the purposes of the ordinance; and they were authorized to make all rules and regulations required to perform their task. Violation of these rules would be punished by a fine of from five to one hundred dollars. The sum of $50,000 was placed at the disposal of the committee. The ordinance was to take effect from its passage and remain in effect until the committee of public health considered the epidemic ended.[38] The board of delegates gave approval to the ordinance at a meeting at 8 P.M. on June 27.

This ordinance effectively turned over to a group of private citizens the temporary operation of city government, including its legislative, executive and financial responsibilities and powers.

Whatever its motivation,[39] the decision of the city council to commission the citizens' committee to wage the war on cholera was a wise one. During the six months when the council had carried the responsibility, its efforts had been unimaginative and ineffective. The committee of public health was a carefully selected and extremely able group. Gantt, Blennerhassett and Polk were prominent lawyers. Chambers, editor of the St. Louis *Missouri Republican,* was the best informed person on public health matters in town. Kennett was a retired merchant, a member of the board of aldermen from the Fourth Ward, and the future mayor of St. Louis for three terms beginning in 1850. Hedges was an agricultural machinery manufacturer; Field, a writer and actor; Bach, a tavern owner; and Clarke, the operator of a sawmill.[40] These men had not only knowledge and administrative ability but also the dedication to the public welfare which motivated them to accept a job that would bring them into close contact with a mysterious and terrifying disease which killed its victims in a matter of hours, that would require them to neglect their own businesses or professions for an unpredictable length of time, and which might involve them as defendants in individual or collective legal suits or actions.

The committee of public health was created near the peak of the epidemic. During the week ending Sunday, June 24, there were 752 deaths, 601 from cholera.[41]

Without waiting for official notification that the city council had completed action on the emergency ordinance, the committee of public health met at the Planters' House, on the evening of June 27, to begin their work. Each morning thereafter — and occasionally in an extra evening session — they assembled to plan and supervise the campaign against the pestilence.

The committee established in each ward, usually in a public school building, a temporary hospital, with two physicians and a staff of nurses in constant attendance. All destitute persons suffering from cholera were sent to these centers. Most of the nurses were from the order of the Sisters of Charity. Later a corps of young male volunteer nurses was organized. In each ward a medical supply depot was set up to provide outpatient care.[42] The Sisters' Hospital, the city hospital and the hotel for invalids were available for cholera patients able to pay for their treatment.

The two members of the committee of public health from each ward were made responsible for the appointment of physicians and inspectors and the carrying out of sanitary measures in their wards.[43]

The committee published a notice to the citizens of St. Louis to clean up their premises and to have the collected filth and decaying matter deposited in the street next to their lots by 10 A.M. Friday, June 29, in order to be picked up by the city's scavenger and slop carts. Neglect to comply with the order was punishable by a fine. On the assumption that cholera was an air-borne disease, the committee recommended the burning at dusk each day of wood shavings, coal, tar and sulphur, hoping that the fumes of hundreds of fires would fumigate the atmosphere. The extensive use of lime and other disinfecting agents also was urged.[44]

In their daily sessions, the committee listened to reports from representatives of the wards concerning sickness and mortality statistics, staffing problems, supply requirements, the public reaction to their measures and the abatement of nuisances. These reports revealed the intolerable living conditions of the poor which provided the social basis of the cholera epidemic. The report of the Third Ward at the committee meeting on Saturday, July 7, described one of the city's nuisances called "Shepherds' Graveyard:"[45]

A man has been employed to prevent emigrants from occupying the vacated houses in the "Graveyard," and persons from casting filth there. Dr. Alleyne, who had been specially employed in said district, reported that his examination fully confirmed what had been previously communicated to the Committee with reference to said infected region, between Eighth and Twelfth streets, Pine and Clark Avenue. Many tenements consist of shanties unfit for occupants, partly buried in the mud, and wholly uncomfortable.

The cleansing and disinfecting of the city's yards, streets and alleys and the establishment of a system of temporary hospitals for the sick were two major portions of the committee's campaign against the epidemic; the third part was the institution of an effective quarantine to prevent the landing of shiploads of diseased emigrants on the wharfs.

On July 3, a subcommittee of the committee of public health, accompanied by Mayor James G. Barry, selected Arsenal Island, several miles south of the city as the quarantine headquarters. The system of control was expeditiously put into effect with the stationing of Dr. Henry Carrow as quarantine officer at the Montesano House, on the west bank of the river, with instructions to board and inspect all vessels arriving from the south. Boats carrying diseased passengers were placed in quarantine and the sick persons taken off for medical care. Temporarily, the steamship *St. Louis,* berthed next to the western shore of the island, was used as a hospital. Within several weeks, four large frame houses, able to accommodate 600-800 persons, were built. The committee appointed Drs. Ferdinand Haussler and H. Owens as resident physicians. Dr. Richard Barrett served as chief quarantine officer and visiting physician.[46]

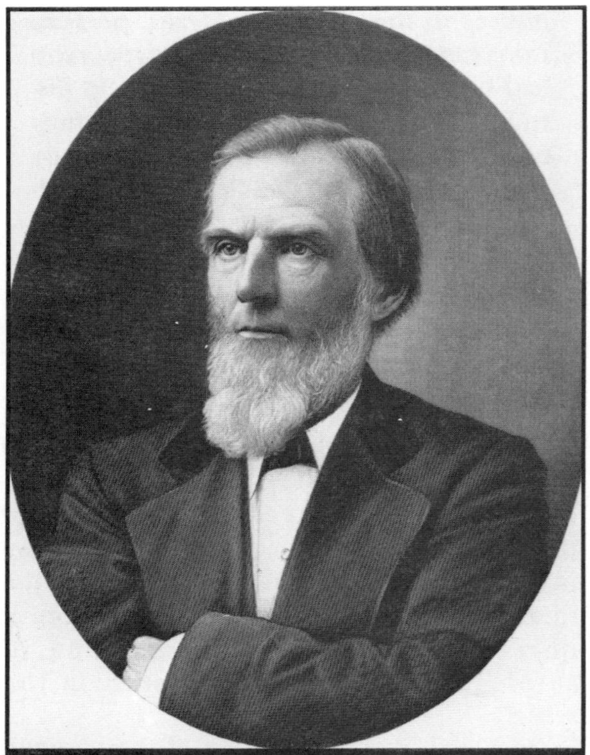

Dr. William M. McPheeters. Coutresy of the State Historical Society of Missouri.

Twenty-six boats were boarded and examined by the quarantine officer; of these nineteen were placed in quarantine for varying periods of time. A total of 1,700 persons were provided medical treatment.[47] For the first time in months, they had the opportunity to bathe, change their clothes, rest and eat nutritious food. Those who were financially able made a contribution to the cost of their rehabilitation. The poor paid nothing.

The cholera epidemic in St. Louis reached a peak on July 10 with a total of 145 deaths. From that point it declined, so that on July 30, 1849, the board of health was able to announce that the epidemic was ended.[48] Dr. William M. McPheeters, who had charge of the Sisters of Charity Hospital during the epidemic, reported that the number of cholera deaths in St. Louis for June 1849 was 1,799, and for July 1849 stood at 1895. For the whole year he reported 4,557 cholera deaths.[49]

That the subsidence of the epidemic was due more to the practical measures of the committee of public health than to the medical skill of the doctors was admitted by Dr. McPheeters:[50]

> That although no skeptic as to the powers of medicine, my experience in the treatment of cholera has taught me how impotent is our art when the disease is malignant — that the result of medication depends vastly more on the character of the case than on the nature of the treatment, and that while mild cases will yield to opposite plans of treatment, nineteen-twentieths of all the worst cases will die in spite of all the doctors and all the medicine in the universe.

Dr. McPheeters reached this conclusion after trying a wide range of medical specifics including opium, morphine, calomel, blood letting, salt and mustard emetics, musk powders, carbonate of ammonia solution, astringent injections and blisters on the abdomen.[51] It is obvious that Dr. McPheeters, as well as his medical colleagues, were treating the symptoms of cholera, e.g., vomiting, cramps and loss of body heat, rather than the cause.

The committee of public health, as its last official duty, prepared a report which revealed that careless municipal housekeeping, at least in part, was responsible for the fact that St. Louis suffered more severely than any other American city in the 1849 epidemic.[52] The report formulated recommendations for improving the health of the city.

Assisted by its special ward and block inspectors, the committee had conducted the first comprehensive survey of living conditions in St. Louis. The findings were shocking as the following description   indicates:[53]

There were not in the employ of the city when we entered upon our duties, six slop carts throughout our limits, at least we were unable to find out the existence of so many upon diligent inquiry. Three-fourths of the city in surface and population is never visited by a slop cart to carry off the liquid filth which accumulates at every dwelling, nor by a scavenger cart to remove more solid impurities. The consequence is, that such parts of our city are exposed, except where the population is of such habits as to need no supervisory care, to the worst consequences of the neglect which we have named. It unfortunately happens that lots of imperfect drainage, and ineligible by reason of want of elevation for the erection of the better sort of residences, lie contiguous to the ordinary places of business of a large class of our laboring population. They are sought for and crowded with tenements constructed with almost a single eye to cheapness in the first instance. In this manner whole blocks are built up and occupied by laboring men and their families, chiefly of foreign extraction. The alleys dividing the blocks are unpaved. Very often the cross streets and sometimes the numbered streets are in the same condition.

Because they were lower than street level, cellars in the poorer districts were frequently filled with stagnant water. With no adequate collection system, householders deposited their garbage and human wastes in the unpaved streets and alleys where these materials decayed and permeated the soil. Under these environmental handicaps, personal cleanliness and health were difficult to maintain.

The committee recommended the following measures: (1) an adequate system of sewers that would drain the whole city and prevent the accumulation of water in cellars and low-lying areas; (2) the paving of every street and alley; (3) the improvement of the system of street cleaning, to assure that the scavenger crews collected the refuse and human wastes in the whole city on a regular schedule; (4) the establishment of a permanent and effective quarantine.[54]

The cholera paid St. Louis a return visit in 1850. By proclamation on May 3, Mayor Luther M. Kennett, who had served with distinction on the committee of public health the previous year, instituted a quarantine requiring all incoming boats "to touch at the quarantine station on Arsenal Island, and land all emigrants and others recently from shipboard, and all sick, diseased or unclean persons, with their stores and baggage."[55] The immediate cause of the mayor's action was the arrival of the *St. Louis* and *Missouri* at the local wharf a few hours previously. On both boats a number of cases of cholera, with some fatalities, had occurred on the passage up the river from New Orleans.[56] Within several days a total of approximately twenty cases of the disease had been reported among St. Louis residents.[57]

On May 5, the steamer *Alvarado* was stationed at Arsenal Island as a temporary hospital, and the quarantine was put into full effect. Construction of the necessary housing was expedited.[58] The mayor sent notice to New Orleans that if boats arrived in St. Louis with an excessive number of emigrants in relation to their tonnage, they would face a long detention in quarantine.[59]

The prompt enforcement of quarantine regulations was the major factor in reducing deaths from cholera in St. Louis from 4,557 in 1849 to 865 in 1850. Cholera continued to claim victims in St. Louis during the 1850s, with epidemic levels of 696 deaths in 1852 and 1,351 fatalities in 1854. Only one cholera death was registered for 1860.[60]

Smallpox, typhoid fever and consumption, three diseases endemic in St. Louis, persisted through the 1850s. Vaccination kept the average death rate for smallpox to approximately 27 a year. Typhoid fever and consumption, for which the doctors had no preventives or cures, claimed a heavy toll. The average annual death rate for typhoid fever was 166 and for consumption 300 persons.[61]

3. Beginnings of a Sewer System

One of the recommendations of the committee of public health was that a system of public sewers, that would drain the whole city and prevent the accumulation of water in cellars and low-lying areas, should be built. The inauguration in April 1850 of Luther M. Kennett as mayor enabled him to implement this recommendation. In his message to the city council in May 1850, he urged completion of the Biddle Street sewer in northwest St. Louis and the construction of a sewer to drain Chouteau's Pond in the southwest part of town. He proposed that the areas covered by these two bodies of water be purchased by the city and transformed into public parks.[62]

Already a start had been made toward the construction of a sewer system for St. Louis. On March 12, 1849, the general assembly passed an act directing the St. Louis municipal authorities to have the city laid off into districts to be drained by principal and tributary sewers, in accordance with a master plan for the whole city. The act further provided that when a majority of owners of real estate within any district petitioned for the construction of sewers in that district, the city council would be empowered to collect a special levy on the real estate in the district for the liquidation of the costs of the district sewers.[63]

The sewer system authorized by the general assembly consisted of three classes: (1) public sewers along the main drainage courses, which would be financed from general revenue; (2) district sewers, the expense of which would be assessed against lots in the district in proportion to area; (3) private sewers, built by permission of the municipal board of public improvements at the cost of the owners of the lots.[64]

On July 30, 1849, the same day that the board of health had declared the cholera epidemic at an end, the city council authorized the building of a trunk line sewer under Biddle Street to drain "Kayser's Lake" into the river.[65] This project had been first proposed by the city's German-born engineer, Henry B. Kayser, in 1840.[66] The council rejected the sewer plan as too expensive and chose a scheme to utilize a number of sinkholes to drain the area. In time the sinkholes became clogged with rubbish and filth, creating a body of stagnant, foul-smelling water. During the 1849 cholera epidemic when it was generally believed that disease were caused by exhalations from decaying matter and polluted water, the elimination of "Kayser's Lake" became a civic improvement of top priority.

Early in April 1850, Kayser began the construction of the Biddle Street sewer by removing the water pipes from the path of the project. The sewer was designed in the shape of a horseshoe twelve feet wide with an arch twenty feet high. At this stage of the construction, Mayor Kennett, a Whig, appointed

Samuel R. Curtis of Keokuk, Iowa, to replace Kayser as city engineer. Curtis supervised the completion of the city's overall sewerage plan. He later won fame as commander of the Union forces which defeated the Confederates at the battle of Pea Ridge, Arkansas, March 6-8, 1862.[67]

The drainage of Chouteau's Pond presented certain legal problems which were not involved in the Biddle Street project. The owners, members of one of St. Louis's wealthy and prestigious families, had shown no willingness to sell to the city, so the power of eminent domain might have to be exercised. A letter from a concerned correspondent, published in the St. Louis *Missouri Republican* of April 27, 1850, described how badly the pond had deteriorated from its former status as St. Louis's favorite recreational area:[68]

I would like to enquire whether the new city administration have it in contemplation to adopt any measure calculated to abate or ameliorate this disgraceful nuisance in the heart of the city. In its present condition it is the receptacle of the washings of contiguous streets, of the rubbish of manufacturing establishments, of the offal of slaughter pens and all around the upper end of the pond numbers of the dead carcasses of dogs and horses are left to be exhaled by the sun and to infect the atmosphere. It is doubtful whether there is, in our midst, any one local cause so prolific of disease as this much complained of pond.

Amendments to the St. Louis charter, approved by the general assembly March 3, 1851, cleared the way for the completion of the city's first area-wide sewerage project.

The amendments granted power to the St. Louis City Council to "drain and keep drained Chouteau's Pond, whenever they deem it best so to do for the general health."[69] The city was also given authorization to increase its bonded debt to finance its sewerage program.[70]

This program consisted of five main sewers. The first was the Biddle Street sewer, running from Ninth Street to the river. The second was a sewer on Poplar Street, from Ninth to the Mississippi waterway. This would empty Chouteau's Pond. Three north-south sewers were planned; one on Seventh Street, running north to intersect the Biddle Street drainage system; and two on Ninth Street, one extending south to meet the Poplar Street conduit, and the other, on North Ninth Street, north of Biddle, coursing south to the Biddle sewer.[71]

The area bounded north by Biddle Street, south by Poplar Street, east by the Mississippi River, and west by Ninth Street, was subdivided into thirty-three districts, each to be drained by a district or common sewer.[72]

The Biddle Street sewer was completed and put into service on August 14, 1851.[73] The construction of the Poplar Street sewer and the elimination of Chouteau's Pond were accomplished by the end of 1853.[74]

Within the period 1850-1853, corresponding roughly with the three administrations of Mayor Kennett, major contributions to the improvement of public health in St. Louis were made. The quarantine against incoming boats bringing epidemics to the city, which in 1849 had been instituted and operated on a temporary basis by a committee of private citizens, was put on a permanent footing, under the constituted city authorities. The advantage of having the quarantine station at Arsenal Island ready and plans made for its speedy use was demonstrated in May 1850, when cholera revisited St. Louis.

During this period, two notorious nuisances and threats to public health, i.e. Kayser's Lake and Chouteau's Pond, were eliminated. The belief that these ponds emitted miasmata which caused disease was perhaps unfounded. But they certainly were breeding places for mosquitoes which spread malaria. Boys, who swam or fished in the polluted waters, risked cholera, typhoid or dysentery.

A start was made on the provision of a sewer system for St. Louis. As the city grew, the system was expanded to cover the new additions. With a municipal sewer system, water could be piped into homes, businesses and factories. Flush toilets, in place of insanitary vaults, could be installed. An abundance of water for bathing, cooking and other household uses could be provided.

4. Shortages at the Waterworks

The expansion of St. Louis's population from 16,469 in 1840 to 77,716 in 1850, placed a heavy burden on the city's waterworks. Besides many new households, there was a sharp increase in business and manufacturing establishments, with their enormous water requirements. Street sprinkling and cleansing demanded great quantities of water. Since consumers paid a flat rate depending on the category in which they were placed, there was no incentive to be economical in water usage. The land on which St. Louis was situated rose in terraces from the river level, with the consequence that the old reservoir on Broadway encountered difficulties in delivering water by gravity flow to the new western suburbs.

In January 1850, a new basin, known as the Benton Street reservoir, located on a ten-acre tract owned by the city in the northwest part of town, was put into operation. The site, which was bounded by the present Twentieth, Twenty-second, Benton, and Madison streets, was almost two miles from the point in the river where the water was pumped. The pipe which connected the pumping station and the reservoir followed street lines and had a number of sharp turns which slowed the velocity of the water. The reservoir was 250 feet square and fifteen feet deep.[75] It had a capacity of approximately 8,000,000 gallons.[76] The ground on which it was situated had the highest elevation of any available site within a reasonable distance from the river.

By 1854, the daily consumption of water, excluding Sundays, was 3,500,000 gallons or 21,000,000 gallons a week. The pumping station was able to deliver 3,000,000 gallons a day to the reservoir. Consequently, the station had to operate twenty-four hours a day, seven days a week, to provide the minimum water requirements.[77] Little time was available in the reservoir for sedimentation to occur.

A second reservoir was put into service in the summer of 1855 at the ten-acre site in northwest St. Louis. This basin was 500 feet long, 250 feet wide, with a depth of 40 feet. Its rated capacity was 32,218,000 gallons. Valves in the floor of the reservoir were designed to drain off the accumulated sand and mud. A third reservoir was planned on the same site.[78] When this became available, the water supply could be passed through the series of three adjoining basins before being distributed through the mains. This process would increase the settling action and produce a clearer and more wholesome product.

The St. Louis water drawn from the merged currents of the Missouri and Mississippi rivers, was reputed to be the finest river water in the world for drinking purposes. It had the quality of remaining fresh and sweet for long periods of time,[79] an important feature in the days before refrigeration. However, its muddy appearance when first drawn from the hydrant made it the subject of frequent citizen complaint and of constant efforts by the city to improve its quality.

By the summer of 1855, a serious cause for concern regarding St. Louis's water had developed. North St. Louis and Bremen, suburbs upstream from the city's pumping station, were filling up with people and industries. Their refuse and wastes were draining into the river. Besides, the St. Louis wharf officially had been extended to a point considerably above the water intake, with the result that ships at dock were dumping their garbage and human wastes into the harbor from which the city drew its water supply. The suggestion was made by the city engineer that the new engine house, scheduled to be erected at the Bates Street site, be moved north several miles to the neighborhood of Bissell's Ferry Landing — a site well beyond contamination by urban discharges. The proposal, in the form of a resolution, passed the board of delegates and was sent to the board of aldermen, with a letter of support from the mayor.[80] The measure failed to win approval in the upper house. It was not until more than twenty years later that this important move was finally made.

5. Health Department Matters

A revision of the ordinance establishing and regulating the Health Department was approved by the city council on April 1, 1850. Despite the fact that the board of health had not distinguished itself in coping with the cholera epidemic of 1849, no major changes were made in its organization or responsibilities. The board continued to be composed of the health officer and one alderman from each ward,[81] as according to the earlier ordinance of 1843.

The revised ordinance permitted the board of health to have a clerk who would establish an office in city hall and carry on the business of the board between its scheduled meetings. In addition to attending the board's sessions and recording the proceedings, the clerk was to examine applicants for admission to the city hospital and grant permits to persons entitled to this privilege. Previously, the mayor or the city register had granted these permits. The clerk was not required to be a trained medical person. His salary was $600 a year,[82] which was $100 more than the compensation of the health officer.

The board of health was authorized to establish temporary hospitals.[83] The need of this power was demonstrated during the 1849 cholera epidemic. Since the work of the resident physician at city hospital had increased, he was granted permission to employ two assistants.[84] The number of consulting physicians on the staff of the city hospital was enlarged from four to six.[85] The health officer's term of office was lengthened from six months to a year. Students of medicine, when accompanied by a professor of any of the medical colleges of Missouri, were to be admitted to the wards and lecture rooms at city hospital for clinical instruction.[86]

In 1853, the city council passed an ordinance making it the duty of police officers to notify the mayor or the city register regarding insane persons found wandering unattended on the city streets. The mayor would then request the county court to take charge of these persons and provide for them the proper medical care.[87] At first the St. Louis city officials had sent insane persons found within its limits to the Sisters' Hospital for treatment at the municipality's expense. However, legislation enacted by the general assembly made the county courts responsible for this class of sick persons.

The board of health in early May 1855 announced steps to make its services more readily available to the public. Regular hours were established when its office in city hall would be open; further, the city hospital staff was instructed to have a wagon at the office of the board during business hours to transport sick persons to the hospital.[88]

6. *The Crisis of the Medical Profession*

During the 1840s and 1850s, a loss of faith by the doctors themselves in the usual drugs and practices of internal medicine occurred. This originated in France, the leader in medical research. This attitude known as "clinical nihilism," involved a conviction that it is nature not medicine that cures. In St. Louis this defeatist spirit was strengthened by the inability of the physicians to treat with any success their thousands of patients in the 1849 cholera epidemic. Despite their skepticism, most doctors persisted in their commitment to the Rush system of purging and bleeding.[89]

Only in the cases of smallpox and malaria did the doctors have effective preventives or remedies. Dr. Antoine Saugrain had introduced vaccination in St. Louis in 1809. Despite this reliable agent, the St. Louis health authorities were not able to effect a sufficiently complete inoculation of the population to keep the disease from flaring up periodically.[90]

The usefulness of cinchona bark as a specific for malaria had been recognized as early as the seventeenth century in Peru and other regions of the Andes where the tree was a native. A large supply of the bark was carried

in the medicine chest of Lewis and Clark on their transcontinental voyage of discovery. It was not until 1820 that the alkaloid quinine was isolated from the bark in a Paris laboratory. Quinine was available in St. Louis in the 1830s and 1840s in the forms of powder, pills and a tonic. The pills of Dr. John Sappington of Arrow Rock, Missouri, who was influential in establishing the use of quinine in treating malaria, were sold in St. Louis through the firm of Jarrett and Ferguson, grocers and commission merchants.[91] Dr. Sappington recommended the use of his antifever pills at all stages of treatment of malaria. The standard practice of the times was to use quinine as a stimulant or tonic in the later stages, following the usual depletion procedures.[92]

In reaction to the "heroic" remedies of allopathic medicine, various sectarian systems flourished. The most popular was homeopathy. The first homeopathic physician in St. Louis was Dr. J. G. Rosenstien who opened an office in April 1842. Dr. John T. Temple, a graduate in medicine of the University of Maryland, came two years later. Dr. B. H. Peterson, another homeopathic practitioner, arrived in July 1848, followed in 1849 by Dr. J. T. Vastine from Pennsylvania.[93]

The New School physicians in 1851 formed a society under the name of the St. Louis Homeopathic Medical Society. The local group sent delegates to the organizational meeting of the Western Medical Association (Homeopathic) which assembled in Chicago the first week of June 1851.[94] The heavy German migration to St. Louis in the late 1840s provided both practitioners as well as patrons of homeopathic medicine.

One of the best trained of the local homeopathic fraternity was Dr. Thomas Griswold Comstock who graduated at the St. Louis Medical College and took post-graduate work in Philadelphia and at the finest medical

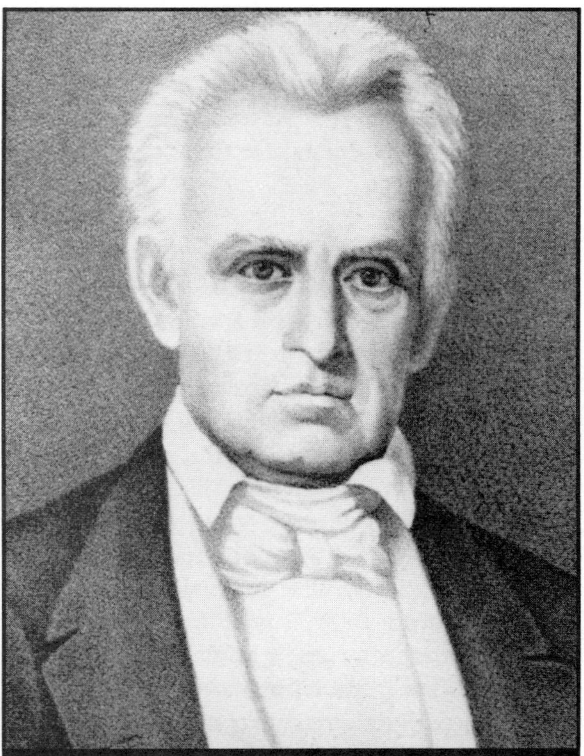

Dr. John Sappington. Coutresy of the State Historical Society of Missouri.

schools of Europe. In 1857, the local doctors founded the Homeopathic Medical College of Missouri.[95] Drs. Augustus H. Schott and E. C. Franklin served for a number of years on the college faculty. Dr. William Tod Helmuth, after a long period of service in St. Louis, went to New York City where he acquired fame as a surgeon.[96]

A correspondent , in a letter entitled "A Sociable Talk about the Doctors," published in the St. Louis *Missouri Republican* of February 28, 1853, listed the different competing schools of medicine: allopathy, homeopathy, hydropathy, Eclectic, steaming, and herb and root practice. He quoted a number of noted authorities attesting the ineffectiveness and often damaging effects of medicines prescribed by the allopathic physicians. In summing up his argument for homeopathy, he stated:[97]

> To Homeopathy, is generally conceded this advantage, that if it does not cure, it cannot kill, and notwithstanding the ridicule which is most liberally bestowed upon it, for its minute doses, it gains ground in every quarter of the civilized world. Even in Philadelphia, which city has been the most celebrated in the nation for her medical institutions, and where, but a few years since, Homeopathy was treated with contempt, there are at this time nearly one hundred Homeopathic physicians, many of them distinguished for talents and learning, and a Homeopathic Institute established under the supervision of able and scientific professors.

The Missouri legislature made no effort to raise the level of the medical profession by showing a preference for any one system of practice or by requiring certain standards of professional training. "An Act to Sustain the Credit of the State," approved by the general assembly on February 16, 1847, declared that "every person or co-partnership of persons in this State, who shall follow the practice of medicine for a livelihood in whole or in part is hereby declared to be a physician." The only requirement for becoming a doctor in Missouri was to pay a small fee for a license.[98]

The allopathic, or regular physicians, of St. Louis mounted a strong counter-offensive. They possessed a number of advantages in their competition with the new medical sects. The regulars were the inheritors of the long medical tradition, dating back to Galen and Hippocrates. Many had benefitted from the finest medical education available in the United States and Europe. They generally were members of the wealthy and conservative upper-middle class of the city. Some were active and influential in politics and business affairs. In February 1850, they formed the St. Louis Medical Society which took the place of the earlier Medical Society of Missouri.[99]

On November 4, 1850, under the leadership of the local medical society, an organizational meeting of the State Medical Association convened in St. Louis. The next day standing committees were set up on the following subjects: practical medicine; medical literature and science; surgery; obstetrics; medical topography, endemics and epidemics; publication; indigenous plants; and medical education.[100]

The afternoon session of November 5 was given over to the discussion of petitions and resolutions. The issues brought up were to constitute the agenda of the state organization for the next fifty years.

Dr. Adam Hammer of St. Louis, a recent emigre from Germany who had studied medicine at Heidelberg and Paris, sponsored a resolution petitioning the legislature to enact a law providing "that no person be permitted to practice medicine, surgery or midwifery, unless he shall be a graduate of some medical college, faculty or university of this State." He also urged the establishment of screening procedures for licensing physicians from other states and Europe. These proposals were approved.[101]

Dr. J. B. Johnson called attention to the legislation passed by the general assembly on February 16, 1847, conferring the status of physician on every person in the state practicing medicine for a livelihood. He advanced the following resolution which won the convention's support;[102]

Resolved, That this Association regard said interference in pronouncing upon the qualifications of physicians, uncalled for, and unjust to the medical profession, who are supposed to be the best judges of its own fellows, and their abilities. Resolved, That this Association memorialize the next Legislature for the repeal of said enactment.

A resolution was introduced petitioning the legislature to establish a uniform system of registration of births and deaths. Another called on the legislature to alter the laws of Missouri so that physicians in suits to collect fees need prove only the fact of general attendance on a patient and not the specific items and services.[103]

A jurisdictional issue between apothecaries and physicians, which had developed in St. Louis particularly, was aired on the floor of the convention. In St. Louis, the apothecaries, following the practice in England, were in the simpler cases prescribing and administering drugs to individuals who consulted them. The convention adopted two resolutions which attempted to limit the role of the apothecary in the treatment of patients:[104]

Resolved, That the business of the Apothecary is to provide himself with the purest drugs and to compound them according to prescribed formula.

Resolved, That the Apothecary has no just right to interfere with what strictly belongs to the physician.

Dr. William M. McPheeters submitted a resolution calling for the state association to urge the physicians of Missouri to form county and district societies to work as auxiliaries of the state organization. A committee of three members of the state group was appointed to assist in this undertaking.[105] In 1847, the American Medical Association had been established in Philadelphia. The organizational efforts of the state Medical Association were in line with the plans of the national organization to extend its support to the level of local medical groups.

At the convention of the State Medical Association in St. Louis, opening April 19, 1853, Dr. Charles A. Pope, dean of the St. Louis Medical College, moved that an invitation be extended to the American Medical Association to hold its 1854 annual meeting in St. Louis. The motion was approved. Delegates from the state organization were appointed to attend the assembly of the national association in New York beginning May 3, 1853 and personally convey the invitation.[106]

The American Medical Association, in acceptance of the invitation, assembled in St. Louis May 2, 1854.[107] The gathering of delegates was made possible by the development of a rail network with terminals in St. Louis. The delegates from the older states who must have had some misgivings about meeting in the land of Indians and buffaloes, found St. Louis a bustling city with its wharves crowded with ships and commerce and its bankers planning a railroad to the Pacific. They might have been surprised to find that the St. Louis doctors had attended the same medical schools in the United States and France as they had.

The meeting in St. Louis had the intended effect of bringing the doctors of Missouri into close working relations with those of the rest of the country. This professionally was beneficial and stimulating to the local doctors. It also had the effect of strengthening the national association as a major pressure group in behalf of allopathic medicine.

One of the first acts of the association at the May 2 session was the election of officers.

Dr. Charles A. Pope of St. Louis was chosen president.[108]

The reading and discussion of scientific papers usually constitutes the most important part of the business of the association's meeting. For the 1854 gathering, the papers were disappointing; many which had been scheduled were not ready for presentation or were given only in abstract form. The influence of the 1849 visit of cholera was seen in the presentation of a number of papers on epidemics in various parts of the country.[109]

The tendency of doctors of that day to engage in medical speculation rather than in scientific research was exemplified by several incidents at the convention. When called to express his views on the pathology of yellow fever, Dr. Moses L. Linton, one of the editors of the St. Louis *Medical and Surgical Journal*, declared[110]

that vegetable decomposition was not necessary to the production of the autumnal diseases of this country. He considered yellow fever nothing more than an aggravated type of bilious fever caused by the retention of hidro-carbonaceous substances in the blood. In other words, the agencies producing yellow fever were Northern blood subject to the heat of Southern latitudes.

A resolution was offered on the floor of the convention by Dr. Paul F. Eve of Nashville. "That a committee of three be appointed by the chair, to report at the next meeting of the Association, the best means of preventing the introduction of disease by emigrants into our country."[111] Dr. Linton, without waiting for the committee to make its investigation and report at the meeting the following year, offered a proposal aimed at predetermining the committee's findings:[112]

Resolved, That in the opinion of this Association, quarantine establishments afford no protection to states and cities against the invasion of cholera and yellow fever.

Dr. Linton's resolution directly was contradicted by the experience of St. Louis in the cholera epidemic of 1849 when the quarantine established and operated by a citizens' committee saved the city.

The fact is that no serious medical research or investigation was being conducted in St. Louis during the 1850s. The medical profession then consisted of doctors and medical school professors. The task of the doctors was to treat patients either in private practice or in the hospitals. The medical school professors, through the fees of their students, were paid to deliver lectures. The role of pathologist or medical researcher had not yet emerged in the American medical profession. A few doctors, despite the demands of their practice, did manage to find time for scientific study, as a recreational or hobby interest. In St. Louis, the scientific hobby was usually not medicine, but botany, zoology, geology, ethnology or some other natural science. The reasons were several. The doctors were not equipped, through training in organic chemistry, bacteriology and other life sciences to do medical research.

The attraction of the West, an uncatalogued new world, lured many doctors from the eyepiece of the microscope. St. Louis at this time was the point of departure for expeditions traveling westward on various missions. Military units, exploring parties, and hunting or fur trapping expeditions were usually accompanied by scientists to prepare maps, inventory mineral resources, study geological formations, and identify and classify plant, bird and animal life. Drs. George Engelmann,

Adolph Wislizenus and Hiram A. Prout participated in these scientific exploratory missions.[113] Other St. Louis doctors pursued their scientific interests without going so far afield.

The interest in science was widespread enough to justify the formation on March 10, 1856, of the Academy of Science of St. Louis. The academy established a natural science museum, published transactions, and prepared and discussed research papers.[114] Doctors formed the majority of members. Army officers and fur traders were next in importance.

At the annual meeting of the academy on January 2, 1860, Dr. Hiram A. Prout was chosen president; Dr. George Engelmann, first vice president; and Dr. Charles A. Pope, second vice president. Dr. Prout followed Dr. Wislizenus in the presidential office.[115] The outgoing president's report provided a statement of the aims of the academy:[116]

> With larger means . . . a great deal more might be accomplished here in the center of the Mississippi Valley, in the cultivation of the natural sciences, in developing the natural resources of the Great West, and in stimulating young men to habits of observing the wonders and studying the laws of nature, which must result in the increase of human knowledge and the improvement of mankind.

The academy experience provided invaluable training for the St. Louis physicians. Their previous medical education had been mostly a course of indoctrination in the dogmas of traditional medicine. In the deliberations of the academy, they were introduced to the scientific method of inquiry which is basically the search for truth in an intellectually free atmosphere. In their stated commitment to "observing the wonders and studying the laws of nature," the physician members of the academy would be led to question, and later to reject, many of the basic concepts and assumptions of their profession. Particularly vulnerable to scientific attack were the prevailing ideas of disease causation: the humoral thesis, Rush's concept of capillary tension and the miasmatic theory. The bleeding of patients and the administration of large doses of calomel in the depletion stages of treatment also came under scientific scrutiny. Through the services of the academy, its members were able to make the transition from dogmatic medicine to the scientific system pioneered by Louis Pasteur, Robert Koch and other European researchers.

7. *Hospital Expansion*

Although St. Louisans differed in their choices of methods of medical care, they apparently agreed in regard to the city's need for more hospitals. St. Louis had increased in population almost five-fold from 1840 to 1850. The Sisters' Hospital and the half-completed city hospital were obviously inadequate. The need existed not only for more general hospitals but also for institutions serving special patient constituencies.

One of the first steps taken was the completion in 1855 of the city hospital in accordance with the original plan. In 1846, only half of the architect's design for a three-story structure with two wings had been built. The completed hospital was in service only a year when on May 15, 1856, it was completely destroyed by fire. It was rebuilt the following year at a total cost of $62,000.[117]

The United States Marine Hospital for the care of sick and disabled river boatmen finally became a reality. The start of construction had been delayed for many years by objections to the original sites proposed because of the

great distance from the river. On March 10, 1850, it was announced that a sixteen-acre tract on Marine Avenue and Miami Street, near the arsenal in South St. Louis, had been selected as the location for the hospital, and that $30,000 had been appropriated for its construction.[118] At this site a two-story brick building, which was opened for patients in 1858, was erected.[119] The hospital ideally was located near the river bank so that patients could be brought to it by boats.

In the spring of 1848, the city council bought the "Old County Farm" from the county court for $6,000.[120] The farm at the time was on loan from the court. The city was using it as the site of a smallpox hospital. The neighbors objected, citing the large increase of the disease in the vicinity following the operation of the pesthouse there. In October 1852, the board of aldermen recommended that the smallpox hospital be moved from the Old County Farm to Quarantine (Arsenal) Island.[121] The city engineer drew up plans for a hospital at the proposed new site. This arrangement was abandoned when on July 7, 1854, the council purchased from Augustus Langkopf fifty-eight acres of land on the shore of the Mississippi River, a mile and a quarter south of Jefferson Barracks and about twelve miles south of St. Louis. On the western part of the grounds, away from the river, wards for the treatment of smallpox patients were erected.[122]

The quarantine station, located on Arsenal Island, was also moved to the Langkopf site. A large stone house on the property was refitted as the residence of the superintendent of quarantine. A number of wooden buildings were constructed near the river for hospital use.

A city ordinance, approved December 8, 1855, amended and consolidated the legislation governing the operation of a permanent hospital at the quarantine station. The hospital was to be staffed by a physician, assistant physician, steward and matron, appointed on a yearly basis. The board of health was empowered to exercise management and control of the hospital.[123]

Boats coming to St. Louis from the south had to stop at the quarantine station and discharge all emigrants and others recently from shipboard, and all sick, diseased and unclean passengers. During the period from April 1 to November 1, any steamboat with more than twenty deck or steerage passengers for each 100 tons register of the boat, coming from New Orleans or any point below Memphis, would be detained at quarantine for cleansing and purification for not less than forty-eight hours or more than twenty days.[124]

The Anne Biddle Infant Asylum and Lying-In Hospital was organized, in May 1853, and began operations at a temporary site at the corner of Menard and Marion streets. Its permanent home was at Tenth and O'Fallon streets. Funded by a bequest from Mrs. Anne Biddle, daughter of John Mullanphy, the institution was incorporated March 5, 1869, by its managers, the Sisters of Charity. It accepted abandoned children and provided obstetrical services for unmarried as well as married women.[125]

The Good Samaritan Hospital was founded, in 1858, and opened shortly afterwards in a small house at the corner of Sixteenth and Carr streets. It was supported by contributions from the Protestant churches and charitably inclined citizens of St. Louis. The hospital board purchased property on Jefferson Avenue at the head of O'Fallon Street upon which they erected a building that was completed shortly after the start of the Civil War. It was rented to the government to be used as a military hospital for almost two years.[126]

The hospitals of the 1850s were quite different from modern hospitals. They were hardly more than boarding houses or hotels where doctors could visit and treat their charity patients. Most were small in size, beginning often in a former private residence. They lacked laboratories and diagnostic equipment.

The nursing profession was in its infancy. Most of the nurses in the St. Louis hospitals were members of Catholic religious orders, especially the Sisters of Charity. Nursing was a form of Christian service, rather than a profession pursued for financial rewards. Much of the patient care provided by doctors in the hospitals was freely given. The doctors too were under the influence of the tradition, going back to medieval Europe, that treating the sick was a Christian obligation. The founding of hospitals in St. Louis appears to have been motivated in part by rivalry between the different religious denominations.

Once a hospital had acquired its building, the costs of operation were fairly low and relatively stable for the last half of the nineteenth century. It was not until the first decade of the next century that expensive equipment such as the X-ray came into use.

Most middle class families avoided the hospitals and had their medical treatment provided and their operations performed in their homes. There were sound reasons for this preference. Because of overcrowding and the neglect of simple principles of sanitation and ventilation, the early hospitals were unable to prevent the spread of infections within their own walls. Before the adoption of aseptic and antiseptic precautions, the danger of post-operative complications in surgery and obstetrics was high, particularly in hospitals.[127]

8. Progress at the Medical Colleges

The fall terms of the Medical Department of the University of the State of Missouri ("McDowell's College") and of the Medical Department of St. Louis University ("Pope's College") opened in late October 1849 in new buildings.[128] McDowell's new quarters, located at Eighth and Gratiot streets, consisted of an octagonal stone edifice seventy-five feet in diameter and one hundred and ten feet high. Attached to this main unit was a brick building, fronting for ninety feet on Eighth Street and extending back a distance of seventy-five feet.

The octagonal building contained three stories. The first housed a dispensary where poor patients might receive free medical advice, treatment and surgical operations. The second floor provided a reception room and a private library for the professors. The anatomical amphitheater was on the third floor. It was seventy feet in diameter and fifty-two feet high. The amphitheater was lighted by Gothic windows and skylights. High above the seats, encircling the room, was a gallery where anatomical representations were exhibited. The room and gallery provided seating for 2,000 persons.

The attached brick building had three floors and an attic. A chemical laboratory and lecture room occupied the first level. A lecture room and a library filled the second floor. A natural history museum monopolized the third floor. The dissecting rooms were located in the attic. The use to which a two-story wing on the opposite side of the octagonal tower was put is not known.

The major financing for the building was furnished by Dr. Joseph N. McDowell.[129] His fees as a lyceum lecturer, as a medical college professor and as a surgeon of wide reputation were the sources of his apparently ample income.

The new building of the Medical Department of St. Louis University was located at the corner of Seventh and Myrtle streets. It was financed by the munificence of Colonel John O'Fallon, father-in-law of Dr. Charles Pope. The building fronted on Myrtle a distance of sixty feet, and extended to the rear for ninety feet along Seventh Street. The height was seventy feet. Just inside the main entrance on Myrtle Street was a lecture room capable of seating 600-800 students. Behind the lecture room were laboratories for chemistry and other sciences.

On the floor above the lecture room was the amphitheater, forty-five feet in diameter and forty-eight feet high. It was illuminated by a domed ceiling and surrounded by a gallery in which a museum collection was exhibited. The amphitheater and gallery seated 1,500 persons. The library also was on the second floor above the science rooms. On the third and fourth floors, in the rear of the building, were four dissecting rooms. The offices of the professors were arranged around the circle of the amphitheater. Many of the medical illustrations in the gallery were drawn by Dr. Pope, an artist as well as a surgeon.[130]

The two buildings reflected the contrasting personalities of McDowell and Pope. McDowell's was Gothic in style, monumental and fortress-like in shape. Pope's was classically influenced and was more attractive from an artistic viewpoint. It mirrored his love of the arts through long residence in Paris and other European centers.

Since its organization in 1842, the Medical Department of St. Louis University had made excellent progress. One hundred and two students attended the 1848-1849 term; twenty-four of these graduated. The next year, attendance reached 112. Graduation requirements were approximately the same as in other similar institutions. The annual announcement for 1849-1850 stated that no institution in the country devoted more time to clinical instruction than Pope's College.[131] These opportunities were described in the St. Louis *Missouri Republican* of September 8, 1850:[132]

> There are in the city two large hospitals — the one under the charge of the Sisters of Charity, and the other belonging to the city. The faculty of the St. Louis University have the entire control of the Charity Hospital, and their students are admitted to it. The City Hospital is open to both the Medical Schools. In the latter, an hour is spent each day by the students, in company with the Professor, visiting the patients, and becoming familiar with the characteristics of diseases and the mode of treatment. On Wednesdays and Saturdays, the entire mornings are devoted to Hospital exercises, examinations, lectures, the witnessing of operations, etc. In each of these hospitals, there always are a large number of patients laboring under a variety of diseases, wounds, etc.

The medical staff at Pope's College for 1849-1850 numbered nine, almost double the faculty of 1842, and comprised the following professors: Dr. M. L. Linton, practice and principles of medicine; Dr. Charles A. Pope, principles and practice of surgery, clinical surgery, and dean of the college; Dr. A. Litton, chemistry and pharmacy; Dr. M. M. Pallen, obstetrics and diseases of women and children; Dr. James Blake, general and descriptive surgical anatomy; Dr. Thomas Reyburn, materia medica and therapeutics; Dr. R. S. Holmes, physiology and medical jurisprudence; Dr. W. M. McPheeters, clinical medicine and pathological anatomy; and Dr. Charles W. Stevens, demonstrator.[133]

The professorship of clinical medicine and pathological anatomy was an important addition to the medical program at Pope's College. Its aim was to correlate the symptoms observed by the physician at bedside with later autopsy findings in order to get a more complete picture of each disease entity. This was a pioneering endeavor that was being carried out with marked success in the research centers in France.

When ranked on the basis of the number of students enrolled and the number graduated for the year 1849-1850, the Medical Department of St. Louis University placed 17th and the Medical Department of the University of Missouri 18th. The combined totals of students enrolled and students graduated at the two local medical schools entitled St. Louis to the honor of being the fifth most important medical center in the country.[134]

In 1854, the medical faculty renewed their request for a separation from St. Louis University. This time, by mutual agreement, the break was effected. The Medical Department, having secured an independent charter, became St. Louis Medical College.[135]

9. Care of the Insane: From Local to State Control

On February 16, 1847, Governor John C. Edwards signed a bill establishing the State Lunatic Asylum, later renamed State Hospital Number One, at Fulton, Missouri. Four hundred acres of land in and near Fulton were acquired as the site of the institution.[136] The

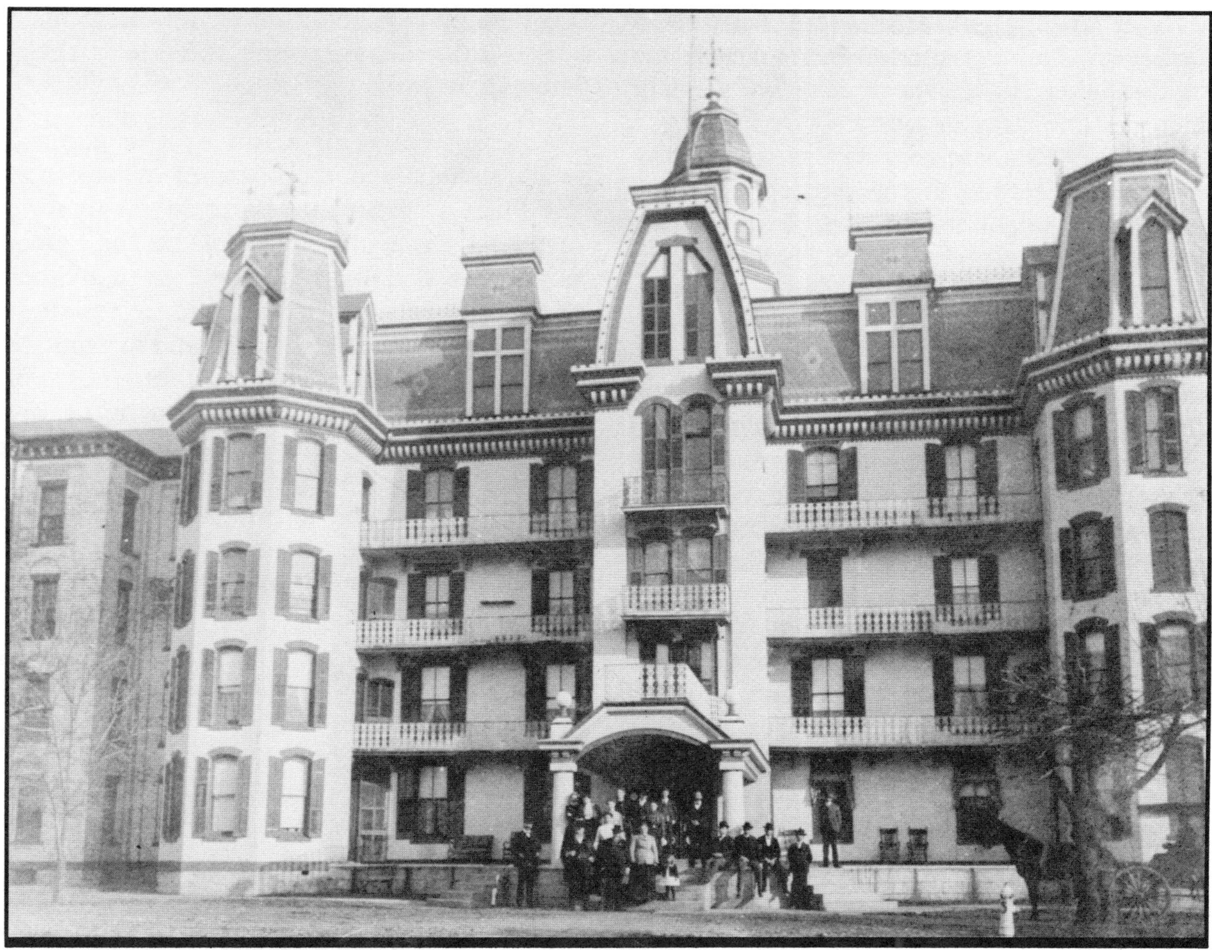

Fulton State Hospital (original portion). Courtesy of the Hospital staff.

hospital was opened for patients in 1851. Control of the institution was vested in a board of managers consisting of seven members serving four-year terms. The managers were instructed to appoint a superintendent who should be a "physician of knowledge, skill and ability in his field, and of experience in the management and treatment of the insane."[137]

Fulfillment of the latter part of this requirement posed some problems. Fulton was the first public mental hospital west of the Mississippi. The only institutions in the state which had acquired any experience with this class of patients were two Catholic hospitals in St. Louis, the Sisters of Charity Hospital and the St. Vincent Insane Asylum. They, for a number of years, had accepted a limited number of mentally deranged persons sent to them at the city's expense.

The first superintendent was Dr. T. R. H. Smith, a physician who had been in general practice in Columbia for the previous eleven years. He was born in Kentucky, February 21, 1820. His medical apprenticeship began in 1838 under Dr. W. H. Richardson, a professor in the Transylvania Medical School in Lexington. Smith graduated from Transylvania in 1840 after slightly more than two years of medical school training.[138]

The establishment of a state mental hospital represented an important step forward. Previously the county court, under the general assembly's act of March 3, 1835, had appointed a guardian to look after a person adjudged insane. Unless the guardian was a relative or friend, the level of service he rendered was probably minimal, since he took the job for the monetary allowance the court granted him. In many cases the insane person was kept shut up without social contacts and provided the bare essentials of food and clothing. Even in the Sisters' Hospital in St. Louis, the insane were kept in the building's basement.

The trend in American psychiatry between 1820 and 1860 involved the provision of humane, institutional care for mental patients. The philosophical background of this movement was the general humanitarianism of the period as exemplified by the teachings and activities of Dr. Benjamin Rush and Dorothea Dix.[139]

The Wooster State Lunatic Hospital in Massachusetts set the pattern of "moral treatment" which was followed by most of the nation's mental institutions, including that at Fulton, Missouri. Gerald N. Grob, in his valuable study *The State and the Mentally Ill,* describes this enlightened method:[140]

> While susceptible to many interpretations, moral therapy meant kind, individualized care in a small hospital with occupational therapy, religious exercises, amusements and games, and in large measure a repudiation of all threats of physical violence and an infrequent resort to mechanical restraint. In brief, the new therapy implied the creation of a healthy psychological environment for the individual patient as well as the group.

Subsequent legislation by the general assembly enlarged the board of managers of the Fulton institution from seven to nine members, three of whom must be competent physicians. The managers were given authority to appoint a superintendent, assistant physicians, treasurer, steward and matron. To assure that the state mental institution did not become filled with senile and incurable patients, the superintendent was authorized to limit admission to those persons whose condition could be improved by treatment, and to discharge patients unlikely to be helped by a longer stay in the asylum.[141]

Chapter III

St. Louis: Gateway to the West, 1849-1860

1   St. Louis *Missouri Republican*, Nov. 4, 1845, p. 4:1.

2   *Ibid.,* Jan. 11, 1850, p.2.

3   James Cox, *Old and New St. Louis* (St. Louis, Central Biographical Publishing Co., 1894), p.15.

4   St. Louis *Missouri Republican*, Aug. 3, 1850, p. 3:1; *ibid*, Jan. 6, 1851, p. 2:2.

5   Marcus Lee Hansen, *The Atlantic Migration 1607-1860: A History of the Continuing Settlement of the United States* (Cambridge, Mass., Harvard University Press, 1941), pp. 263, 266.

6   Terry Coleman, *Going to America* (Garden City, N.Y., Anchor Press/Doubleday, 1973), p. 216.

7   In response to the news of the overthrow of King Louis Philippe in France and the outbreak of revolutionary movements in other European countries, Mayor John M. Krum by proclamation designated Monday, April 24, 1848, for a massive demonstration of sympathy with the nations of Europe struggling for freedom. The large German colony in St. Louis, mostly recent emigres, took a leading part in the parades and speechmaking. St. Louis *Missouri Republican*, Apr. 24, 1848, p. 5.

8   William B. Faherty, *Dream by the River: Two Centuries of St. Louis Catholicism 1776-1967* (St. Louis, Piraeus Publishers, 1973) p. 80. Faherty pointed out that the successive western boundaries corresponded to elevation changes: "Laclede chose the location for St. Louis precisely because it rose in terraces back from the river. Third Street formed the first terrace. As the city grew, Eighteenth Street ran along the second terrace, Ewing just west of Jefferson along the third, and Grand Avenue along the fourth." *Idem*. The progressively higher terraces determined the location of the early water reservoirs.

9   St. Louis *Missouri Republican*, Sept. 6, 1843, p. 4:2-3. The entire 1843 city ordinance was published on the page cited.

10   *Ibid.,* July 13, 1857, p. 2:2.

11   *Ibid.,* May 10, 1853, p. 2:4.

12   Ibid., Nov. 7, 1846, p. 2:2.

13   Charles E. Rosenberg, *The Cholera Years: The United States in 1832, 1849 and 1866* (Chicago, The University of Chicago Press, 1962), p. 101.

14   St. Louis *Missouri Republican*, Sept. 14, 1848, p. 2:3. Dr. Barbour gave the following description of the symptoms exhibited by his patient: "On Saturday [Sept. 9] he went over to Belleville, Ill. to attend to some business and returned the same day, late in the evening, apparently very well, with the exception of fatigue. He retired at a late hour, in consequence of the indisposition of his child, still feeling no other indisposition than a sense of weight and oppression at his stomach. About 2 o'clock he was awakened with a pain in his stomach and bowels, and was seized with, as he supposed, common diarrhea. These symptoms become rapidly, more severe, and in rapid succession. Violent vomiting and purging of limpid rice water discharges, and general cramps of the muscles ensued. At 4 o'clock when I [Dr. Barbour] saw him, the vomiting, purging and cramps, still continued, and became more intense; the discharges from the stomach and bowels, almost colorless, were fearfully copious, and seemed to pour from him in involuntary gushes; the muscular spasms were indescribably painful; his pulse was extinct; his skin cold, clammy, livid, and, upon the extremities, greatly shrivelled; his countenance sunken and ghastly." After several short periods of recovery, the patient died in great agony on Wednesday morning, Sept. 13. *Idem*.

15   *Ibid.,* Sept. 15, 1848, p. 2:3.

16   *Ibid.,* Dec. 21, 1848, p. 2:1.

17   *Ibid.,* Dec. 27, 1848, p. 2:1.

18   *Ibid.,* Jan. 28, 1849, p. 2:6.

19   *Ibid.,* May 2, 1849, p. 2:1.

20   Hansen, *opus cit.*, pp. 242-251, 266-269; Coleman *opus cit.*, pp. 111-116.

21   Coleman, *opus cit.*, pp. 111-116.

22   St. Louis *Missouri Republican*, June 29, 1849, p. 2:1.

23   *Ibid.,* Nov. 30, 1842, p. 2:3.

24   Hansen, *opus cit.*, p. 188.

25   Coleman, *opus cit.*, p. 215.

26   St. Louis *Missouri Republican*, May 8, 1849, p. 2:1.

27   *Ibid.,* Apr. 7, 1849, p. 2:2; *ibid,* Apr. 10, 1849, p. 2:2.

28   *Ibid.,* May 16, 1849, p. 2:1.

29   *Ibid.,* May 14, 1849, p. 3:1.

30   *Ibid.,* May 12, 1849, p. 2:1.

31   *Ibid.,* May 17, 1849, p. 2:1.

32   *Ibid.,* June 18, 1849, p. 2:2.

33   *Ibid.,* June 24, 1849, p. 2:1.

34   *Ibid.,* June 26, 1849, p. 2:6.

35   *Idem*.

36   *Ibid.,* June 27, 1849, p. 2:2.

37   *Idem*.

38   *Idem*.

39   The St. Louis *Missouri Republican* sharply criticized the city authorities for shirking their duty: "At a time when the city authorities have abandoned their posts, and have shuffled off from themselves the responsibility which justly and properly attaches to their official position, it is eminently demanded and required, that all good men should come up and assist in carrying out such sanatory provisions as may be suggested by the committee...This committee, although they have been placed, unexpectedly and undesired, in the most responsible position which any twelve men could have been placed, are determined not to do, as the city fathers have done, desert their posts or shrink from any responsibilities which the emergency of the times may require." St. Louis *Missouri Republican*, June 29, 1849, p. 2:2.

40   *Green's St. Louis Directory for 1851* (St. Louis, Charles and Hammond Printer, 1850, *passim*.

41   St. Louis *Missouri Republican*, June 26, 1849, p. 2:1.

42   *Ibid.,* June 28, 1849, p. 2:2.

43   *Idem*.

44   *Idem*.

45   *Ibid.,* July 8, 1849, p. 2:5.

46   *Ibid.,* Aug. 2, 1849, p. 2:6.

47   *Idem*.

48   St. Louis *Daily New Era*, July 30, 1849, p. 2:1.

49   E.J. Goodwin, *A History of Medicine in Missouri* (St. Louis, W. L. Smith, Publisher, 1905), p. 79.

Unfortunately for history, St. Louis was the only city in the state which kept disease and mortality statistics. The newspapers, however, published accounts of the incidence of cholera in outstate areas. In the spring and early summer of 1849, the cholera raged on the Mississippi and Missouri river boats loaded with European emigrants, in communities along the two rivers, particularly the Missouri from St. Louis to Kansas City, and also in the camps near Kansas City and St. Joseph of the California-bound gold seekers. Thirty-five deaths occurred among the Mormom emigrants on the steamboat Mary on her passage from St. Louis to Kansas City in the second week of May. The Kansas traveling upriver to Independence about the same time, lost seven or eight passengers. The steamer Monroe, having suffered a number of deaths from cholera, was placed in quarantine at Jefferson City; there the passengers, officers and crew deserted ship. The steamers Timour, Alex Hamilton, and Highland Mary, bound upriver from St. Louis, were reported to have suffered illness and deaths from the disease. (St. Louis *Missouri Republican*, May 12, 1849, p. 2:1.) Among the river towns, Brunswick was hard hit, and business partially was suspended. Some of the inhabitants of Brunswick fled to Glasgow and Boonville, possibly carrying the seeds of cholera with them. (St. Louis *Missouri Republican*, June 25, 1849, p. 2:1.) The pestilence wrought havoc among the population of Arrow Rock, an important river crossing. The crowded camps of the gold seekers on the western border of the state did not suffer as severely as might have been expected. The adventurers were mostly healthy young men; and their camps were out of the path of the hordes of diseased European emigrants. A few cases of cholera occurred in Independence and St. Joseph during the final week of April. The cholera epidemic in Independence was waning by the end of the third week of May. Most of the California-bound miners had departed. It was estimated that no more than twenty to twenty-five local citizens of Independence had died of cholera. (St. Louis *Missouri Republican*, May 29, 1849, p. 2:1.) The number of emigrants who died in the miners' camps was unknown. The death rate in these camps and along the continental trails rose as the available water sources became contaminated with disease germs from heavy and careless usage.

50 *Ibid.*, p. 88.
51 *Ibid.*, pp. 89-92.
52 St. Louis *Missouri Republican*, Aug. 7, 1949, p. 2:2.
53 *Ibid.*, Aug. 3, 1849, p. 2:5.
54 *Ibid.*, Aug. 3, 1849, p. 2:5-6.
55 *Ibid.*, May 3, 1850, p. 2:3; *ibid.*, May 4, 1850, p. 2:1.
56 *Ibid.*, May 4, 1850, p. 2:1.
57 *Ibid.*, May 6, 1850, pp. 2:1.
58 *Idem.*
59 *Ibid.*, May 13, 1850, p. 3:1.
60 Max A. Goldstein, ed., *One Hundred Years of Medicine and Surgery in Missouri* (St. Louis, St. Louis Star Publisher, 1900), pp. 84-85.
61 *Idem.* The mortality statistics for St. Louis for the period 1850-1900 were compiled by Dr. Walter B. Dorsett. He remarked that the figures for typhoid fever were probably underestimated. Typhoid fever was so common that many doctors failed to report it. *Idem.* (Translate these figures into deaths per 1000)
62 St. Louis *Missouri Republican*, May 14, 1850, p. 2:6.
63 William Hyde and Howard L. Conard, *Encyclopedia of the History of St. Louis.* Vol. IV. (New York, The Southern History Company, 1899), pp. 2041-2042.
64 *Ibid.*, p. 2041.
65 John P. Dietzler, "Major General Samuel Ryan Curtis — City Engineer," *Missouri Historical Review*, Vol. LI, No. 4 (July 1957), p. 357.
66 St. Louis *Missouri Republican*, June 25, 1840, p. 4:2. Kayser proposed that the sewer run to the river along Wash Street, two blocks south of Biddle.
67 Dietzler, *opus cit.*, p. 355-358.
68 St. Louis *Missouri Republican*, Apr. 27, 1850, p. 2:3.
69 *Ibid.*, Mar. 25, 1851, p. 4:4.
70 *Idem.*
71 Hyde and Conard, *opus cit.*, Vol. IV, p. 2042.
72 *Idem.*
73 Dietzler, *opus cit.*, p. 360.
74 Faherty, *opus cit.*, p. 80.
75 St. Louis *Missouri Republican*, Jan. 22, 1850, p. 2:1.
76 *Ibid.*, July 21, 1854, p. 2:6.
77 *Idem.*
78 *Ibid.*, July 21, 1854, p. 2:6.; *ibid.*, Aug. 16, 1855, p. 2:2.
79 *Ibid.*, Aug. 16, 1855, p. 2:2.
80 *Ibid.*, Aug. 7, 1855, p. 2:1.
81 *Revised Ordinances of the City of St. Louis*, Revised and Digested by the City Council in the Year 1850 (St. Louis, Chambers and Knapp, City Printers, 1850), p. 223.
82 *Ibid.*, pp. 223-224.
83 *Ibid.*, p. 225.
84 *Ibid.*, p. 230.
85 *Idem.*
86 *Ibid.*, pp. 229-230.
87 *Revised Ordinances of the City of St. Louis*, Revised and Digested, in the year 1853, by the City Council (St. Louis, Keemle and Hagar Printers, 1853), pp. 452-453.
88 St. Louis *Missouri Republican*, May 11, 1855, p. 3:1.
89 Richard Harrison Shryock, *Medicine and Society in America 1660-1860* (New York University Press, 1960), pp. 148-149; Charles E. Rosenberg, *The Cholera Years: The United States in 1832, 1849, and 1866* (Chicago, The University of Chicago Press, 1962), pp. 154-155. Rosenberg comments on the low prestige enjoyed by doctors in the period 1830-1860; "Doctors, like lawyers, had always served as a target for the resentment and humor of the cynical. But never, it seemed, had public unanimity and bitterness been as great. Physicians were, in the words of one popular saying, the nutcrackers used by angels to get our souls out of the shells surrounding them." *Idem.*
90 Goldstein, *opus cit.*, pp. 84-85.
91 St. Louis *Missouri Republican*, Dec. 7, 1839, p. 1:4.
92 David D. March, *The History of Missouri.* Vol. I New York, Lewis Historical Publishing Co., 1967), pp. 706-707.
93 St. Louis *Missouri Republican*, Apr. 18, 1842, p. 2:6; *ibid.*, July 8, 1848, p. 4:2; Walter B. Stevens, *St. Louis:*

The Fourth City, 1764-1909 Vol. I (St. Louis, The
S. J. Clarke Publishing Co., 1909), p. 610.

94 St. Louis *Missouri Republican*, May 15, 1851, p. 3:1.

95 Stevens, *opus cit.*, Vol. I, p. 610.

96 *Ibid.*, p. 611.

97 St. Louis *Missouri Republican*, Feb. 28, 1853, p. 2:2.

98 *Laws of the State of Missouri*, Passed at the First
Session of the Fourteenth General Assembly, Held at
the City of Jefferson on Monday, November 16, 1846
and Ended on Tuesday, February 16, 1847 (Jefferson
City, James Lusk, Public Printer, 1847), p. 124.

99 St. Louis *Missouri Republican*, Jan. 11, 1853, p. 3:2.

100 *Ibid.*, Nov. 6, 1850, p. 3:1.

101 *Idem.*

102 *Idem.*

103 *Idem.*

104 *Idem.*

105 *Idem.*

106 St. Louis *Missouri Republican*, Apr. 19, 1853, p. 2:3.

107 *Ibid.*, May 3, 1854, p. 2:4-7.

108 *Idem.*

109 *Ibid.*, May 4, 1854, p. 2:3-4.

110 *Idem.*

111 *Ibid.*, May 5, 1854, p. 2:4.

112 *Idem.*

113 Dr. Eugelmann's botanizing trips took him to Arkansas
and Louisiana, Texas, Colorado and New Mexico,
Oklahoma, and North Carolina and Tennessee. William
Bek, "George Eugelmann, Man of Science," *Missouri
Historical Review*, Vol. XXIII, No. 2 (Jan. 1929), p. 184.
Dr. Wislizenus traveled in the Northwest as far as Ft.
Hall, Oregon, and in the Southwest, by the Santa Fe
Trail and connecting Mexican roads, to Chihuahua,
Mexico. Hyde and Conard, o*pus cit.*, Vol. IV, pp.
2515-2516.

114 St. Louis *Missouri Republican*, Jan. 5, 1860, p. 2:4.

115 *Idem.*

116 *Idem.*

117 William Hyde and Howard L. Conard, *Encyclopedia
of the History of St. Louis*. Vol. II (New York,
The Southern History Co., 1899), p. 1052.

118 St. Louis *Missouri Republican*, Mar. 10, 1850, p. 2:3.

119 *Idem.*

120 *Ibid.*, Mar. 20, 1848, p. 2:5.

121 *Ibid.*, Nov. 1, 1852, p. 3:1.

122 Hyde and Conard, *opus cit.*, Vol. II, pp. 1010, 1052.
The Ordinances of the City of St. Louis, Missouri,
Digested and Revised by the City Council of Said City,
in the Years 1855-56 (St. Louis, George Knapp and Co.,
Printers, 1856), pp. 611-612.

123 *Ordinances of the City of St. Louis 1855-56*, p. 612.

124 *Ibid.*, pp. 612-613.

125 St. Louis *Missouri Republican*, May 9, 1853, p. 1:6;
Hyde and Conard, *opus cit.*, Vol. II, pp. 1052-1053.

126 Hyde and Conard, *opus cit.*, Vol. II, p. 1053.

127 *The Encyclopedia Americana*, 1953 edition. Vol. XIV,
"The Modern Hospital," (New York, Americana
Corporation, 1953), p. 428.

128 St. Louis *Missouri Republican*, Oct. 20, 1849, p. 2:2.

129 *Idem.*

130 St. Louis *Missouri Republican*, Oct. 14, 1849, p. 2:2.

131 William Frederick Norwood, *Medical Education in
the United States Before the Civil War* (Philadelphia,
University of Pennsylvania Press, 1944), p. 357.

132 St. Louis *Missouri Republican*, Sept. 8, 1850, p. 2:6.

133 Norwood, *opus cit.*, p. 357, footnote 16.

134 St. Louis *Missouri Republican*, Nov. 2, 1850, p. 2:5.

135 Norwood, *opus cit.*, pp. 357-358.

136 Floyd C. Shoemaker, *Missouri and Missourians.* Vol. I
(Chicago, The Lewis Publishing Co., 1943), pp. 658-659.

137 *Revised Statutes of the State of Missouri*, Revised and
Digested by the Eighteenth General Assembly, During
the Session of 1854 and 1855 (Jefferson City, James
Lusk Public Printer, 1856), pp. 219-231. (Vol. I) *Note*

138 J. W. Hodge, ed., *The United States Biographical
Dictionary.* Missouri Volume (New York, United States
Biographical Publishing Co., 1878), pp. 93-94.

139 Shryock, *opus cit.*, p. 130.

140 Earl A. Collins and Albert F. Elsea, *Missouri, Its People
and Its Progress* (St. Louis, Webster Publishing Co.,
1940), pp. 284-286; Gerald N. Grob, *The State and the
Mentally Ill; A History of the Worcester State Hospital
in Massachusetts 1830-1920* (Chapel Hill, University
of North Carolina Press, 1966), p. 62. Counties sending
patients to the Fulton hospital were required to
provide them with an outfit of clothing, also
replacements when necessary. The expense of getting
patients to and from the asylum and of burying them
if they died there had to be paid by the counties.
The Revised Statutes of the State of Missouri, Revised
and Digested by the Eighteenth General Assembly,
During the Session of 1854 and 1855 (Jefferson City,
James Lusk, Public Printer, 1856), Vol. I, pp. 226-227.

141 *General Statutes of the State of Missouri*, Revised by
Committee Appointed by the Twenty-Third General
Assembly (Jefferson City, Emory S. Foster, Public
Printer, 1866), pp. 304-307.

Chapter 4

St. Louis in the Civil War Period

1. Importance of Missouri to the Union Cause

WITH THE OUTBREAK of the Civil War in the spring of 1861, the question of which side Missouri would choose became of great importance. The state lay astride the main rail, highway and river routes between the industrial East and the farming and mining states of the Middle West and Far West. It was a populous state with an impressive pool of military manpower. Missouri was a leading producer of livestock, particularly horses and mules. Based at St. Louis was a numerous fleet of river steamers, whose officers and crews were experienced in navigating the Missouri-Mississippi rivers system. St. Louis was fast becoming an industrial center, with shipyards, foundries, flour mills and other manufacturing plants.

Although Missouri was traditionally a slave state, recent immigration from the Northern states and from Europe, particularly Germany and Ireland, had tended to weaken its ties to the South. The development of the east-west railroad system operated to this same end. Public opinion in Missouri in the winter and early spring of 1861 favored some compromise to appease the seceding states of the Deep South. Once war broke out, many Missourians would have preferred a policy of

armed neutrality and non-involvement.[1] But the indispensability to the Union of the trafficways through the state doomed this option.

On May 10, 1861, General Nathaniel Lyon, Union commander of the Department of the West, captured Camp Jackson in Lindell Grove in the western suburbs of St. Louis where units of the state militia were in training. In the pro-Southern legislature in Jefferson City, a bill was hastily enacted providing for the recruitment and arming of large military forces whose oath of loyalty would be to the state of Missouri rather than to the United States.[2]

Following an unsuccessful effort at the Planters House in St. Louis on June 11, 1861, to achieve a compromise and a status of neutrality for Missouri, with Governor Claiborne Jackson and General Sterling Price representing the Southern point of view, and General Lyon and Francis P. Blair as spokesmen for the Union, Jackson and Price departed by the Union Pacific Railroad for Jefferson City. On June 12, Governor Jackson issued a call for 50,000 state troops.[3]

The governor and his staff, with such soldiers as had assembled in Jefferson City, then evacuated the capital and fled west to Boonville where he determined to make a stand. General Lyon with 2,000 volunteers and regulars moved out of St. Louis by boat on June 13. The force disembarked four miles above Rocheport, and about two miles from the camp established by the state militia. The battle of Boonville, the first in Missouri during the Civil War, involved an encounter on the morning of June 17 between the poorly organized and equipped state troops and General Lyon's column. The state militia was routed in a fight that lasted about thirty minutes.[4]

The Union government quickly followed up the military successes at Camp Jackson and at Boonville. General Lyon, before he left Boonville, established a system of armed patrol boats on the Missouri River to prevent volunteers for Price's army crossing that water barrier. The Columbia *Missouri Statesman* reported on June 21, 1861, that during the previous week, federal troops had been pouring into Missouri from several directions and that they had taken complete occupation of St. Louis, Jefferson City, Boonville, Independence, Kansas City, St. Joseph, Chillicothe, Macon, Hannibal, Rolla and Springfield. It was estimated that within a few days 30,000 Union troops would be on duty in Missouri.[5]

2. St. Louis as a Military Headquarters

On July 3, 1861, the federal government created the Western Department, comprising Missouri, Illinois, Iowa, Kansas, Minnesota, Arkansas, Nebraska Territory, Colorado Territory, Dakota Territory and a part of Kentucky.[6] General John C. Fremont with headquarters in the Brant mansion at Chouteau Avenue and Eighth Street was put in charge.

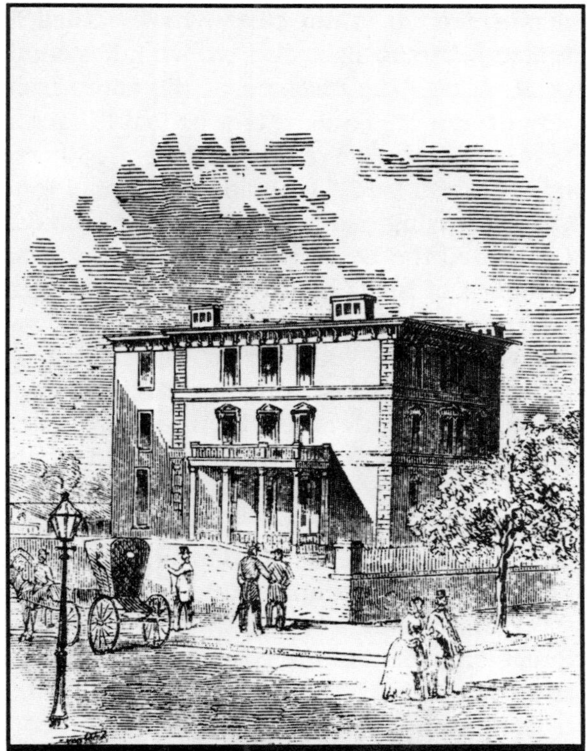

General Fremont's headquarters in St. Louis Coutresy of the State Historical Society of Missouri.

St. Louis became the center for the production and distribution of supplies to the Western armies. Depots for fuel, lumber, food, clothing and medicine were established. Remount stations for purchasing horses and mules were set up.[7]

In the late summer of 1861, the War Department contracted with James B. Eads to build seven ironclad gunboats, to be ready by October 10. Four of these were constructed at shipyards at Carondelet in South St. Louis, the other three at Mound City, near Cairo, Illinois.[8] These boats rendered important service in General Ulysses S. Grant's capture of Forts Henry and Donelson in February 1862.

One of General Fremont's first moves was to establish a training camp for his extensive department. It is not clear why he failed to utilize Jefferson Barracks, twelve miles south of St. Louis. The distance of the camp from downtown St. Louis was a probable factor. Instead, General Fremont chose a 150-acre tract of farm land, belonging to Colonel John O'Fallon, lying just west of the fairgrounds.[9] He named the new camp "Benton Barracks," in honor of his father-in-law Senator Thomas Hart Benton. On this site, construction was started in the summer of 1861, and by autumn a number of buildings had been completed. The quarters for the troops consisted of two half-mile long rows of wooden sheds, facing each other across a wide space. The sheds were divided lengthwise into two separate apartments, each section holding about 200 men. The occupants slept on wooden trays, in three tiers on the walls. A bunk held four men.[10] Behind the barracks were stables and cooking huts.

Conditions were chaotic – and decidedly unhealthy – when volunteer regiments from all over the military department began to arrive in August before preparations for their accommodation had been completed. The camp was built on cultivated land, so became a sea of mud in rainy weather. There were no permanent-type roads. The barracks were built of a single layer of boards and were drafty and difficult to heat. The camp site was beyond the western limits of St. Louis's water system.[11] It had to depend on a limited supply from wells. This was not enough to enable the troops to maintain a minimum standard of cleanliness.[12]

The bringing together of thousands of men, most from small towns and rural areas, exposed them to diseases they had not before encountered and for which they had developed no immunity. The army lacked an immunization program, except for smallpox. The cramped living and sleeping arrange-

ments facilitated the spread of contagion. Because of the fear of fresh air, which was suspected of transmitting noxious miasmata, the living quarters were not properly ventilated.[13] With large numbers of men untrained in camp discipline, enforcement of sanitary methods of disposing of human and kitchen wastes was next to impossible. The new camp quickly became contaminated with filth.

In the peacetime army, no medical organization for units larger than the regiment existed. There was no precedent to guide the organization of medical and hospital services for a military camp of more than 20,000 persons, such as Benton Barracks. Time was required to develop plans and facilities and to recruit doctors to provide this service.

Under these conditions, measles, pneumonia, typhoid fever and diarrhea became epidemic at the camp in the winter of 1861-1862. Three hundred men, out of a single cavalry regiment, were reported sick, most with measles. Many of the measles patients were attacked later by pneumonia and died. In another unit, 1,000 out of 1,300 men were suffering from coughs and colds. Smallpox also made its appearance on a significant scale, necessitating a special hospital.[14]

3. St. Louis as a Military Hospital Center

A large group of wounded soldiers numbering 721 arrived in St. Louis following the battle of Wilson's Creek on August 10, 1861. These soldiers had received their first medical treatment in a field hospital, set up in a farmhouse or barn near the scene of battle and consisting of an improvised operating table and a few surgical instruments and medical supplies. At the field hospital, the doctors probed and bandaged wounds and amputated shattered limbs. No facilities, except perhaps a tub of well water, were available for cleansing the doctor's hands and sterilizing his instruments. A high incidence of post-operative infections occurred.[15]

The wounded from the Wilson's Creek battle had been carried by army wagons to Rolla where they were loaded on railway cars and transported over the Pacific Railroad to St. Louis. This method of moving the wounded was so expeditious and satisfactory that General Fremont ordered the fitting out on the Pacific Railroad of two hospital cars with nurses, berths and cooking facilities. These were probably the first specially equipped hospital cars in the United States.[16]

The advanced party of the Wilson's Creek casualties numbering 100 arrived at the St. Louis railway station on 14th Street at night and were moved in furniture wagons to the New House of Refuge Hospital, situated in the open country about two miles south of St. Louis. The New House of Refuge, an asylum for abandoned or mistreated children, had been requisitioned by the army, and officially opened on August 6. But neither beds, bedding, stoves, food, medicines or nurses were actually ready when the first patients arrived. Dr. Bailley, the physician in charge, obtained cooked food for supper from families in the neighborhood. The men slept on the bare floors.[17] Gradually the necessary equipment, supplies and personnel for a functioning hospital were acquired and conditions improved markedly. Within a week, three or four hundred more sick and wounded from the Wilson's Creek encounter were received.

Later arrivals were sent to the Sisters of Charity Hospital and to the city hospital. These two institutions, which together had space for perhaps 350-400 persons, were already partially filled with civilian patients.

Since the wounded from a single battle were overtaxing existing accommodations, it was obvious that something must be done to increase St. Louis's medical and hospital resources. On September 5, 1861, General Fremont, in response to the appeal of several concerned citizens, created the Western Sanitary Commission.[18] The general's order defined for the new organization a comprehensive mission embracing "the selection and furnishing of buildings for hospitals, the finding of nurses, the visiting of camps, the inspection of food, the suggestion of better drainage, the obtaining from the public of means for promoting the moral and social welfare of soldiers in camp and hospital."[19]

General Fremont appointed to the commission James E. Yeatman, Carlos S. Greeley, Dr. John B. Johnson, George Partridge and the Reverend William G. Eliot. Yeatman who was chosen chairman was a former Tennessee plantation owner. As an idealistic young man, he had sold his estate and freed his slaves. He moved to St. Louis where he engaged in banking. [20] The impressive accomplishments of the commission during the four years of its existence were in large part due to Yeatman's leadership, his administrative skill, his knowledge of the nation's problems and their possible solutions, and his deep sympathy for those for whom the war had caused loss and suffering.

Carlos S. Greeley and George Partridge were successful and public-spirited merchants. The Reverend William G. Eliot was a Unitarian minister, civic leader and educator. He was the founder of Washington University and of Mary Institute. During his long illustrious career, he served as the conscience of St. Louis.[21] With a medical degree from Berkshire College, an honorary degree from Harvard University and a year of internship on the staff of the Massachusetts General Hospital,

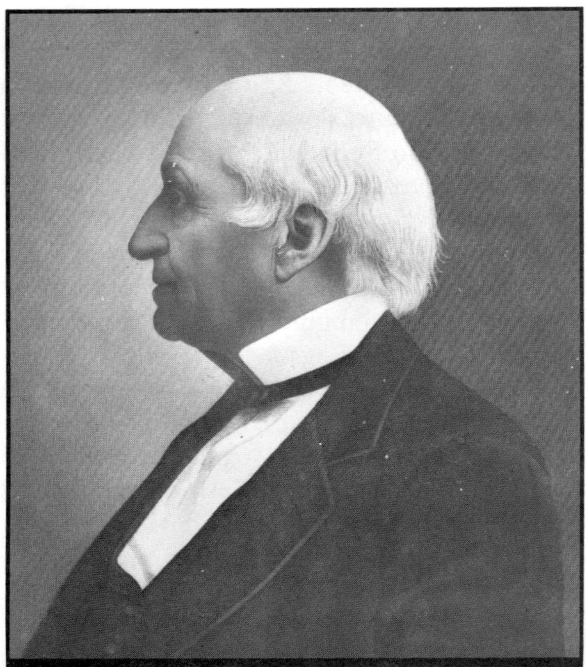

James E. Yeatmen

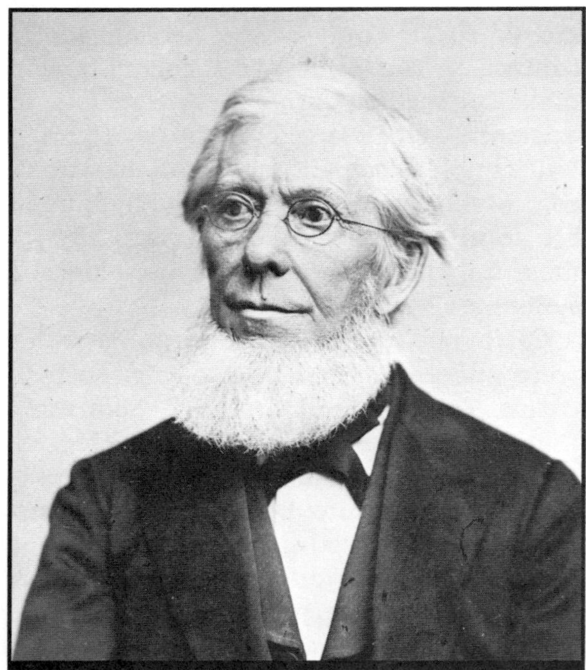

William Greenleaf Eliot, D. D.

Dr. Johnson arrived in St. Louis in 1841. He married into a prominent St. Louis family. By his professional competence, he gained an extensive patronage and the recognition of his peers.[22]

General Fremont thus defined the relationship between the Western Sanitary Commission and the established military organization: "This Commission is not intended in any way to interfere with the Medical Staff, or other officers of the army, but to cooperate with them, and aid them in the discharge of their present arduous and extraordinary duties."[23] The commission was able from its inception to establish close working relations with the local medical director, Surgeon DeCamp, and the assistant surgeon general of the United States Army, Colonel R. C. Wood, a member of General Fremont's headquarters staff and chief of the Medical Department of the West.[24] The title "surgeon" was equivalent to the civilian term "doctor."

One of the first actions of the commission was to establish a new hospital large enough to accommodate 500 patients. A spacious five-story building at Fifth and Chestnut streets was secured and outfitted with beds and bedding, diet kitchens and bathing arrangements. A local physician, Surgeon John T. Hodgen of the United States volunteer corps, was put in charge of the staff of assistant surgeons, nurses and other service members. This institution was designated the "City General Hospital." Situated in downtown and convenient to the railroad depots and to the river landings, it became the receiving center for the most severely wounded or ill patients, where they were given immediate attention and from which they were later distributed to other hospitals.[25]

In this building, the Western Sanitary Commission made its headquarters. It occupied a small room on the second floor as an

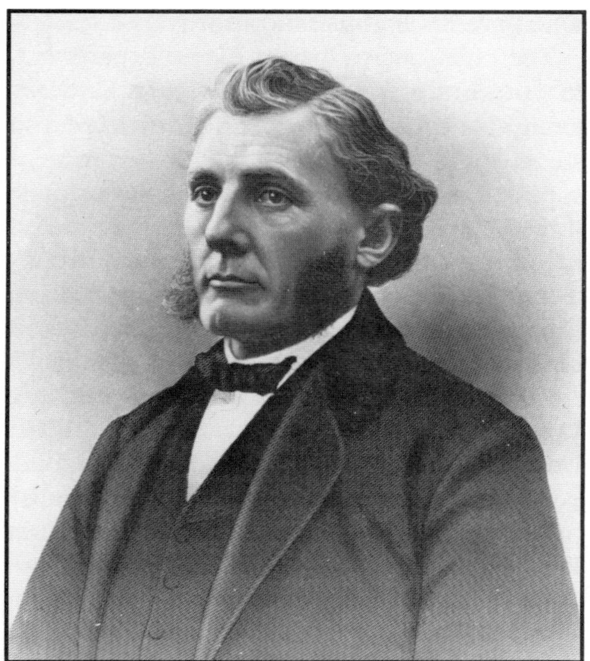

Dr. John T. Hodgen. Courtesy of the State Historical Society of Missouri.

office and a store room in the basement for its sanitary supplies. Yeatman devoted his whole time to the work and had a cot in the office. The entire committee met each day. The only paid employee was a man who served as clerk and porter. Much of the work of opening and inventorying incoming shipments, making up orders for units in the field, keeping records and answering correspondence was done by the commission members themselves.[26]

During the third week of September, the siege of Lexington occurred. Some 300 wounded men from this battle were brought to St. Louis hospitals.[27]

On September 13, a post hospital and two convalescent hospitals were opened at Benton Barracks. Two days later the Good Samaritan Hospital at Pratte and O'Fallon streets was converted into a military facility. On October 20, a smallpox hospital with a

capacity of 250 patients was established on Duncan's Island in the Mississippi River opposite the arsenal. A new hotel building on Fourth Street was taken over by the commission and transformed into a hospital. November 4 on Spruce Street between Seventh and Eighth streets the structure used by the commission as a center for the reception of supplies was converted into the "Pacific Hospital." The Hickory Street Hospital in south St. Louis consisted of two adjoining three-story residences. It was opened on February 1, 1862, for the use of reserve corps personnel.[28]

From February 13-15, 1862, the battle of Ft. Donelson on the Cumberland River in West Tennessee was fought in a swirling snowstorm between the Union forces under General U. S. Grant and the Confederate troops commanded by General S. B. Buckner. The Confederates suffered 231 killed and 1,007 wounded; the Union losses were even greater.[29]

When the news of this encounter reached St. Louis, the Western Sanitary Commission made preparations to assist in the care of the sick and wounded. A member of the commission, accompanied by physicians, nurses, members of the Ladies' Union Aid Society and by Surgeon J. H. Grove of the United States volunteer corps, proceeded to Paducah, Kentucky, at the mouth of the Cumberland River where the wounded from the battle had been brought. The medical director at Paducah placed the steamer *Ben Franklin* at their service and instructed that a load of the wounded be placed in their charge to be brought to St. Louis. One hundred and fifty-five wounded were selected from the Paducah hospitals to make this first trip.[30]

Each morning the ladies attended to the bathing and grooming of the patients.

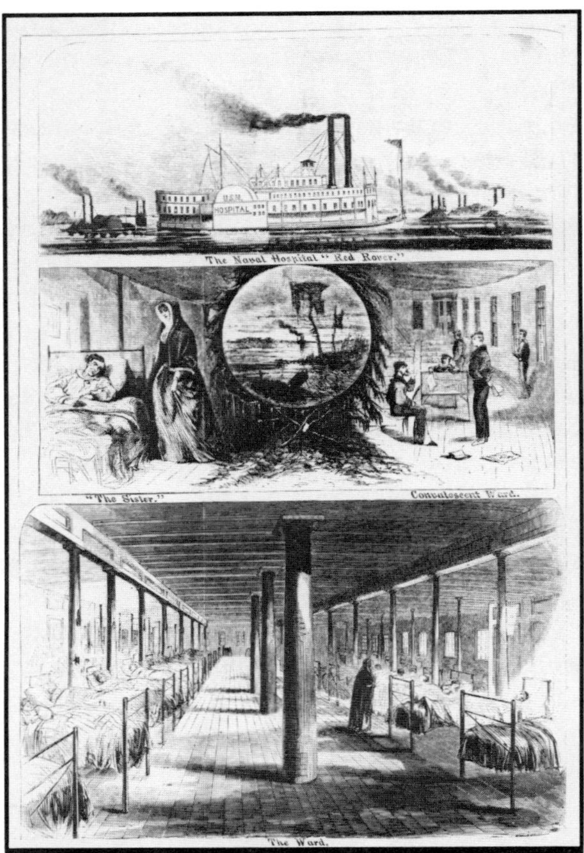

Civil War hospital steamer. Courtesy of the State Historical Society of Missouri.

Breakfast followed. Then the surgeons made their rounds examining the patients and dressing their wounds. After supper, there was group singing, scripture reading and prayer. [31] The comfortable circumstances of the boat and the kind attentions of the ladies contributed to raise the spirits and improve the health of the wounded.

The successful trip of the *Ben Franklin* gave rise to the proposal to outfit a fleet of hospital steamers to accompany the Union armies in their campaign on the western rivers. The plan was forwarded to Major General Henry W. Halleck, commander of the Department of the Missouri, who gave his enthusiastic approval. [32]

The chief quartermaster of the department, in cooperation with the Western Sanitary Commission, chartered and outfitted the steamer *City of Louisiana.* The government supplied it with beds and commissary stores; the Western Sanitary Commission completed the equipping. The commission also furnished the assistant surgeons, the apothecary, the male and female nurses and a full stock of sanitary supplies. [33]

On April 6-7, 1862, the battle of Pittsburg Landing was waged. On that battlefield, 1,735 Union soldiers were killed and 7,882 wounded. The latter were brought to St. Louis by boat. [34] The first load of wounded from Pittsburg Landing reached St. Louis on April 14, 1862, on board the steamer *Crescent City.* They numbered approximately 400. [35] As the wounded arrived at the St. Louis wharf, a volunteer corps of stretcher bearers – businessmen, clerks, manufacturers, artisans and professional people – carried them up the steep half-mile climb to hospitals in the vicinity of Fifth Street. [36]

The heavy casualties from the battle of Pittsburg Landing and the prospect of mounting losses as General Grant continued his campaign against Vicksburg, prompted the opening of two new major hospitals. The first was the Jefferson Barracks Hospital on the Mississippi River about twelve miles south of St. Louis. To make room for the hospital, all training activities of the regular army at Jefferson Barracks were discontinued and the entire encampment converted to hospital use. The enlisted barracks consisted of long rows of one- and two-story houses, surrounding on three sides a large parade grounds with the east end of the quadrangle open to the river. These and the post hospital, a three-story frame building with wide porches, were utilized. [37]

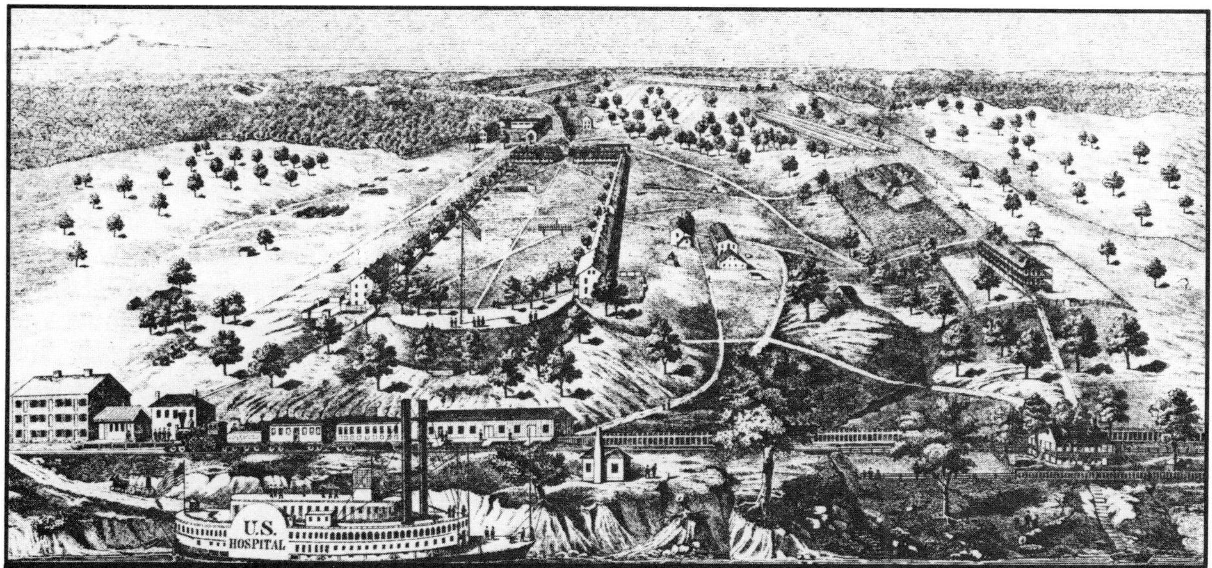

Jefferson Barracks General Hospital (in upper right corner). Courtesy of the State Historical Society of Missouri.

On higher ground to the west of the barracks area, an extensive new medical development was carried out. Three triple rows of buildings 600 feet long, divided into wards of 300 feet each, were erected at considerable distances from each other. These buildings were so arranged that in each group of three adjoining structures the central row was devoted to a dining room and quarters for surgeons, nurses and stewards. A system of waterworks was installed by which all buildings were amply supplied. The hospital complex with accommodations for 2,500 patients was one of the largest and finest in the country. The institution was opened April 30, 1862. It was in the charge of Surgeon J. F. Randolph, United States Army, assisted by Surgeon J. H. Grove, United States volunteer corps, six assistant surgeons, a post chaplain and a hospital chaplain.[38]

The United States Marine Hospital was also converted to military service. This institution in peacetime served the medical needs of boatmen on the western rivers. It was located on the bank of the Mississippi River a half mile below the arsenal. Built of stone and brick and four stories high, it had a capacity of 150 patients.[39] It was opened under military management on May 4, 1862. Its accommodations were increased during the war by the construction of two frame pavilions.[40]

In order to provide for sick and wounded Confederate soldiers captured at Pittsburg Landing, a hospital was opened July 1, 1862, in a section of the McDowell Medical College on Gratiot Street which was used during the war as a military prison.[41]

The losses suffered by the Union forces in the Vicksburg campaign were responsible for another program of hospital construction, the major feature of which was the Benton Barracks Hospital. This structure was built according to the popular pavilion plan. The former amphitheater of the fair grounds was enclosed, floors were provided and the space gained was divided into five wards, radiating like spokes from the central arena.[42] Each ward was 140 feet long and 46 feet wide.

Large halls separated the wards. Under each ward was a dining room, also space for commissary stores, surgeons' quarters, baggage rooms and bathing facilities. Stairs from the center of the ward descended to the dining room.[43]

The completed structure constituted "a circular building, one thousand feet in circumference, and three hundred and thirty feet in diameter, with a large circular space in the center, open to the sky and air."[44] This hospital was opened on March 1, 1863, and took the place at the camp of the former Benton Barracks Post Hospital and the two convalescent hospitals. The capacity of the new hospital was ordinarily 2,000; but 2,500 patients could be accommodated in emergencies.[45]

A former seven-story hotel at Broadway and Carr Street was converted into the Lawson Hospital and opened for operations on January 17, 1863. It had accommodations for 600 patients. The Western Sanitary Commission provided an elevator for the structure. The hospital was in the charge of Surgeon C. T. Alexander, United States Army, with five assistant surgeons and a chaplain.[46]

The Schofield Barracks Post Hospital on Chouteau Avenue went into service on February 19, 1863. This hospital was in the neighborhood of the military headquarters of the Department of Missouri and probably served the personnel of the headquarters detachment. It had accommodations for forty-three patients and was staffed by a surgeon and an assistant surgeon.[47]

The addition to the available hospital space in St. Louis and vicinity of the Benton Barracks Hospital, the Lawson Hospital and the Schofield Barracks Post Hospital made it possible for the army medical department to discontinue the use of the Fourth Street Hospital, the Pacific Hospital, the St. Louis Hospital and the city hospital. As of the summer of 1863, the hospitals of St. Louis and its general area had a capacity of 8,000 patients, but could easily accommodate 10,000 in an emergency.[48]

A number of floating hospitals were outfitted and commissioned to transport sick and wounded soldiers from the armies of Generals Henry W. Halleck and Ulysses S. Grant along the Tennessee and Mississippi rivers to general hospitals in St. Louis and other cities in the zone of the interior. The first of these was the *City of Louisiana*, later renamed the *R. C. Wood* in honor of the assistant surgeon general of the United States. Other hospital steamers which plied regularly to St. Louis were the *City of Memphis*, the *Empress*, the *Imperial*, the *City of Alton*, the *Crescent City*, the *Stephen Decatur*, the *D. A. January* and the *Continental*.[49]

An analysis of the passenger list of the *Stephen Decatur* which arrived at Jefferson Barracks May 29, 1862, from Pittsburg Landing, indicates the tremendous role which sickness played in depleting the ranks of the Union Army. Out of a total of approximately 280 military personnel, 120 were suffering from diarrhea, 56 from debility, 18 from rheumatism, 13 from typhoid fever, 12 from malaria, 56 from various other diseases and only 5 from battle wounds.[50] The high incidence of diarrhea was attributed to the lack of fresh fruits and vegetables in the standard army ration which consisted basically of hardtack, beans, salt pork and coffee. Another contributing factor was the practice of troops in the field to drink from any stream, lake or pool they encountered.[51]

Following the capture of Vicksburg, July 4, 1863, the Western armies directed their drive toward Atlanta. As the fighting moved away from the Mississippi River, the flow of wounded to St. Louis by hospital steamers declined. New military hospitals were established in Memphis, Nashville and Chattanooga.[52] Hospital trains brought the wounded to general hospitals in these cities. The role of St. Louis became mainly that of a convalescent center.

Up to May 1, 1864, the total number of military patients treated in hospitals of St. Louis, including those at Jefferson and Benton Barracks was 61,744. Of this number 5,684 died with a fatality rate of 9 1/10 percent.[53]

4. Regional and National Activities of the Western Sanitary Commission

The activities of the Western Sanitary Commission, although at first mainly concerned with providing adequate hospitals for St. Louis as the medical headquarters of the Western Department, assumed a wider scope as the Civil War proceeded. This expansion involved providing hospitals and sanitary supplies for the Western armies in all their campaigns, the establishment of a number of soldiers' homes, and the planning and execution of programs for dealing with the problem of refugees – white as well as black – created by the war.

An appeal by the commission, published in the St. Louis *Missouri Republican* of August 12, 1862, gives a description of its widespread activities;[54]

The Western Sanitary Commission of St. Louis is under the necessity of again appealing to the patriotic citizens of the loyal States for the contribution of money and hospital stores . . .

The demands upon the Commission are as great as at any previous time, and the field of its labors is daily enlarged. An army of not less than 150,000 men in Tennessee, Kentucky, Arkansas and Missouri, and the Gunboat Flotilla, looks to St. Louis for nearly all its sanitary supplies, and must continue to do so through the war, as the most convenient and accessible place at all seasons of the year. Heretofore, the Commission has been able to meet all requisitions. It has never refused to send, liberally and promptly, to any point, whatever has been needed to alleviate suffering, and to cure or prevent sickness. At the present time arrangements are in progress to supply regiments in the field with vegetables and other articles of food for sick and convalescent soldiers. At Corinth and Columbus this will be done by cooperation with Dr. Warriner, Agent of the United States Sanitary Commission, and elsewhere by the Western Commission alone.

Acting in concert with the regular medical staff of the army, the commission established hospitals in all the principal cities captured by the Union Armies along the Mississippi River.[55] The Western Commission sent sanitary supplies to general and post hospitals in Illinois, Kentucky, Tennessee, Mississippi, Alabama, Arkansas and Louisiana. [56]

In addition to hospitals, the commission set up a system of soldiers' homes. The first was opened at 29 South Fourth Street in St. Louis on March 13, 1862.[57] The homes were the Civil War equivalents of the U.S.O. centers established during World War II in various American cities. They served as temporary homes for troops that were on furlough or had been discharged. Food and lodging were free. The staffs provided information; they helped with letter writing and travel arrangements. They lent emotional support to thousands of veterans who were returning to civilian life with disabling injuries. Soldiers needing medical attention could get outpatient care from doctors and nurses who made regular calls at the homes. Newspapers, magazines and books were available; and non-denominational services were held regularly.[58]

As the fighting moved down the Mississippi River, homes were established at Columbus, Kentucky; Memphis, Tennessee; Helena, Arkansas; and Vicksburg, Mississippi. Up to December 1865, 421,616 soldiers had been entertained in these homes, 982,592 meals had been served and 410,252 lodgings provided.[59]

The Western Sanitary Commission was one of the first organizations to tackle the problem of the freedmen. It was estimated that in the region between Cairo, Illinois, and Natchez, Mississippi, at least 40,000 blacks were homeless and destitute. The region for months had been a battle ground. The agricultural economy had been disrupted. Slaves had abandoned the plantations and had fled to Union Army camps, seeking security and employment. They were not always welcomed. Some commanders forced them to work without pay. [60]

In behalf of the freedmen, Yeatman made a special appeal to the country. The generous response made it possible for the commission to take ameliorative action: [61]

The replenished Commission sent to the hungry and ragged freedmen large supplies of both food and clothing; established hospitals for them in different places; provided them with physicians, nurses and medicines; put a stop to the tyranny of inconsiderate or hard-hearted military officers; and established schools for them in which they were taught to read, and write, to add and subtract, and do properly the ordinary work of the kitchen and field. Mr Yeatman went over all the territory where the men and women, sent out by the Commission, were working for the freedmen, and gave to them such suggestions and directions as in his judgment would render their work most beneficent and fruitful. He himself established for the freedmen a system of work on plantations around Vicksburg, which, before the close of the war, yielded the best results. On behalf of his project he appealed to the public through the press; laid it personally before the President and found for it an open ear and thus enlisted the government on its behalf.

White refugees flocked to St. Louis during the war. Some were fleeing from the destruction caused by opposing armies; others from the danger of guerrilla violence in the rural areas. Many, including the wives of soldiers, sought employment to support their families.

The Western Commission established the first home for refugees on Elm Street in St. Louis early in 1862. It was conducted on the same principles as the home for soldiers. Lodging in the home was usually temporary until the guests secured employment or found more permanent quarters with friends or relatives. The Ladies Union Aid Society of St. Louis was active in securing aid and employment for the wives of soldiers. The first home was jointly financed, the commission providing $3,000 and the federal government $2,000.[62]

The problem of white refugees was critical in the entire region south of Missouri on both sides of the Mississippi River and evoked the following response: [63]

There the Commission, as exigencies arose, selected, one after another, ten central points, each of which was made headquarters for all the region contiguous to it. At these centres they founded temporary hospitals, and opened schools for the refugees. They fed, clothed, taught and nursed them, and, so far as practicable, put them to work.

5. Influence of the War on the Provision of Health Services

The role of St. Louis as the medical headquarters of the Western theater of operations had important consequences for the development of health services. The effects were not only in methods of treatment but also in the way medical institutions were organized and operated. During the war, the army's surgeon general established professional standards of medical practice and provided a comprehensive system of guidance and direction. The result was the development of one of the finest systems of medical and hospital care in the world.[64]

With this experience, St. Louis doctors were reluctant to return after the war to the anarchic condition of medical practice in Missouri, where any person could become a doctor by paying a small fee and where there was no agency to coordinate the war against disease. St. Louis doctors took the lead in a campaign to establish a state board with power to raise the standards of the medical profession and to safeguard the public health.[65] Later they worked for the development of national public health agencies and programs.

The war trained St. Louis physicians to operate medical institutions on a mass production basis. Before the war, the typical physician had seen and treated a limited number of patients by driving in his buggy to make house calls. The Sisters of Charity

Hospital and the city hospital were small institutions, each having a capacity of 150 to 200 patients. City hospital was staffed by a resident physician, two assistants and six consulting physicians. The large wartime hospitals required dozens of doctors and immense staffs of nurses and other service people. Specialized areas of hospital administration developed, such as personnel affairs, staff training, record keeping, dietetics, and buildings and grounds. The wartime hospitals demonstrated the economy of having a doctor's patients assembled in one place rather than scattered over town.

The opening of the nursing profession to women was an important and lasting change brought about by the war. Previously in St. Louis, the nurses were mostly members of religious orders who regarded their work as a form of Christian service. They were generally not highly trained. Under the direction of Dorothea Dix, a national nursing corps was recruited. The earlier objections to female nurses, i.e., that they would faint at the sight of blood, that they were physically incapable of doing the heavy work of lifting patients, and that the intimacy of nursing would be an affront to their modesty, were proven without foundation.[66] At Benton Barracks Hospital, with the aid of Emily Parsons of Cambridge, Massachusetts, supervisor of nursing, an efficient staff of female nurses was developed.[67] Women nurses were also employed at other St. Louis hospitals.

An improved classification of diseases, based on the system developed by the British Army, was adopted by the surgeon general's office and became standard in American practice.[68] This eliminated the custom of each doctor making his individual classification scheme and, frequently, of identifying diseases by their major symptoms, rather than by their causes. An example of the new system is the disease report of city hospital for the semi-annual period, ending March 1864.[69]

Several important changes in medical treatment were recommended. In May 1863, Surgeon General William Alexander Hammond banned the use of calomel and tartar emetic (another mercury preparation) in military hospitals. "No doubt can exist," Hammond stated, "that more harm has resulted from the misuse of both these agents, in the treatment of disease, than benefit from their administration."[70] Since calomel was the universal remedy in the medical practice of doctors, particularly in the South and West, the ban was widely disregarded.[71] The surgeon general's office also looked with disfavor on the use of bleeding.

The practice was instituted in general hospitals in the late period of the war to prepare detailed case reports on each patient,[72] giving the nature of the wound or disease, medicine or therapy prescribed, and eventually the success or failure of the treatment. These records were summarized in the multi-volume publication entitled *The Medical and Surgical History of the War of the Rebellion.* This was the most comprehensive description yet produced of the status of American medicine and surgery, and an important milestone toward the development of scientific medicine in the United States.

The war contributed to the expansion of St. Louis as a center for the manufacture and distribution of medical and hospital supplies. It is very probable that a large proportion of the supplies furnished to the Western armies came from local sources. In St. Louis at the time the following firms were in the wholesale drug business: William D'Oench, Pike and Kellogg, J. Matthews and Sons, and A. Leitch.[73]

6. Emergence of the "Social Evil"

The war brought out of the closet a problem — the "Social Evil" — which prudery had previously kept pretty well concealed. Veiled references to venereal disease had appeared in the advertisements of patent medicines,[74] which claimed to cure ailments resulting from youthful indiscretions. Doctors, to avoid embarrassing their patients, did not report cases they had treated. The police, at least, knew that St. Louis had a red light district, including the nest of brothels near the north end of the city's paved levee.

The war greatly magnified the problem of prostitution in St. Louis and increased the number of patients in its hospitals suffering from venereal diseases. Two major factors were responsible. The breakdown of family and community life in the Border States and the South sent armies of refugees, black and white, flocking to St. Louis. Hundreds of young women, unable to find homes or honorable employment, turned to prostitution. The assembling in St. Louis of 20,000 - 30,000 young men in Benton Barracks and other camps created a potential market for their services.

The St. Louis *Missouri Republican* gave this assessment of the magnitude of the problem in an editorial of September 5, 1864:[76]

The evil is tremendous. The extent to which it prevails is awful — far exceeding any ideas which may be formed of it by those whose positions do not give them the means of proper information in respect to it. It is one of the saddest fruits of this war. A foul taint has been carried like a stream of poison into the blood and bones of scores of thousands, who will in many instances transmit that taint to posterity, the effects being felt by generation after generation in leprous diseases which will make life a curse and its victims a burden to society.

The editor, again venturing forth on ground where even angels might fear to tread, proposed a plan which offered hope of providing some alleviation of the problem:[77]

Hitherto, as in England, so in this country, prostitution has been treated as a crime, which had to be suppressed and punished, and not as an evil which called for regulation. One consequence of this necessarily, is that the followers of the vice being left to regulate themselves, have done it so imperfectly as to open the door to the admission and spread of foul diseases, which corrupt the blood of both present and future generations. Were they regulated by stringent laws, which required strict and frequent examinations, this consequence might to some extent be prevented.

This proposal was later tried in St. Louis. It provoked a bitter political fight which pitted the social reformers against the preachers and women's organizations.

7. *Dispersion and Reunion*

The war divided the St. Louis medical fraternity as it did other groups in St. Louis. The majority of St. Louis doctors continued to pursue their private practice, avoiding offense to the military authorities. A number engaged in medical service to the Union cause. The most illustrious member of this latter group was Dr. John Thompson Hodgen, who served as chief surgeon of the Fifth Street Hospital, as surgeon general for the Western Sanitary Commission and as surgeon general of the state of Missouri.[78] Dr. Hodgen is credited with inventing, in 1863, the Hodgen splint, the one important orthopedic contribution of the war.[79]

Dr. Simon Pollack was active in the work of the United States Sanitary Commission and the Western Sanitary Commission, serving as hospital inspector.[80] Dr. J.B. Johnson made a valuable contribution as one of the five members of the Western Commission. Dr. Adam E. Hammer rendered service as surgeon in charge of the New House of Refuge Hospital.[81]

The most prominent defector to the Confederate cause was Dr. Joseph N. McDowell. His action was not surprising since he had been outspoken in defense of slavery.[82] Dr. William M. McPheeters went south in retaliation to assessments levied by the local military government against his family for alleged pro-Confederate sentiments and statements. He was chosen medical director on the staff of General Sterling Price.[83] A group of St. Louisans banished to the South on the steamer *Belle Memphis* on May 13, 1863, included Dr. S. Gratz Moses, who during the remainder of the war served in hospitals of Savannah.[84]

At the close of the war, the St. Louis doctors, who had been in exile in the South returned. In January 1866, Dr. Joseph N. McDowell got back to St. Louis and regained possession of his building at Eighth and Gratiot streets.[85] Classes were resumed at the Missouri Medical College shortly afterwards.

Chapter IV

St. Louis in the Civil War Period

1. William E. Parrish, *A History of Missouri 1860-1875* (Columbia, Mo., University of Missouri Press, 1973) Vol. III, pp. 3, 10.

2 Walter Williams and Floyd C. Shoemaker, *Missouri: Mother of the West* (Chicago, The American Historical Society, 1930), Vol. II, pp. 60-61.

3 *Ibid.*, pp. 63-65.

4 *Ibid.*, pp. 67-69.

5 Columbia *Missouri Statesman*, June 21, 1861, p. 2:3.

6 Alan Nevins, *The War for the Union* (New York, Charles Scribner's Sons, 1959), Vol. I, p. 309, footnote 2.

7 An indication of the volume of supplies maintained in St. Louis depots is provided by a request forwarded to the St. Louis quartermaster by General Grant in the winter of 1861-1862 for a million bushels of coal. Kenneth P. Williams, *Lincoln Finds a General: A Military Study of the Civil War* (New York, The Macmillan Co., 1956) pp. 172-173.

8 Bern Anderson, *By Sea and by River: A Naval History of the Civil War* (New York, Alfred A. Knopf, 1962) pp. 42, 87.

9 J. Thomas Scharf, *History of St. Louis City and County* (Philadelphia, Louis H. Everts and Co., 1883) Vol. I, p. 400.

10 Floyd C. Shoemaker, *Missouri and Missourians* (Chicago, The Lewis Publishing Co., 1943) Vol. I, pp. 901-902. This description of Benton Barracks in the winter of 1861-1862 was based on an eye witness account published by the English writer, Anthony Trollope, in his book *North America*.

11 The St. Louis reservoir was in the vicinity of Eighteenth Street. Benton Barracks were just west of Grand Avenue, which ran along a terrace higher than the reservoir.

12 Regarding Benton Barracks and the soldiers housed there. Trollope reported: "Never in my life before had I been in a place so horrid to the eyes and nose as Benton Barracks. The path along the front outside was deep in mud. The whole space between the two rows of sheds was one field of mud, so slippery that the foot could not stand…The soldiers were mud-stained from foot to sole. These volunteer soldiers are in their nature dirty, as must be all men brought together in numerous bodies without special appliances for cleanliness, or control and discipline as to their personal habits. But the dirt of the men in Benton Barracks surpassed any dirt that I had hitherto seen." Quoted in Shoemaker, *Missouri and Missourians*, Vol. I, pp. 901-902.

13 J. G. Forman, *The Western Sanitary Commission* (St. Louis, R. P. Studley and Co., Printer, 1864), p. 14.

14 *Ibid.*, p. 13.

15 Duane Meyer, *The Heritage of Missouri: A History* (St. Louis, State Publishing Co., Inc., 1973), p. 364.

16 Forman, *opus cit.*, p. 5; Galusha Anderson, *The Story of a Border City During the Civil War* (Boston, Little, Brown and Co., 1908), p. 296.

17 Forman, *opus cit.*, pp. 5-6.

18 Anderson, *A Border City During the Civil War*, p. 288.

19 Walter B. Stevens, *Centennial History of Missouri* (St. Louis, The S. J. Clarke Publishing Co., 1911), Vol. I, p. 784.

20 Anderson, *opus cit.*, p. 289.

21 *Ibid.*, p. 290.

22 Walter B. Stevens, *St. Louis: The Fourth City 1764-1909* (St. Louis, The S. J. Clarke Publishing Co., 1909), Vol. I, p. 599.

23 Forman, *opus cit.*, p. 8.

24 *Ibid.*, pp. 16, 26.

25 *Ibid.*, pp. 8-9.

26 *Ibid.*, p. 9.

27 *Ibid.*, pp. 9-10.

28 *Ibid.*, p. 10; Shoemaker, *Missouri and Missourians*, Vol. I, p. 901; *Report of the Western Sanitary Commission for the Year Ending June 1, 1863* (St. Louis, Mo., Western Sanitary Commission, 1863) pp. 8, 14, 16.

29 Forman, *opus cit.*, p. 23.

30 Forman, *opus cit.*, pp. 23-24.

31 *Ibid.*, p. 24.

32 *Ibid.*, pp. 25.

33 *Ibid.*, pp. 25-26.

34 *Ibid.*, p. 42.

35 St. Louis *Missouri Republican*, Apr. 15, 1862, p. 1:6-7.

36 Anderson, *The Story of a Border City*, p. 291.

37 *Report of the Western Sanitary Commission, 1863*, p. 13.

38 *Idem.*

39 *Ibid.*, p. 12.

40 Forman, *opus cit.*, p. 64.

41 *Report of the Western Sanitary Commission, 1863*, p. 17.

42 *Ibid.*, p. 14.

43 St. Louis *Missouri Republican*, Mar. 1, 1863, p. 3:4.

44 *Report of the Western Sanitary Commission*, p. 14.

45 *Ibid.*, p. 15.

46 *Idem.*

47 *Ibid.*, p. 17.

48 *Ibid.*, p. 9.

49 *Ibid.*, pp. 18-19; Forman, *opus cit.*, p. 106.

50 St. Louis *Missouri Republican*, June 1, 1862, p. 1:7-8. It is likely that the percentage of sick soldiers aboard the *Stephen Decatur* was unusually high. Other hospital ships probably brought a greater proportion of combat casualties.

51 George W. Adams, *Doctors in Blue: The Medical History of the Union Army in the Civil War* (New York, Henry Schumann, 1952), p. 155.

52 Adams, *Doctors in Blue*, p. 155.

53 Forman, *opus cit.*, p. 87.

54 St. Louis *Missouri Republican*, Aug. 12, 1862, p. 1:5.

55 Anderson, *A Border City During the Civil War*, p. 297.

56 Forman, *opus cit.*, p. 104.

57 *Ibid.*, p. 35.

58 Anderson, *A Border City During the Civil War*, p. 292-293.

59 *Ibid.*, p. 300.

60 *Ibid.*, pp. 298-299.

61 *Ibid.*, p. 299.

62 *Ibid.*, pp. 293-295.

63 *Ibid.*, p. 300.

64 Adams, *opus cit.*, pp. 172-173.
65 St. Louis *Missouri Republican*, May 7, 1873, p. 8:1-2;
    ibid, Apr. 20, 1876, p. 5:1.
66 Adams, *opus cit.*, p. 177.
67 Forman, *opus cit.*, p. 73.
68 Adams, *opus cit.*, pp. 37-38.
69 St. Louis *Missouri Republican*, Apr. 12, 1864, p. 4:1.
70 Adams, *opus cit.*, p. 38.
71 *Ibid.*, p. 39. Doctors continued to use calomel and
    similar mercury preparations bacause they were major
    weapons in treating venereal diseases.
72 *Ibid.*, p. 37.
73 St. Louis *Missouri Republican*, Mar. 16, 1863, p. 2:7;
    ibid, Mar. 17, 1863, p. 2:8; *St. Louis Directory for 1864*
    (St. Louis, Richard Edwards, Editor and Publisher,
    1864), p. 59.
74 The manufacturers of Helmbold's "Extract Buchu" used
    the following slogan in their advertising: "Take No
    More Mercury or Unpleasant Medicines for Unpleasant
    and Dangerous Diseases." St. Louis *Missouri
    Republican*, Sept. 5, 1862, p. 1:2.
75 James N. Primm, *Lion of the Valley: St. Louis, Missouri*
    (Boulder Colorado, Pruett Publishing Co., 1981) p. 181.
76 St. Louis *Missouri Republican*, Sept. 5, 1864, p. 2:3.
77 *Idem.*
78 Stevens, *St. Louis: The Fourth City*, Vol. I, p. 603.
79 Adams, *opus cit.*, p. 133.
80 E. J. Goodwin, A *History of Medicine in Missouri*
    (St. Louis, W. L. Smith Publisher, 1905), p. 41.
81 *Report of the Western Sanitary Commission*, 1863,
    p. 10.
82 Goodwin, *opus cit.*, p. 38.
83 *Ibid.*, p. 234.
84 John Rodabough, *Frenchtown* (St. Louis, Mo.,
    Sunrise Publishing Co., Inc., 1980), p. 84.
85 *Ibid.*, pp. 87-88.

Chapter 5

Progress in Public Health Administration, 1866-1883

1. A Professional Board of Health in St. Louis

THE MISSOURI GENERAL ASSEMBLY, by an act approved March 9, 1867, made important changes in the composition and powers of the St. Louis Board of Health.[1] Previously the board had been a political body, staffed by members of the city council. Its ineffectiveness had been demonstrated at the time of the 1849 cholera epidemic. But the council was unwilling to give up its domination of the health board. There was a limited amount of patronage involved, including the position of health officer, the staff at city hospital and the street inspectors. Besides there was possibly some concern that a board staffed by doctors might release information regarding disease epidemics which, though true, would be harmful to the city's commercial interests.[2]

An important factor in bringing about a reform of the board of health was the tragic experience of St. Louis the previous year, when Asiatic cholera claimed a total of 3,527 lives.[3] Following the cholera attacks in 1849 and 1850, St. Louis set up a permanent quarantine station below the city where incoming boats were stopped and examined for evidence of contagious disease. With this precaution, the citizens felt reasonably secure. But the cholera invasion of 1866 overcame St.

Louis's defense system. Refugees from the devastated South, thousands on foot, and returning soldiers, introduced the infection, which found fertile soil in the crowded living conditions of post-war St. Louis.[4]

The failure of the St. Louis Board of Health contrasted with the success of New York City in dealing with a similar threat in the winter and spring of 1866. There a Metropolitan Board of Health, staffed by some of the city's finest physicians and given greatly increased power to clean up the city and to establish quarantines, had kept the toll of cholera victims to a minimum.[5] New York's well publicized achievement pointed the way for other communities to follow.

The 1867 law provided that the board of health should consist of five members, three of which had to be physicians with diplomas from regular[6] medical schools; the other two members would be chosen from persons outside the medical profession. The mayor was authorized to appoint the members of the board; confirmation by the city council was not required. The board was directed to elect a clerk, who would manage the health office. The clerk had to be a medical college graduate. The board of health was vested with authority to appoint all the members of the public health service, including the city health officer, the resident physician at city hospital, the physician at quarantine, and other medical officers and employees.[7] The new board thus began its operations remarkably free of political interference or control.

The board was required to meet twice a week between April 1 and November 1, and oftener if necessary. For the first time, salaries were provided for the board members, $1,000 for the president and $500 for the other members.[8]

The board was charged with the general supervision of the public health of the city. Failure to obey an order of the board to abate a nuisance constituted a misdemeanor, punishable by a fine of not more than $500. The board, to secure speedy execution of its orders, could provide for the abatement at city expense and assess the cost of the work as a lien on the property where the nuisance occurred. In addition to its authority to prosecute a property owner for harboring a nuisance and its power to assess the cost of city abatement as a lien on the property, the board could summarily order a business deemed detrimental to the public health to discontinue or to remove beyond the city limits.[9]

The law gave the board authority to require physicians to report promptly all cases of contagious diseases they had treated as well as all deaths from such diseases that had occurred among patients under their care.[10]

Mayor J. S. Thomas chose the members of the new board wisely. To head the group, he selected Dr. John T. Hodgen, who during the Civil War had served as superintendent of the city general hospital and also as surgeon general of the Western Sanitary Commission and of the state of Missouri. The second medical member was Dr. Elsworth F. Smith. He received his professional education at St. Louis University and at hospitals and clinics in Paris from 1852 to 1854. He had been assistant surgeon in charge of the St. Louis Military Smallpox Hospital and also of the wartime Eliot General Hospital. From 1857 to 1863, he served as health officer for St. Louis. Dr. Joseph Heitzig was the third medical member. Joseph S. Pease, a commission merchant and Constantine Maguire, a drug dealer, were selected to complete the membership of the board.[11]

Drs. Hodgen and Smith brought to their new task wide administrative experience and a thorough understanding of the methods of sanitary science developed by the army. They were accustomed to an expanded role of government health agencies.

A major portion of the time of the board of health was occupied with the investigation and elimination of nuisances. St. Louis, without benefit of a master plan or zoning regulations, had grown from an agricultural village to a commercial and industrial city. Small family-run businesses, such as dairies and slaughterhouses, were scattered through the residential areas. These were in filthy condition and created neighborhood nuisances with their refuse and offal, as the following description of the Mill Creek area by the city health officer in a report dated November 11, 1867, to the board of health indicated:[12]

I have the honor to report that I have examined Mill Creek, from Eleventh Street, to the city limits, west, together with the various slaughter houses and tanneries along its course. Mill Creek takes its origin at a point far beyond the city limits, intersects Grand Ave., between Clark and Chouteau avenues, then taking a tortuous course of three or four miles in extent, through the central part of the city, it empties into the Mississippi at the foot of Rutger Street. It drains a large area on either side of its course, and is the receptacle of a vast amount of filth and refuse material. It is, in effect, an open sewer, running through the heart of the city, which is being sewered as rapidly as the means of the city will permit, but which will not be completed (according to the calculations of the City Engineer) for fourteen years. This stream gathers through its tributaries, the decaying animal and vegetable matter of a large portion of the city and distributes the putrid effluvia to the population along its course. In addition to the vast amount of decomposing material which would naturally find its way into a stream running through a densely populated city there is added the offal and refuse natura from the dairies, slaughter houses and tanneries, above alluded to . . . . There is also a large sewer emptying into this creek at Adolph Street, at the mouth of which is constantly poured out the blood and offal from the slaughter houses in the vicinity of Washington, Christy and Franklin Avenues and in the neighborhood of Twentieth Street.

The slaughter houses situated immediately on the bank of the stream and emptying their waste material into it are seven in number. The dairies so situated are five, and the tanneries two. All these are nuisances and should be abated.

A persistent problem was that of stagnant pools of water, originating with sinkholes or created by the city's street improvement program which often blocked the normal channels of rain runoff. These pools became repositories of refuse and filth.

Newer immigrants, particularly blacks, were forced by poverty to live under crowded, insanitary conditions, in run-down housing that lacked sewer and water connections.

Establishments utilizing the by-products of the slaughterhouses created intolerably unwholesome conditions, as along Horse Creek just beyond the northern edge of town. Dr. William W. Grissom, city health officer, revealed the situation there in a letter to the board of health, following a visit in late August 1867:[13]

At the northern end of the slough there is a large bar which at this stage of the river prevents the water from flowing in or out, rendering the slough a stagnant pond of the most loathsome character. Having been exposed to the sun the past three months with all manner of decayed animal and vegetable matter, it emits a most intolerable stench. In some places the slough has become dry by evaporation which does not seem to improve its condition. As to the grease factories, slaughter houses and bone yards, the article that appeared in the *Dispatch* of August 23rd more fully describes their condition than I could possible do, yet I cannot refrain from stating that I visited the bone yard of the former contractor of dead animals which is situated about 200 yards north of the city limits, between Horse Creek and the river. In the rear of this building there is a low piece of ground about half an acre which is filled to the depth of eight or ten feet, with a putrid and decomposing mass of animal matter, the refuse from this building. I found several wagon loads of the heads of cattle, which had been recently deposited there, but which were in a state of decomposition. There was a number of carcasses on the outside of the building. I have seen many filthy places but I do not think I have ever seen one to equal this. As to the slaughter house and soap and grease factories, they are strung along Horse Creek for some considerable distance, each emptying its refuse matter into the creek, causing a most horrible stench.

This creek in times of high water emptied into the Mississippi River above the intake of the city's waterworks.

The success of the board of health's campaign to eliminate nuisances depended upon full cooperation by various city agencies — the comptroller, the city council, the police and the courts. This assistance was often lacking.

The unwillingness of the comptroller to guarantee that contractors, who received special tax bills for abating nuisances, would get their money, rendered this method of financing improvements unworkable in many cases. The issue came to a head at a meeting of the board of health on July 19, 1869:[14]

The matter originated from the action of the Board had previously. The Board some time ago condemned certain ponds belonging to various parties, as public nuisances, and ordered the owners to fill them up. They failed to comply with the order and the Board instructed the messenger to have the work done as an urgent sanitary measure. It was so done, and for payment the contractors received special tax bills against the parties. These the latter refused to pay, and the contractors applied for payment to the Board of Health. It then came before

the City Comptroller, who hesitates to sign warrants for their payment, doubting whether the proceedings of the Board in connection with the matter have been so regular as to insure the repayment of the money into the City Treasury.

Taking property owners to court yielded meager results. In a few cases the police court judge imposed a token fine of $5 or $10. Other cases were continued from week to week and finally dismissed; some suits were dismissed when first presented.[15]

The ordering of businesses detrimental to health to move produced only temporary benefits. Grease factories, slaughterhouses and boneyards operated out of inexpensive quarters with a minimum of equipment. When ordered to leave, they packed up and moved a few miles north of the city limits, where the county authorities were more hospitable.

Despite these enforcement problems, the board of health was able, in March 1868, to announce that, of 8,645 nuisances found by the sanitary police during its first year of office, it had been successful in abating 5,787 cases.[16]

In addition to its efforts to prevent diseases by cleaning up the environment, the board of health operated several programs for the control of disease through increasing the immunity of persons to infection. These were vaccination and various kinds of quarantine.

Dr. Antoine Saugrain introduced vaccination as a preventive of smallpox in St. Louis in 1809. But with a constantly changing population, it was impossible to completely eradicate the infection of the city. It broke out on a large scale in army camps in St. Louis during the Civil War.

To prevent a recurrence of the wartime smallpox epidemic, the board inaugurated in 1867 a comprehensive medical care program. For each of the city's eleven wards, the board appointed a physician.[17] The first task of the physician was to become acquainted with the people of his ward. Then, instead of sitting in his office waiting for patients, he visited needy families in their homes.[18] He treated their illnesses and provided necessary medicines; he also vaccinated those members of the family who had not been immunized. This plan, based on the generous assumption that the poor are entitled to good medical attention, was very successful. This conclusion was borne out by statistics compiled by the board of health. For 1867, there were eighty-nine cases of smallpox and eighteen deaths. The situation was much improved the next year, with ten reported cases and only one death.[19]

But the battle against the dread disease had been only temporarily victorious. At a meeting of the board of health on September 4, 1869, Dr. Rudolph Rattinger warned that the respite from smallpox was over, and that the city was in the midst of another epidemic. From his considerable experience in dealing with the public, he cited a number of reasons why vaccination programs had failed to wipe out the disease:[20]

There are various causes for the neglect of vaccination. With the mass of the people the cause is simply carelessness. Some have seen or heard of soreness or sickness following vaccination, and are fearful of similar consequences; some have seen or heard of a case of smallpox happening to a person who was previously vaccinated, usually of course unsuccessfully, and consequently do not believe that vaccination gives protec-tion. Some have even religious scruples against vaccination; and some are willing to have their children vaccinated, but they think that they are too young for it when a few months old, and the next three or four years they put it off from time to time because the child is teething, has measles, scarlatina, whooping cough, etc., or because they think the weather or season is not favorable, and when they finally do get ready, it happens usually that their physician has no fresh vaccine virus.

To overcome the apathy of the public, Dr. Rattinger favored a law compelling people to be vaccinated. He estimated that three or four physicians, devoting three months a year, could get a thorough job done. The doctors should be in their offices from one to three in the afternoon and from seven to eight o'clock in the evening. Children should be required to be vaccinated within six months of birth. Provision should be made for older children and grown persons to be successfully vaccinated.[21]

If such a law could not be passed, Dr. Rattinger recommended the appointment of ward physicians who should visit each tenement in their wards at least once each year and would provide general medical care as well as smallpox immunization. This was the system followed with good results in 1867-1868. To appoint ward physicians, who would sit in their offices and would provide only vaccination service, might shield the board of health from censure, he declared, but would not prevent a smallpox outbreak.[22]

The board of health rejected Dr. Rattinger's recommendation and, at its meeting of September 16, 1869, adopted the economy immunization plan, which the following staff was appointed to implement: Dr. Rudolph

Rattinger, 1410 So. Seventh Street, for the southern part of the city; Dr. George Blickbaum, 1026 N. Tenth Street, for the northern part; and the dispensary physician, at the health office, 198 No. Sixth Street, for the central portion of the city.[23]

Closely related to the board's overall campaign against nuisances were the efforts made to assure St. Louis wholesome supplies of water and milk. This objective would require the closing of hundreds of private wells throughout the city and also the drastic changing of the means by which the people were provided with dairy products.

St. Louis doctors, through medical journals and personal contacts with their European counterparts, were undoubtedly acquainted with the research of Dr. John Snow of London and Max von Pettenkofer in Munich,[24] which established the fact that cholera is a contagious disease caused by a poison which reproduces itself in the bodies of its victims. This poison is contained in the excreta and vomit of cholera patients. These substances, by draining into and contaminating water supplies, spread the disease.[25]

The board proceeded against impure wells under its general power to abate nuisances prejudicial to public health. In 1868, the state legislature authorized the board to order persons whose wells had been found contaminated to take out licenses to be supplied with municipal hydrant water.[26] This order met with widespread public opposition. A number of cases regarding refusal to take out water licenses were dismissed in police court.[27]

The order went against certain well-established local customs. Many citizens, especially in summer, preferred the cool, clear water from their wells to the warm, muddy liquid provided by the city waterworks. Wells, particularly those outside of taverns, furnished free water for horse and mule teams. While the animals were refreshing themselves, the teamsters enjoyed a beer or two at the bar. This fact brought the brewing industry to the support of the well owners. The aim of the board to close all wells, not merely those found impure, violated public ideas of fairness and appeared an example of bureaucratic highhandedness.[28]

Although St. Louis in the late 1860s had attained a population of almost 300,000 persons, it still received its milk and other dairy products by the same method employed when it was a small agricultural village. Scattered throughout the post-Civil War city were hundreds of small dairies, with herds ranging from one or two, to fifty cows per dairy. Five of these dairies were on the banks of the notorious public sewer, Mill Creek.[29] The cows were confined in crowded sheds or stables, the floors of which were covered with mud and manure. They were shut off from fresh air and sunshine. Their feed consisted largely of swill from the breweries and distilleries. The small dairies lacked the means to refrigerate their product, which was delivered to families in the neighborhood, and poured from large milk cans into receptacles provided by the customer. Adulteration by the addition of water and lowering of the fat content by skimming were common practices.

The board of health, which operated from 1867 to May 1870, lacked the power to proceed against the dairies on the basis of the unwholesome nature of their product. Its only weapon was to attack as nuisances those that operated in filthy quarters. Since neighborhood dairies were almost universally offensive, Dr. W. W. Grissom, health officer, in November 1867, recommended that the commercial production of milk be prohibited within the city limits.[30]

In April 1870, a revision of the St. Louis city charter by the general assembly provided a new board of health,[31] with greatly expanded powers. The new board consisted of five members, including the mayor, who would act as president, a member of the city council, a member of the board of police commissioners, and two practicing physicians to be appointed by the mayor with confirmation by the council. This arrangement restored city officials to a majority of seats on the board.[32]

The board was empowered to appoint a health officer and resident physicians for the city hospitals. In case of an epidemic, following a proclamation by the mayor, the board could assume emergency powers and take all necessary measures to suppress the disease incursion, without the intervention of the city council.[33] The revised charter extended the authority and jurisdiction of the board for three miles beyond the city limits in all directions.[34] This would give the city power to prevent offensive industries from re-establishing themselves just beyond the municipal borders. The new charter required the board to keep a full record of all births, marriages and deaths within the city.[35]

Taking advantage of the powers conferred by the revised charter, the city council by ordinance authorized the board of health to exercise broad control of the quality of milk sold in St. Louis:[36]

Whoever shall sell or offer for sale any milk adulterated with water or other substance, or any milk produced from diseased cows, shall be deemed guilty of a misdemeanor. The Health officer shall see that this section is properly enforced, and for that purpose shall have the right to enter all places, where milk may be sold, and cause a sample to be analyzed; and the Board of Health shall make a complete registration of all dairies and milk depots . . . .

The board of health, at its meeting of March 20, 1871, adopted stringent rules regarding the sale of milk in St. Louis. Any person selling milk in the city was required to register his name in a book kept by the board of health and to give full details regarding his dairy operation. No person could sell milk without a permit, the issuance of which was conditioned on the dairyman pledging not to sell adulterated or impure milk. The health officer was instructed to inspect periodically all stables where milk cows were kept. He was to examine all milk sold and seize for condemnation any found impure or adulterated; further, he was to report the offending dairyman to the police for prosecution.[37]

It was estimated by the medical members of the board that approximately $2,000,000 worth of milk, from 7,000 cows, was sold annually in St. Louis. Approximately half of this milk was impure, because it was adulterated or was derived from cows fed on distillery swill.[38] Impure milk was identified as a major cause of typhoid fever.[39] St. Louis had a yearly death rate of forty percent of its children under five years of age. It was thought that this rate could be reduced one-half or one-third by a wholesome milk supply.[40]

In September 1870, the Farmers' Pure Milk Association, a St. Louis corporation with a capital of $30,000, had been organized. This was the first modern milk processing plant in the city. It planned to establish purchasing contracts with a network of dairy farms, at first in the neighboring counties of St. Charles and Warren. Farmers selling milk to the association must agree to feed only natural foods — no swill — to their herds. The participating members delivered their milk to ice-houses established along the rail lines entering St. Louis; from these points the milk was shipped into the city. The association, at its headquarters in St. Louis, had equipment for pasteurizing and for testing the milk for fat content and purity, in order to assure a standard quality of product. In this central plant, the milk was bottled and distributed throughout the city. The pure milk group had the support of the board of health, the medical profession and many leading citizens, but it faced determined opposition from the dairy men who profited from feeding swill.[41]

On July 9, 1870, the city council enacted an ordinance regulating prostitution or what was euphemistically called the "Social Evil".[42] Hitherto the council's concern for the public health had been limited mainly to combatting epidemics and abating nuisances. The problem of prostitution had come to public attention in St. Louis during the Civil War when the city served as the military and medical headquarters for the Union armies in the Western theater of operations.

The 'Social Evil' did not disappear with the return of peace. Instead, from well-known red light districts, it moved into old mansions in residential areas, and even into the upper stories of public buildings. After dark, the prostitutes plied their trade on the streets, in places of entertainment and at bars and beer halls. The human wreckage caused by venereal diseases, for which the medical science of the day had no satisfactory remedy, was well known to physicians.[43]

The issue was extensively discussed in the general assembly during February 1868. J. B. Woerner, chairman of the Committee on Criminal Jurisprudence, citing the ineffectiveness of curbing prostitution by arrests and fines of the madames and prostitutes, recommended a program of regulation involving registration and frequent medical examinations of the inmates of bawdy houses.

Opponents declared that this would amount to legalization of what was generally regarded as a crime. A majority of the committee approved regulation and referred the proposed bill to the St. Louis delegation for their reaction.[44]

The matter rested until May 1870, when the revised St. Louis charter gave the city council authority to "regulate or suppress" prostitution.[45] The council chose to try the regulation experiment, though this system had found more favor with European than American cities.

The "Social Evil" ordinance, of July 9, 1870, divided the city into six districts. The police were appointed to carry out the registration of prostitutes, visiting each brothel or place of business. Through personal interviews, they gathered basic information regarding the inmates. This information was sent to the office of the chief of police for tabulation and organization. To each district a physician was assigned. With the information for his district collected by the police, the physician examined the prostitutes to determine which were infected with venereal disease. Those found infected were sent to the city hospital for treatment.[46] Stricken from the original bill as it passed the council were provisions for a separate hospital for the prostitutes and a home where they could live while they were taught skills for making an honest living.

The board of health drew up an elaborate system of rules supplementing the city ordinance, aimed mainly at curbing the means by which the Cyprians attracted their patronage. The rules, for example, prohibited prostitutes from appearing at the windows or doors of their houses or from plying their trade in the streets or public places; also from riding in open carriages in the daytime or visiting taverns and beer parlors. Holding that most of the board's rules were null and void, the city attorney dismissed the complaints against the first group of prostitutes charged under them.[47]

Problems arose from the practice of sending diseased prostitutes to the city hospital. Many female patients objected to sharing accommodations in the wards with the fallen women. There was also the problem of keeping the prostitutes from getting too friendly with the male patients.[48] The method of treatment of venereal diseases consisted of massive doses of calomel or other mercury compounds, which caused excessive salivation, loosening of the teeth and frequently rotting of the soft parts of the mouth and cheeks.[49] Some of the prostitutes, possibly judging that the method of treatment was worse than the disease from which they suffered, secretly left without permission.[50]

With opposition to the program of regulation of the "Social Evil" coming to the surface, Dr. William L. Barrett, health officer, undertook to defend the new system. In a report prepared and published with the approval of the board of health, he cited the success of the program in reducing the incidence of venereal disease.

The number of cases of venereal disease treated in the St. Louis municipal hospitals in the eight months prior to the inauguration of regulation was 599; for the first eight months of regulation, the number dropped to 174, a decline of 425 cases.[51]

To meet some of the objections to the control plan, a revised "Social Evil" ordinance was passed on June 20, 1871. This provided for the establishment of a separate hospital for the prostitutes and also a house of industry, where they would be trained in vocational skills. Funding for these two institutions was provided by a monthly tax of $10 on every bawdy house and $1.50 on each inmate.[52]

This measure passed in the city council by a vote of nineteen to two. The measure had been drafted in the board of health, where city officials outnumbered the medical professionals three to two. Authorization for St. Louis to adopt the regulation plan had been granted by the general assembly after careful consideration. These facts indicate that the "Social Evil" experiment was regarded by both state and city officials as a wise and proper plan for dealing with a serious public health problem.

The board of health chose as the site for the new hospital the Thomas property, comprising a two-story brick house and thirteen and a half acres of land, located in an attractive rural setting about four miles in a southwesterly direction from downtown St. Louis. The tract had an orchard of 1,200 fruit trees and a productive garden. This new hospital was put into operation in the fall of 1872 with Dr. E. M. Powers as superintendent.[53]

Early in 1873 a concerted campaign was launched to discredit St. Louis's program for the regulation of the "Social Evil". The architect of the campaign was the Reverend William G. Eliot, civic leader, Unitarian minister and the founder of Washington University. The opening gun in this campaign was a long letter by Dr. Eliot, attacking the "Social Evil" law, which appeared in the St. Louis *Missouri Republican* of February 18, 1873. The letter was prefaced in the columns of the press by an exchange of notes between Dr. Eliot and St. Louis's Catholic Archbishop Richard Peter Kenrick, in which the archbishop promised his moral support, although refusing to take an active public part. The timing of Dr. Eliot's letter was designed to forestall the inclusion of the "Social Evil" legislation in the new charter, which was being framed for St. Louis.[54]

Anticipating a thunderous "No!" from his readers, he asked if they were willing to have the "Social Evil" system become a permanent part of St. Louis society:[55]

Are we prepared for this? Consider what it is that we are doing. Look at the facts as they now are. We are sanctioning by law the setting apart, the keeping, under city authority, more than a thousand women as prostitutes for the satisfaction of the unbridled lust of men. We register their houses at a stipulated price, we enter their names on the city record, we cause them to be "inspected" every week by physicians appointed for the purpose; we take payment for this from the wages of sin; we send the diseased to a hospital for cure and return them to their vile calling and thus recognize the whole course of their living as a legal arrangement for the "regulation" of vice. Is it not a fearful thing for men who have mothers and sisters and wives and daughters to sanction such degradation as this? In a Christian community, where women are believed to have souls, shall they be deliberately held for such a use? Can Christian women who respect their own sex quietly look on while their sisters, for whom Christ died, are by law recognized and upheld in a pollution so deep?

Continuing his attack against the "Social Evil" regulation system, Dr. Eliot moved to have its legality tested in court. He filed a complaint against Kate Clark, who operated a bawdy house at the northwest corner of Sixth and Elm streets, alleging that her business was in violation of state laws against prostitution. The state of Missouri took responsibility for conducting the prosecution when the case was tried in the St. Louis Court of Criminal Correction, August 16, 1873, Judge John W. Colvin presiding. The city of St. Louis did not intervene, but forced Kate Clark to defend herself, as well as the city ordinance under which she had been given permission to conduct business.[56]

Judge Colvin, in a decision rendered August 23, declared the city's licensing ordinance illegal. He cited three grounds for his judgment: first, the St. Louis ordinance was in violation of state legislation banning bawdy houses and prostitution; secondly, it was discriminatory, since it provided for examination and registration of females engaged in illicit sex but not for their male customers; finally, the charter provision, granting St. Louis authority to regulate prostitution, was a special law for a situation which could have been handled by a general law, applicable to the whole state.[57]

The reaction of the state legislature, following the voiding of the St. Louis licensing system, was to pass in March 1874, another special law, which went to the opposite extreme of removing practically all regulation of prostitution, including that embodied in state law.[58] Had the new legislation been drafted by the bawdy house proprietors, it could not have been more favorable to their interests.

The new law made the mayor and the city council — not the board of health — responsible for the government and maintenance of the "Social Evil" hospital and the house of industry. Funds for operating these two institutions, henceforth, had to come out of the city's general revenue, since the tax on bawdy houses and their inmates, which had previously supported these facilities, had been struck down.[59]

For the section of the former "Social Evil" ordinance providing for weekly medical examinations of registered prostitutes, an inferior new system was substituted. This required every physician, treating a prostitute or suspected prostitute for venereal disease, to report the fact to the board of police commissioners, who would make arrangement by warrant to confine such person in the "Social Evil" hospital.[60] The practical effect of this section was that the actual prostitutes would hesitate to go to a doctor for treatment. And a young female, who contracted venereal disease through indiscretion and went to a doctor, risked being adjudged a prostitute and sent to the "Social Evil" hospital. No opportunity for her to defend herself against the doctor's suspicion was provided.

Two sections of the new law were apparently designed to cripple the efforts of the police to curb prostitution. Any police officer found in a bawdy house, except in discharge of his duty, would be considered guilty of a misdemeanor.[61] This restriction would tend to eliminate all routine surveillance of bawdy houses by the police.

A final provision made it unlawful for the police to arrest any proprietor or inmate of a bawdy house except upon a warrant based on the affidavit of some reputable person that the house was a place of ill fame. The police could not make raids based on their own knowledge but had to wait for a citizen complaint.[62]

In order to place some restraints on the freedom accorded prostitutes by the special state law of March 1874, the city council drafted a stringent new "Social Evil" ordinance, which was passed June 22, 1875. Unlike its predecessor act of July 9, 1870, this ordinance was aimed at suppressing — not regulating — prostitution; and the earlier idealistic plan of rehabilitating the fallen women was abandoned.[63]

The law branded as illegal the various operations involved in commercialized sex, including the keeping of a bawdy house; the visiting or frequenting by anyone of a house of ill fame; the renting of property for purposes of prostitution; the wandering about the streets at night of prostitutes; and the plying of trade by bawds in public places.[64]

Although a great deal of the time and effort of the board of health in the early 1870s was devoted to the "Social Evil" issue, other problems also required attention. Smallpox posed a continuing threat, which from time to time was met with halfway measures. In November 1871, nine vaccinating physicians were appointed, whose special mission was to visit public and private schools and insist that all scholars be immunized. [65] An epidemic broke out in January 1873, sending 254 persons with the disease to the Grand Avenue smallpox hospital.[66] In December 1874, physicians were appointed for each ward to vaccinate all who would permit it. [67] But a short while later, their services were terminated because of widespread public indifference and opposition to their efforts.[68]

Under the rules governing the sale of milk passed by the board of health on March 20, 1871, Dr. John Bryson was named dairy inspector with the responsibility for checking for adulteration and impurity. At that time, the question whether swill was a wholesome cattle food had not been settled conclusively by political and judicial determination. Dr. Bryson stated, at a meeting of the board of health on September 28, 1871, that out of 270 St. Louis dairies, he found only four which did not use swill. These were all large dairies; some of them supplied milk shipped in by railway.[69]

To eliminate the nuisances created in residential areas by some 400 small enterprises, Dr. William L. Barrett, health officer, in October 1871, recommended the establishment of abattoirs for the slaughtering of animals.[70] Two years later, a company was formed to erect a general slaughterhouse near the Pacific Railway stockyards. A large number of local butchers signified their intention to locate there.[71]

In order to enable the board of health to analyze samples of water and milk, Dr. D. V. Dean was appointed in 1871 to the newly-created post of city chemist. His field of responsibility was expanded to include the ice supply sold in the city, much of it from impure ponds.[72] This office was later involved in the inspection of meat and other food products.

On March 14, 1872, the board of health upheld its clerk in refusing to register for practice in St. Louis Dr. Solomon S. Wehr, who claimed a degree from a college suspected of being a diploma mill.[73] This was the first attempt of a governmental body to establish qualifications for the practice of medicine in Missouri. In late May 1873, Dr. Emma R. Still, with a diploma from an Eclectic and also a homeopathic college, applied to be enrolled on the doctors' register in the office of the board of health. The board, after investigation, granted that request. She was the first woman physician in St. Louis thus recognized.[74]

By an act passed on March 27, 1874, the state legislature joined the city of St. Louis in placing certain restrictions on the medical profession. No one was permitted to practice medicine or surgery in Missouri without a degree of doctor of medicine from a duly established college or university. Every prospective doctor had to file a copy of his diploma in the office of the clerk of the county where he intended to work; the clerk thereupon would enter his name on the roll of physicians. Physicians practicing in Missouri, who entered their names prior to September 1, 1874, were not required to file copies of their diplomas.[75] This provision permitted doctors, who registered before the deadline, to continue to practice without a diploma.

2. St. Louis's First Commissioner of Health

The state constitution of 1875 effected a major change in the government of St. Louis. It provided for splitting off the city of St. Louis from the adjacent county. St. Louis, as a separate political entity, was furnished a completely new charter, which went into effect in 1876. An important feature was the substitution of strong administrative heads, in place of committees, to direct various municipal departments. In the field of public health, e.g., a health commissioner was appointed.[76] The new administrative posts were full-time, long-term, salaried positions, affording the incumbents opportunity to develop professional expertise. These assignments concentrated responsibility and provided the means for meeting situations with prompt, decisive action.

Mayor Henry Overstolz appointed Charles W. Francis as the city's first health commissioner. Francis was born in the state of Delaware in 1836 and educated at St. Mary's College in Wilmington. He came west and, for a number of years, engaged in fur trading on the upper Missouri River with the Northwestern Fur Company. Having moved to St. Louis, he was employed in local mercantile enterprises until 1873. He served as a member of the city council from 1874 to 1877.[77]

The powers and responsibilities of the health commissioner were as follows:[78]

He has general supervision over the public health of the city, and over the enforcement of the regulations, laws and ordinances in relation thereto. He may make rules and regulations with the approval of the board of health, for the protection and promotion of the public health, and may enter buildings, lots and places of every description in the city, to make examinations and abate nuisances. He provides for the registration of births, deaths and marriages within the city, and has charge of the city hospitals, quarantine, insane asylums, morgue and city dispensary; appoints the subordinate employees in the city hospital, female asylum, insane asylum and quarantine; and in the prevalence of an epidemic may take measures to abate, avoid, mitigate and suppress it, with the approval of the board of health.

The health commissioner was the chief executive officer of the board of health, which consisted of the mayor, the president of the city council, a member of the board of police commissioners, the health commissioner, and two practicing physicians. He was appointed by the mayor, with the approval of the council, for a term of four years.[79]

Prominent among the problems facing the health commissioner was the swill milk issue. The board of health had the power to prohibit the sale in St. Louis of impure milk. But there was disagreement whether milk from swill-fed cows was impure. The owners of hundreds of small dairies, that used swill, contended that it was not. They had the support of the brewery and distillery lobby, which benefitted from the sale of their by-products as cattle feed.

The board of health appointed a sub-committee to investigate the matter. Dr. D. V. Dean, former city chemist, headed the sub-committee, which presented its report at a public meeting of the board on February 12, 1877, when testimony from both sides of the controversy was aired. Dr. Dean cited an impressive array of published American, British and French authorities to back his claim that swill or slops fed to cattle impaired their health and contaminated the milk they produced. Testifying to the same conclusion were E. D. Richardson, a pork packer; J. C. Cabanne, a large-scale dairyman; and Mr. Tolkacz, a former veterinary-surgeon in the Prussian army.[80]

The pro-swill group introduced a medical witness to affirm the wholesomeness and nutritiousness of their products. They also sought to prove that the prejudice against milk from swill-fed cows was created by the Farmers Pure Milk Association in order to gain a competitive advantage in the St. Louis market. The board took no immediate action as a result of the public meeting.[81] Uncertain how to proceed, the board of health, at its meeting of September 20, 1877, asked for a legal opinion regarding its power to prohibit the sale of swill milk.[82] The city counselor, in reply, denied that the board had the authority to ban the sale of swill milk in the absence of a city ordinance to that effect. Apparently at the time, the swill milk lobby and its allies were able to block the passage in the council of such an ordinance.

Stalled in its efforts to get the council to act, the board of health decided upon a different approach. At its meeting of March 6, 1879, the board requested Commissioner Francis to present the names of dairy owners within the city limits who fed swill, as the basis for prosecution.[83] This would throw upon the courts the responsibility of deciding if swill milk was impure, and thus banned for sale in St. Louis.

The special act passed by the state legislature, in March 1874, halted the compulsory registration and examination of prostitutes, thus drastically reducing the number of diseased women being sent to the "Social Evil" hospital. The law, however, required that the city continue to maintain the institution at its own expense. Because of the diminished demand for the specialized medical services of the "Social Evil" hospital, a plan was developed to transform it into a general hospital for women. This idea gained favor because the city hospital was an old, poorly ventilated and overcrowded building, while the "Social Evil" hospital was a modern structure, located in an attractive suburban setting. The transfer of female patients began in June 1875, at which time the new structure was renamed the Female Hospital.[84] The policy of segregation by sex continued under Commissioner Francis, with the city hospital serving males, the Female Hospital the gentle sex.[85]

A serious health problem for St. Louis was created by the fact that hundreds of homes, because of the refusal of landlords to install hydrants, were without access to city water. This forced tenants to use water of uncertain quality from wells and cisterns or to obtain city water surreptitiously from the hydrants of neighbors. The 1876 charter authorized the board of health to order the installation of hydrants in homes and tenements whenever it decided that such action was necessary for the preservation of the health of the occupants of such buildings.[86]

Proprietary medical schools proliferated in St. Louis in the period between 1865 and 1900. Although public confidence in the efficiency of medical science was low, [87] the field was attractive to young men ambitious to achieve professional status. One result was an oversupply of physicians. Some doctors, finding private or hospital practice only marginally remunerative, sought to supplement their income by becoming proprietors or faculty members of medical colleges.

It was a fairly simple matter to start a medical school. The major requirements were a building in which to conduct lectures and a skeleton teaching staff. Laboratories, libraries and teaching exhibits could be acquired gradually if the school succeeded.

Missouri law, at least at first, posed no serious obstacles. The statute, of March 27, 1874, recognized as valid the diploma of any medical school, which had been "duly established".[88] This general requirement was subject to judicial and legislative interpretation. At first it meant little more than that the promoters had applied for and received a charter of incorporation from the secretary of state.

Much of the litigation regarding medical schools and diplomas arose in St. Louis, where the board of health attempted to look beyond the diploma of a candidate for registration to the credibility of the school, which had issued the certificate. Did the school have an adequate faculty of qualified teachers? What was the length of training required for graduation? How stringent were the examinations? Answers to these questions would enable the board to distinguish between reputable medical schools and fly-by-night diploma mills.

In 1874-1875, Dr. George H. Field established the St. Louis Eclectic Medical College, with its lecture hall at 319 North Market Street. At a meeting of the board of health on February 14, 1878, Dr. Field presented two of the school's graduates — Dr. L. C. Washburn and Dr. C. A. Gibbs — and asked that they be officially registered. Commissioner Francis pointed out the city ordinance, providing for the registration of doctors, required that they be graduates of colleges "in good standing." To prove that the college was not in good standing, Francis introduced Dr. J. E. Dunbar, who testified that without attending the St. Louis Eclectic Medical College or passing any comprehensive examination, he had bought a diploma for $25. Evidence was produced that not all the doctors, who signed the diplomas, were actually teachers at the school. On the basis of the negative testimony, the board refused to register the two doctors.[89] The board also denied to the faculty and students of the St. Louis Eclectic Medical College access to the city hospital for clinical study, because its professors were not registered as physicians under city ordinances.[90] A plan to seek a writ of mandamus to force the board of health to recognize the college was vetoed by Dr. Field's counsel, since the board, as an administrative body, had a discretionary power the courts would not override.[91]

St. Louis had a frightening encounter with yellow fever in 1878 and 1879. Its previous acquaintance with the disease had been acquired from indirect sources. St. Louis newspapers gave extensive coverage to the yearly ravages of the plague in New Orleans and other cities of the Deep South. Each summer a sizable migration to St. Louis of citizens of the South took place in order to avoid infection. St. Louisans, serving on the city's fleet of river boats and barges, traversed the danger zone of the disease on their trips southward.

Experience had proved that Missouri was reasonably immune to local epidemics of yellow fever.[92] The mosquito *Aedes aegypti,* which transmitted the disease, could not ordinarily survive the Missouri winters.

The 1878 and 1879 yellow fever epidemics were different from earlier ones. Instead of being centered on New Orleans, they focused on Memphis, Tennessee, a city in close contact with St. Louis by river steamers as well as by railroads. Gerald M. Capers, in his history

of Memphis, described the 1878 scourge as "one of the most severe fever epidemics in American urban history."[93]

The first yellow fever death in Memphis in the 1878 epidemic occurred on August 13. Within ten days, the death toll was numbered in the hundreds. Within two weeks of the first death, twenty-five thousand persons abandoned the city in a mad exodus by rail, by river, by wagon and on foot. Many neighboring towns established shotgun quarantines against the refugees.[94] Before the frost in mid-October put an end to the epidemic, the total mortality stood at 5,150 out of the population of 20,000, which remained in Memphis throughout the pestilence.[95]

Following the discovery of a case of yellow fever in St. Louis about the middle of July, Commissioner Francis reactivated the quarantine hospital on the river several miles below Jefferson Barracks. He appointed Dr. Henry C. Davis, then assistant physician at the Female Hospital, as superintendent. Dr. Davis's responsibility was to stop incoming boats for the medical examination of passengers and crews. The sick were removed to the hospital; the other passengers were permitted to continue to St. Louis.[96] Vessels carrying freight from the South were fumigated.

As the number of refugees, and also the patient load at the hospital increased, the work became more than one doctor could handle. Commissioner Francis asked for volunteers from the staff of young physicians at city hospital. Dr. F. T. Outley, Dr. Jacob Friedman and Dr. Walter B. Dorsett responded and were sent to assist Dr. Davis. But months of overwork and exposure to disease had broken the health of the courageous doctor, who died October 15, 1878.[97]

One hundred and fifty-one cases of yellow fever were treated in St. Louis, its suburbs and at quarantine during 1878; of these eighty recovered, while seventy-one died.[98]

Memphis experienced a return of the yellow fever in the summer of 1879, and once more thousands of its citizens fled the city. St. Louis reinstated its quarantine, this time in the form of a total blockade. On July 25, Mayor Henry Overstolz sent the following notice to the board of health in Memphis:[99]

Send no more passengers or freight by boats. We shall not permit any boat coming from Memphis with freight or passengers to come above quarantine grounds, and will compel them to return without landing freight or passengers.

To provide for refugees who might be stranded at the St. Louis Quarantine, Mayor Overstolz planned to establish a temporary camp, well away from the city. To implement this plan, he wired the National Board of Health for tents and rations for 1,000 persons for thirty days.[100] The request was relayed to the secretary of war, the only government official whose department stocked the requested supplies.

The yellow fever epidemics of 1878 and 1879 were not confined to the Mississippi Valley. Eastern coastal cities also suffered severely. Yellow fever epidemics usually began in Cuba or other Caribbean countries. They were spread within the United States by the interstate flight of refugees. These aspects of the epidemic justified the establishment of a national health organization — something that had not existed since the army medical service during the Civil War.

The first agency set up was the National Board of Health. Its original role was to make recommendations to state and local authorities regarding plans for preventing the spread of contagious diseases. The board aimed to supplement rather than supplant local initiative. It later became active in the provision of relief supplies.[101]

The National Board of Health began the establishment of a quarantine system. Previous quarantines were imposed by individual cities which felt threatened by epidemic disease. In early August 1878, Dr. John H. Rauch, Chicago health commissioner, and a member of the Illinois Board of Health and of the National Board of Health, set up a quarantine station at Island No. 1, five miles below Cairo. This was a national, as well as an Illinois, post. It was planned to establish national inspection stations in New Orleans, Vicksburg and at a point eight miles below Memphis.[102]

The National Board of Health found an ally in its war against disease in the recently organized American Public Health Association. At its meeting in Richmond, Virginia, November 22, 1878, the association attempted to condense what was known about yellow fever into six short propositions. One statement agreed upon was that "yellow fever of 1878 was a specific disease," not the advanced stage of malaria as some doctors maintained.[103] By 1878, Louis Pasteur's discovery that for every disease there exists a specific cause, i.e., a microbe or germ, was widely known in medical circles. The association recommended the establishment of a national commission of experts to investigate the cause of yellow fever and the methods of preventing its introduction in the United States.[104] On July 3, a four-member commission appointed by the National Board of Health sailed from New York for Havana to carry out this investigative mission. The group consisted of three physicians and a sanitary engineer.[105] The search, unsuccessful at first, culminated in the discovery in 1900 by Dr. Walter Reed's medical team that yellow fever is not contagious but is transmitted from a yellow fever patient to its next victim by the mosquito *Aedes aegypti.*

3. Public Utilities

With the completion in 1855 of the 32,000,000 gallon reservoir at the Benton Street site, the needs of St. Louis for decades appeared to have been well provided for. But the growth of population and the westward expansion of the city dashed this expectation. The smaller Benton Street reservoir had to be abandoned because it could not deliver water to the higher elevations of the city. This threw the full load of providing water upon the newer 32,000,000 gallon basin.[108] Since there was no back-up source, the large reservoir could not be taken out of operation for cleaning, with the result that it began to fill with mud and sand at the rate of three feet a year.[107]

The water that was delivered during the late 1850s and 1860s was pumped from the old river site at the foot of Bates Street, which by this time was part of the busy St. Louis harbor. Upriver from the pump house were a number of creeks, the banks of which were lined with grease factories, slaughterhouses and bone yards, which poured their filth into the same current from which the city drew its water supply.[108]

In February 1863, a bill authorizing the borrowing of three million dollars for the construction of new waterworks was prepared and approved by the St. Louis Council. The bill was then forwarded to the state legislature with the request that it be enacted. A second bill, for a two million dollar authorization, was introduced in the council by a minority of its members. This plan provided for a separate financial and technical administration of the works. It also was sent to the legislature accompanied by a memorial signed by seventy of the city's largest taxpayers, asking for its passage.[109] At issue were the amount of the waterworks funding and also the method of control, whether by the city council or by an independent board of water commissioners.

The state legislature, on March 23, 1863, approved its own bill which provided for the appointment by the St. Louis City Council of a board of water commissioners, consisting of four members with the mayor as a member ex officio. The law empowered the council to float a three million dollar bond issue to finance the expansion of the works.[110] The council, however, whether due to a preoccupation with the issues of the Civil War or because of a continuing division of opinion among its members, failed to exercise the powers granted it.

Meanwhile dangerous fissures developed in the Benton Street reservoir. By 1864, the accumulation of sediment had reached the level so that only three or four feet of water were regularly available.[111] To satisfy peak demands, the water was pumped directly from the river into the distribution system. The widespread public complaint was expressed in the following editorial from the St. Louis *Missouri Republican* of August 7, 1864:[112]

> For many weeks past we have been drinking mud, eating mud, bathing in mud, and washing in mud, until it has become past all endurance. What does it mean? Badly as the Water Works have been managed in past years, and under half a dozen administrations, we never have had such a condition of things as now. And the Water Works Department treat all representations of

the sufferings of the people with the most supreme indifference.

By an act approved January 18, 1865, the general assembly empowered the governor to appoint the four commissioners of the board of St. Louis Waterworks, who would be solely responsible for directing the improvement program. The law continued the authorization of the city to issue $3,000,000 of bonds to finance the works.[113]

At a meeting of community leaders, city officials and members of the state legislature, held at the Southern Hotel on December 28, 1866, the following statement expressing approval of the general assembly's action in the waterworks issue, was ratified:[114]

> Resolved, That, in the sense of this meeting, it is desirable that the control and management of the waterworks be separated from the City Council, and placed in the hands of a Board of Water Commissioners.

A committee was appointed at the citizens' meeting to draw up a detailed statement of the mission and also the powers and responsibilities of the board of commissioners.[115]

In order to expand the city's scanty water supply, a small auxiliary reservoir was built on the St. Charles Road between Dayton and Gamble streets. The new basin was 210 feet square, with a depth of 21 feet, and a capacity of 2,000,000 gallons. It was put in operation early in 1868. With the auxiliary basin in place, the city could proceed with the long-delayed cleaning of the Benton Street reservoir.[116]

The commissioners constructed the main works of the new water system at Bissell's Point, almost three miles upriver from the old pumping station at the foot of Bates Street. At this new location four settling basins, each 300 by 600 feet with a depth of 21 feet, were built. The main reservoir for supplying the city was constructed in the southwestern part of the city on Compton Hill, at the corner of Grand and Lafayette avenues, about five miles from the settling basins.[117]

The water entered an inlet tower in the Mississippi River, about 250 feet from the shore on which the basins were located, and was forced by the low-service engines into the settling basins. After settling for three days, the water was pumped by the high-service engines into the Compton Hill reservoir.[118] In order to regulate the speed of water through the mains, and also to get it moving again following a temporary stoppage of the high service engines, a water tower seventy-five feet high was built on East Grand Avenue and Twentieth Street.[119]

The waterworks began providing the city with water in June 1871. The two high-service engines were capable of pumping 32,000,000 gallons of water into the Compton Hill reservoir every twenty-four hours. By 1873, the city was using about 20,000,000 gallons daily.[120]

The new system did not provide for any filtration or chemical treatment of the water. With the growing contamination of the river by residential, commercial and industrial wastes. St. Louis's water, though clearer than before, was far from being a completely safe and wholesome beverage.[121]

The healthfulness of St. Louis has been favorably affected by its excellent system of drainage. The gradual rise in terraces of the land on which St. Louis is situated made it feasible to drain the original town directly into the Mississippi River. This stream, with its swift current and large volume of water, served as the city's master sewer.

The first area provided with artificial sewers was bounded by Biddle Street on the north, by Ninth Street on the west, Poplar Street on the south and by the river on the east. To assist in draining this area, the city constructed five main, publicly financed sewers. The total area was divided into thirty-three sewer districts, in each of which the property owners were assessed to pay for their sewers. Sewer bonds were issued by the city to finance the construction, and they were paid off gradually by the tax on the benefiting property owners. This program began in 1849 with the Biddle Street and the Poplar Street sewers.[122]

In 1859, the annual tax to pay off the sewer bonds was abandoned. A new system was instituted by which, upon the completion of a district sewer, the whole cost was assessed upon the property owners in proportion to their holdings in the district. The contractors were given special tax bills in compensation and had the responsibility of making their own collections.[123]

With the change of government occasioned by the charter of 1876, the city adopted a policy by which large districts of 100 to 600 acres, embracing entire watersheds, were established. These districts included the main sewers as well as the district sewers.

Under this plan the involved property owners were assessed to pay the cost not only of the local district sewers but also of the public sewers in the expanded districts.[124]

Before the establishment of the sewer system, human wastes were collected from residential vaults and privies and transported in scavenger boats below the city before being dumped into the river. With the use of water closets and sewers, these materials were deposited in the same current from which the city took its water supply.[125] This created the danger of epidemics of typhoid fever, cholera and other diseases.

4. Diseases and Methods of Treatment

The pattern of disease in St. Louis following the Civil War differed from that of the prewar period. In the earlier era, malaria was endemic and affected a large portion of the population. Cholera periodically visited the city with devastating force, as in 1832, 1849 and 1866. Following the war, consumption, typhoid fever and smallpox were the major killers, with diphtheria, croup, scarlet fever, measles and cerebro-spinal fever also taking an annual toll of victims.[126]

Complete statistics regarding the incidence of disease in St. Louis prior to 1867 are lacking. The records kept by the board of health prior to 1850 were destroyed in the 1849 riverfront fire. From 1850 to 1867, the weekly reports prepared in the board's office were not compiled into a permanent statistical account. Better record keeping was maintained by the professional board of health headed by Dr. John T. Hodgen, beginning in 1867.[127]

A report prepared by the National Board of Health for the period of thirteen weeks, ending April 1, 1862, showed St. Louis with a mortality rate of twenty persons per thousand, the lowest among the major American cities.[128] This achievement was attributable mainly to the city's vigorous program of sanitary science.

Unfortunately, therapeutics had not kept pace with developments in the field of public health. Only modest advances had been achieved in private medical practice. The experience during the Civil War had discredited the use of calomel and bleeding, two stand-bys of antebellum medicine. Quinine had taken the place of calomel as the doctor's panacea. Diagnosis of disease remained largely guess work, based on the doctor's superficial examination at bedside. Many doctors overmedicated, in order to be sure to prescribe some pill or powder that would work. But aside from quinine used in treating malaria, the doctor had nothing comparable to modern antibodies. The best doctors relied on the body's own recuperative powers, aided by rest, proper diet and a minimum of medicine.[129]

Advances in the new science of microbiology were being made in Europe by Louis Pasteur and Robert Koch, which were destined to revolutionize the science of medicine. Their researches revealed that fermentation, putrefaction and various diseases are caused by germs or bacteria.[130] This new theory of disease causation was brought to the attention of St. Louisans by Dr. P. V. Schenck, resident physician at the St. Louis Female Hospital, in an article on "Preventable Diseases," written for the June 3, 1877 issue of the St. Louis *Missouri Republican*. Quoting from a lecture delivered by professor John Tindall at Glasgow, Scotland, October 19, 1876, Dr. Schenck stated "that the conviction is spreading and growing daily in strength, that reproductive and parasitic life is at the root of epidemic diseases."[131]

Even before Dr. Schenck's announcement, the St. Louis Board of Health was employing microbiology in its work. In November 1867, Dr. Hiram S. Leffingwell, in making a routine post-mortem examination, had discovered, through the use of the microscope, the symptoms of trichinosis in the muscles of a deceased patient.[132] In 1871, the office of city chemist was officially established in the Health Department.[133]

In the field of surgery, important progress was being made. The growing employment of anesthesia obviated the necessity of completing an operation quickly and hurriedly. Many St. Louis surgeons had enlarged their skill and experience through service in army field and general hospitals during the Civil War. The adoption of Joseph Lister's teachings regarding antiseptic surgery reduced the incidence of post-operative infections and complications.[134]

Surgeons were handicapped by the lack of any method of seeing within the body to guide operative procedures. When President James Garfield was shot on July 2, 1881, the bullet from the assassin's small caliber pistol remained in the president's body. A team of surgeons using long probes, like knitting needles, punched in the abdomen region in an effort to locate the foreign object. They failed. The laceration of tissue by the probing as well as by the bullet resulted in blood poisoning from which Garfield died on September 15, 1881.[135]

5. *The Medical Profession*

The period during and immediately following the Civil War witnessed the passing of a number of the greatest physicians in the St. Louis profession. Among the deceased were William Carr Lane, mayor of St. Louis, state legislator, soldier and beloved physician; Joseph Nash McDowell, founder of the Missouri Medical College and an outstanding surgeon and medical lecturer; Charles A. Pope, trained in the finest European schools and medical institutions, and dean for many years of the St. Louis Medical College; John Hodgen, surgeon general of Missouri during the Civil War and later chairman of St. Louis's first professional board of health.[136]

These doctors, who had reached the peak of their careers before the war, generally practiced medicine as well as surgery. A number had been very active in politics. Some, as Drs. George Engelmann, Adolph Wislizenus and Hiram A. Prout, were nationally recognized for their pioneer work in botany, zoology, ethnology and other natural sciences.

The generation of physicians, which succeeded these pioneers, tended to specialize. They were either doctors or surgeons. Within these broad categories, various specialties had emerged. These physicians generally avoided active participation in politics and confined their research to medical matters.

The financial success of American doctors of today was not enjoyed by these former practitioners. On the contrary, the latter experienced hard times, as the following letter from a local doctor, published in the St. Louis *Missouri Republican* of February 3, 1878, indicated:

> For a series of years the medical profession has been distressed by a variety of causes. The financial troubles of the country, the almost absolute suspension of all kinds of business, the withdrawal of money from circulation, etc., have affected the community at large and the physicians especially. For the want of means diminishes the number of patients. Chronic cases are forced to temporize . . . It is almost impossible to estimate the reduction of professional income. Some of our friends say it is more than 50 per cent. It is thus seen that the profession has had a very sickly time of it.
>
> Very naturally, a general dissatisfaction prevails in our ranks and in vain many look round for effectual relief. Some think legislation should interfere in our behalf, and some of the states have actually tried the experiment, Missouri included. Let us see what legislation can do for the medical profession. It cannot give the money to the needy to employ physicians. It cannot infuse the confidence in professional aid into the public mind when it is entirely wanting or shaken. It cannot prevent quacks from advertising their nostrums and from attracting the credulous by fraudulent promises. It cannot prohibit the stupendous sale of patent medicine. Nor can legislation change the superstitious belief of people in miracles and supernatural aid in their distress. It cannot deter people from applying to druggists for so-called "simple remedies," and the latter from carrying on lively doctoring business. It cannot interfere with the nefarious employment of "wise old women," to torment their neighbors with all sorts of trash and taking their money for it. In fine, legislation cannot give sense where there is none, and prevent people from being their own doctors.[137]

The allopathic or regular physicians were challenged also by the practitioners of various sectarian systems. Homeopathy, which had made its appearance in the St. Louis market place in the early 1840s, had grown into a serious rival of the established system. There were twenty, possibly more, homeopathic physicians practicing in St. Louis in 1879. The new system of therapeutics had its own medical college at Tenth and Carr streets and published two medical journals. The Good Samaritan Hospital was staffed by doctors of the homeopathic system.[138] Since homeopathy had originated in their homeland, it had a special appeal and strong support among the large German population of St. Louis.[139]

The Eclectic system of medical treatment had many patrons in St. Louis. The eleventh annual meeting of the National Eclectic Medical Association was held in St. Louis in the middle of June 1881. From 350 to 500 physicians were expected to attend. The Eclectics had two medical colleges in St. Louis.[140]

Women, who had gained entrance into the nursing profession during the Civil War, were knocking at the doors of the medical schools. But at first they got a cold reception. The official position of the male members of the profession on the issue was stated by Dr. L. Ch. Boisliniere in his commencement address delivered at the St. Louis Medical College on March 7, 1883 and reported in the St. Louis *Missouri Republican* the following day:[141]

> A great portion of his address was devoted to the discussion of the question as to whether women were adaptable to the medical profession, and his conclusion was most positive that they are not, and that they should stay out of it. The character of the doctor's views is best illustrated by his declaration that ladies should not attempt to become mathematicians, mental philosophers or psychologists, that the muses never found husbands, and of necessity remained single, and that genius and motherhood were simply incompatible. Women could properly become pharmacists, dry goods clerks, telegraph operators and barbers, but they should let physic alone, except when prescribed by a male physician.

There were no women among the thirty-nine graduates.[142]

Most of the pioneer women doctors in St. Louis entered the profession with degrees from homeopathic or Eclectic colleges. Of the twenty St. Louis physicians who attended the May 1879 convention of the Missouri Institute of Homeopathy, four were women.[143]

The philanthropic element was strong in the medical profession. Many doctors served without pay on the staffs of city hospital and of denomination-connected hospitals of the city. Some kept no account books but depended upon their patients to pay something if they were able.[144] The doctors made house calls, delivered babies and performed minor operations in the homes.

6. Proliferation of St. Louis's Hospitals

Following the close of the Civil War, the network of hospitals, which had made St. Louis one of the leading medical centers of the country, was dismantled. The Jefferson Barracks Hospital, with a capacity of 2,500 patients, was converted to its former role as a United States Army training center. The Benton Barracks Hospital, of similar size, was closed and the land restored to its owner Colonel John O'Fallon. A number of smaller military hospitals, which had been conducted in hotels, office buildings and residences, ceased their operations. St. Louis's civilian hospitals, which at times had been requisitioned for military use, were released to serve their normal constituencies. The service they were able to provide was not of the highest quality, at least by modern standards.

The key institution in St. Louis's civilian hospital system was the city hospital. This had been completed in 1855 and rebuilt the next year following a destructive fire.[145] The hospital building had many defects and shortcomings. It was too small and was usually overcrowded with patients. The temperature control and ventilation were poor. The lavatories and toilets were located at some distance from the patients' quarters, making access difficult.[146] Recreational facilities for convalescents were lacking.

The nonrestrictive admission policy of the hospital kept its rooms filled with a wide range of charitable cases, many of which could have been taken care of in a workhouse, insane asylum or at the county farm.[147]

The hospital was administered by the resident physician, who was responsible for business affairs as well as for medical and surgical services. He was aided by a small staff of assistants, usually recent graduates of local medical schools. With a patient load of more than 300 cases, it was impossible for the resident physician to give adequate personal care to each case.[148]

A controversial reorganization of the staff at the hospital was effected in 1874. Upon the resignation of Dr. T. F. Prewitt, the two medical members of the board of health were able to block the appointment of a successor.[149] The duties of the resident physician were then divided. The position of warden was created to handle administration, including discipline, cleanliness, supplies and food service. The provision of medical and surgical services was assigned to a board of visiting physicians, working without pay. The routine twenty-four hour a day medical care was performed by two classes of assistants, the more experienced group of which was compensated. This system, according to its proponents, was in successful use in public hospitals in large Eastern cities.[150] The plan, which had been put into operation in St. Louis by a divided board of health, was criticized in the press and also in medical circles.[151] It came to an end when the board, on January 15, 1875, appointed Dr. George Homan as acting resident physician at city hospital.[152]

To remedy the serious overcrowding at city hospital, the council, at its meeting of July 5, 1872, voted to build a new hospital on the site of the existing one. An appropriation of $25,000 was made for the construction of the first wing.[153] This was ready for occupancy about a year and a half later.

The architectural plan of the new hospital was regarded as unsatisfactory by Dr. Louis Bauer, a leading physician. He cited the experience in French, English and German hospitals where the death rates were frightfully high due to overcrowding and post-operative infections. Instead of building a large multistory hospital in a crowded section of the city, Dr. Bauer proposed the development of a pavilion type of institution. This style of construction consisted of one-story frame buildings, with plenty of intervening space.[154] It had been used successfully during the Civil War at the army hospitals at Jefferson Barracks and Benton Barracks.

At the time of the 1849-1850 cholera epidemic, the city established a permanent hospital on Arsenal Island to house the sick passengers taken from vessels which had been stopped for inspection. In 1854, the quarantine station had been moved to a fifty-eight acre site on the western bank of the Mississippi River, about a mile and a quarter south of Jefferson Barracks. In 1867, four large buildings on Arsenal Island were transferred to quarantine and a first-class hospital was established there. The Quarantine Hospital was used to house the overflow from city hospital, particularly convalescent cases, also feeble-minded and insane patients.[155] The Smallpox Hospital was located several hundred yards west of the Quarantine Hospital. Although at times attendance there was low, the institution was kept in constant readiness for possible outbreaks of the disease.[156]

In 1875, the Social Evil Hospital was transformed into a general hospital for women. With this added space, it was possible for the board of health to close the Quarantine Hospital. The distance of this hospital from the city posed difficult problems of supervision and of supply. It was opened again, however, on an emergency basis during the yellow fever epidemic.

In addition to these hospitals, the board of health operated a dispensary, where free medical service was available to the poor. Patients seeking admission to city hospital had to report to the dispensary, where they were given a preliminary examination by the physician in charge. On the basis of this examination, the physician could himself treat the patient and provide him with medicine and medical advice. For serious cases he rendered first aid and then sent the patient by ambulance to city hospital along with a permit which would gain him admission.[157]

For the week ending March 31, 1876, the St. Louis municipal hospitals reported the following attendance: city hospital, 379 patients; Female Hospital, 140; Smallpox Hospital, 9. The dispensary physician for the week reported 140 new cases and 165 old cases treated.[158]

A study conducted by the board of health in late February 1873 revealed that approximately one half of the patients treated in St. Louis's public hospitals were not legally entitled to the services provided them. St. Louis incurred an expense of $60,000 annually to provide medical care for the rest of the state. The city council presented a memorial to the general assembly asking for the establishment of a general hospital, with 1,000 beds, to be jointly financed and operated by St. Louis and the state.[159] The petition was not granted.

Although St. Louis got no immediate help from the state in handling its patient load, a number of private hospitals were organized to assume part of the burden. These were founded generally by local religious denominations, particularly those having a diocesan form of organization. As these religious associations increased in membership and financial resources, they were able to reach out to the community in implementing the requirements of the social gospel.

In July 1874, the Sisters' Hospital moved from its three-story brick building at Fourth and Spruce streets into a new home on Montgomery Street near Grand Avenue. The main structure with its east and west wings, was four-stories high and of red brick with white facings. The area for patients was divided into wards as well as private rooms. The hospital was designed to be self-sustaining, though it accepted a high proportion of charity patients. A chapel formed an essential part of the whole medical complex. The normal capacity of the hospital was 300 patients. Because of its almost fifty years of service and its excellent staff and accommodations, it was the most popular of the church-related hospitals.[160]

The Good Samaritan Hospital, on Jefferson Avenue at the head of O'Fallon Street, which had been rented in the early part of the Civil War by the Union army, was restored to its owners in 1863. The hospital was a four-story brick structure with a usable attic. It contained forty rooms and had a capacity of 120 patients. At times during the war, 250 soldiers were hospitalized there. The hospital was served by a staff of homeopathic physicians consisting of Doctors E. Kellerer, William Tod. Helmuth, T. G. Comstock and George S. Walker. The hospital originated largely through the efforts of the Reverend Louis E. Nollau of the Evangelical church. It was open, however, to persons of all religious faiths and members of all races. The recovery of the hospital to a condition of maximum usage was slow. In August 1871, only twenty-five patients were in its care.[161]

St. Luke's Hospital began operations in April 1866, under the auspices of the Episcopal Church in St. Louis. Its first building was on a lot between Ohio and Sumner streets. In March 1870, the hospital was moved to the corner of Sixth and Elm streets; three years later, it was relocated on Pine Street, between Ninth and Tenth streets. On June 26, 1881, the cornerstone of a new home for the hospital was laid at the corner of Washington Avenue and Nineteenth Street. The land had been donated by Henry Shaw. Nursing service was provided by the Sisterhood of the Good Shepherd. Doctors J. A. Pottinger, Charles A. Todd, M. A. Pallen, Louis Bauer and John T. Hodgen served as visiting physicians, without compensation. Regularly scheduled religious services were conducted at the hospital. In line with the practice at the Sisters' Hospital, no cases of contagious diseases were accepted.[162] Persons with such diseases were treated at the municipal hospitals or in their homes by private physicians, under strict quarantine regulations.

The Alexian Brothers, an order devoted to the care of the sick and insane, in 1873 constructed at the corner of Carondelet Avenue and Osage Street a new hospital, which they named in honor of St. Joseph. The edifice was of three stories, with a front of 241 feet and two wings. It had a capacity of 200 patients. Adjoining the hospital was a church with seating for 300 persons.[163]

The Sisters of Mercy, an Irish order, conducted St. John's Hospital, located at the corner of Twenty-third and Morgan streets. It conformed to the basic design of a main building and two wings. An infirmary for black women and girls was maintained. The medical and surgical departments of St. John's Hospital were controlled by the faculty of the Missouri Medical College.[164]

In 1872, six members of the order of Sisters of Mary came to St. Louis and established themselves in quarters opposite St. Mary's Church at Third and Mulberry streets. Smallpox was raging in the city, and these sisters tended victims of the malady, day and night, for several months. One year after their arrival, they built a three-story home for their order on the property of St. Mary's Church. During the yellow fever epidemic in Memphis in 1878, thirteen of the Sisters went there to nurse the sick; only eight returned, the others having fallen victim to the disease. The Sisters in 1877 purchased the Felix Coste residence at Sixteenth and Papin streets, where they continued the operation of their hospital.[165]

The Sisters of Mary differed in several ways from other nursing associations: (1) the rules of their order forbade them to exact any charge for their services; (2) they were not confined to their own hospital but went wherever there was a pressing need for their ministrations; (3) they were willing to attend victims of the most dangerous and contagious diseases.[166]

In addition to the city dispensary, the medical colleges and also the private hospitals operated dispensaries which, on an outpatient basis, provided free advice, treatment and medicine for indigent patients.

7. *Post-war Recovery of St. Louis's Medical Schools*

St. Louis's medical colleges during the Civil War had struggled to stay alive. The demand for doctors, both in the civilian and military society, was an encouragement to continue this type of training. Although the building of the Missouri Medical College had been taken over by the Union authorities and converted into a military prison, a skeleton staff continued to operate the college for a while.[167] Dr. Joseph N. McDowell returned to St. Louis from the South in 1866 and reorganized the college. His building had suffered damage during the occupation by the military, and the valuable physiological and pathological exhibits had been destroyed. The college in 1868 moved to a location at Sixth and Elm streets. Several years later, it transferred to a new building at the corner of Twenty-third Street and Lucas Avenue, in close proximity to the Sisters of Mercy Hospital for which the college faculty provided medical and surgical services.[168]

St. Louis Medical College suffered no interruption during the war and quickly returned to normal operations with the restoration of peace. It conferred diplomas on forty-six graduates in March 1868. [169] The Missouri Homeopathic Medical College closed during the conflict but reopened in the fall of 1866. Twenty-one doctors were graduated in 1868.[170]

New medical colleges appeared in an already crowded field. The St. Louis College of Physicians and Surgeons began operations in 1869, with a strong faculty which included the following members: Louis Bauer, M.D., professor of surgery and president of the college; Montrose A. Pallen, M.D., professor of gynecology; Augustus F. Barnes, M.D., professor of obstetrics; T. F. Prewitt, M.D., professor of surgical anatomy and diseases of the skin; J. K. Bauduy, M.D., professor of diseases of the mind and nervous system; John Green, M.D., professor of ophthalmology; G. Baumgarten, M.D., professor of general pathology and pathological anatomy; G. W. Steedman, M.D., professor of clinical surgery and diseases of the genito-urinary organs; Warren B. Outten, M.D., professor of descriptive anatomy; A. J. Steele, M.D., professor of military and minor surgery, fractures and dis-

locations; J. M. Leete, M.D., professor of physical diagnosis and diseases of the chest; J. M. Scott, M.D., professor of practice of medicine; Charles E. Briggs, M.D., professor of physiology; William L. Barrett, M.D., professor of diseases of children; James F. Johnson, M.D., professor of materia medica and toxicology; F. H. McArdle, M.D., professor of chemistry; William T. Mason, LL.D., professor of medical jurisprudence.[171]

Two students received their diplomas at the first commencement exercises at the college in March 1870. In view of the small student enrollment during the beginning year, it is likely that not all of the announced professors actually conducted classes. However, the publication of the names and specialties provides evidence of the extent to which medical practice had become diversified. Twenty-five years previously, three or four professors handled the entire medical curriculum.

In the spring of 1872, the Humboldt Medical College was organized. This, like the St. Louis College of Physicians and Surgeons, taught in the regular or allopathic tradition. The leading spirit behind the founding of the new school was Dr. Adam Hammer, who was born in Germany and educated in famous universities there. He was a brilliant physician and surgeon, but of a contentious nature that kept him at odds with many of his colleagues. Hammer held the chair of surgery and also served as dean of the college. Lectures were held in a building in close proximity to city hospital.[172]

St. Louis had two Eclectic medical institutions. Of these American Medical College was the most successful. It was a joint stock company with capital of $50,000. It held its eleventh regular commencement, February 27, 1879, when thirty-five graduates received their diplomas.[173] The progress of St. Louis Eclectic Medical College was hampered by a protracted controversy with the St. Louis Board of Health over accreditation.

The Jefferson College of Medicine and Dentistry, which started issuing diplomas before acquiring a faculty and classroom facilities, was exposed by a reporter of the St. Louis *Missouri Republican* as a diploma mill.[174]

Missouri Medical College and St. Louis Medical College enjoyed marked success in the years following the Civil War. Missouri Medical College graduated its largest class in 1879 when eighty-two doctors received their diplomas.[175] St. Louis Medical College conferred fifty degrees in 1877.[176]

Dr. Herman Tuholske, in his commencement address at the Missouri Medical College on March 2, 1877, mingled with his warm congratulations to the graduates a few grim words of warning. The St. Louis *Missouri Republican* of March 3, 1877 thus summarized his speech:[177]

> The graduates were welcomed as brothers to the profession — a profession already overcrowded as a natural result of the increase in educational facilities and the consequent greater number who have deserted the trades and sought a livelihood in professional life. The new-made physicians were reminded that in a profession so crowded the laws of natural selection would prevail and only the fittest would survive.

The issue of survival also confronted the medical schools, particularly the weaker ones. Success of the various schools depended on the access of the faculty and students to the lectures and bedside observations at city hospital. Although there were a number of small denomination-related hospitals in St. Louis, these were basically nursing homes for the elderly. They generally accepted no cases of contagious disease. Consequently, the opportunity to observe pathology there was limited. City hospital was the only institution in St. Louis where a wide range of diseases could be studied.

In 1874, following the failure of the board of health to appoint a resident physician, the wards and patients in city hospital were assigned to the faculty and students of the Missouri Medical College and the St. Louis Medical College.[178] Internships at city hospital were limited to graduates of these two colleges. The two medical members of the board of health were usually graduates of these two local institutions.

The faculties of the Eclectic and homeopathic colleges waged an unceasing battle to gain admission to the clinical opportunities available at city hospital. Their failure in many instances arose from the fact that their faculty members were not qualified physicians according to state and St. Louis legislation.

The basic state legislation consisted of the acts of March 27, 1874 and April 28, 1877, which specified that no person could practice medicine or surgery in Missouri without a diploma from some duly established medical school. But a provision of the 1874 law allowed a doctor who lacked a diploma, but had begun to practice before September 1, 1874, to register his name with the county clerk and continue to practice.[179]

St. Louis, under the provisions of the 1877 constitution known as the "Scheme and Charter," was given express authority to regulate various professions and avocations, including physicians. Under this grant, the St. Louis City Council, on October 20, 1877 enacted Ordinance 10,386, which placed restrictions on the practice of medicine. Every person who should thereafter engage in the practice of medicine or surgery in St. Louis was required to file a copy of his diploma in the office of the health commissioner, at which time he would be registered on the roll of accredited practitioners. The commissioner was authorized to refuse to register any doctor whose diploma was fraudulently obtained or which had been issued by a reputed diploma mill.[180]

The board of health regularly turned down requests from Dr. Field of the St. Louis Eclectic Medical College to recognize his college and permit its students to enjoy the clinical opportunities at city hospital. The basis of the board's refusal was that the college was not staffed by registered physicians. A petition from the Homeopathic Medical College of Missouri, asking that a ward in city hospital be set aside for patients preferring care under homeopathic doctors and student assistants, was rejected.[181] But the homeopaths won a partial victory when Judge Horatio M. Jones of Circuit Court No. 5 ordered the board of health to admit faculty and students of the Homeopathic Medical College to visit city hospital for clinical study.[182]

The board of health suffered another defeat when Judge Elmer B. Adams of Circuit Court No. 1 ordered Commissioner Francis to register Dr. Raband who, though lacking a diploma, had practiced in St. Louis for the previous twelve years and had registered his name on July 23, 1874 in the office of the county clerk, under the provisions of the general assembly's act of March 27, 1874.[183] At its meeting of November 22, 1880, the board informed Dr. John Stolz, who had a diploma from the Eclectic Medical College in Philadelphia, a suspected diploma mill, that he could practice in Missouri under state law, but under the St. Louis ordinance No. 10,386 could not be enrolled among the city's physicians.[184]

On November 27, 1880. Commissioner Francis, in order to settle the controversy over which colleges would enjoy the clinical benefits of city hospital announced a visitation schedule for the faculty and students of all seven local medical colleges.[185] The board, in late September 1881, assigned lecturing privileges at city hospital to professors of St. Louis Medical College, Missouri Medical College and American Medical College, but not to the St. Louis Eclectic Medical College or the two homeopathic colleges.[186]

8. *State and Local Cooperation in the Care of the Insane*

The State Lunatic Asylum at Fulton, which had begun operations in 1851, was one of the casualties of the Civil War. In the spring of 1861, the legislature diverted the state asylum tax to military use. Payments by private patients and by the counties for the support of their people were insufficient to cover the hospital's expenses. In September 1861, the institution suspended operations and sent the patients back to their home counties, to be housed in jails, prisons and outhouses. Rebel raiding parties plundered the building of bedding, clothing and other furnishings. Further damage was done by the quartering of a Union cavalry detachment on the asylum grounds.[187]

The asylum reopened in late 1863, following the appropriation by the legislature of $10,000 for repairs and refurnishing.[188] The institution was designed for 100 persons. With no major increase in capacity, it was accommodating 500 inmates by December 1868. Dr. Charles H. Hughes, who succeeded Dr. Smith, was superintendent and physician from 1866 to 1872. Dr. Hughes graduated from the St. Louis Medical College in 1859. He served as surgeon in charge of a number of Union hospitals and camps during the Civil War.[189] Under his administration, water reservoirs, gas works and a sewerage system were installed.[190]

The increase of the patient population from 100 to 500 reduced the services the institution was able to provide. Previously, the superintendent had conducted the institution as a comfortable home, in which he could give each patient individual attention. Involvement in the housekeeping operations and on the hospital's farm had made employment available to most of those able to work.

Legislation enacted by the general assembly in 1870 gave the probate court concurrent jurisdiction with the county court in conducting sanity inquiries. The law also gave the county court the authority to appoint a guardian for any person found by a jury to be so addicted to drunkenness as to be incapable of managing his affairs.[191]

On March 28, 1872, the legislature appropriated $200,000 for the construction of a second insane asylum, to be located in either the northwestern or southwestern part of the state. The factors determining the exact location were thus described:[192]

No location containing less than 120 acres of land shall be considered, and in determining upon a proper location, said commissioners shall have special regard to the following matters: first, salubrity of location, cheapness and excellence of building material, and convenience of access from different parts of the state; second, an abundant supply of pure water, and cost of land for the institution.

The commissioners chose a site near St. Joseph. Construction was started shortly, and the hospital was ready to open in 1874. The architectural design of the St. Joseph hospital was similar to that of the Fulton institution, with a three-story central or headquarters building, to which wings were attached at each end. As the need for more space grew, new units could be added. The building, designed originally for 200 patients, was constructed at a cost of $250,000.[193] This figure was close to the national average of cost for mental institutions of similar capacity. The plan was to build a mental institution in each of the four quarters of the state.

Caring for the insane was a particularly serious problem for St. Louis. As the gateway to the West, and as the only city in Missouri operating a system of hospitals, St. Louis acted as a magnet, attracting thousands of physically and mentally sick persons, many of which were abandoned in cheap boarding houses or on the streets. State law made the county responsible for the care of insane persons within its limits. But St. Louis County, by means of stringent residence requirements, was able for a long while to defeat efforts to get it to assume responsibility.[194]

While the number was small, St. Louis sent insane persons found wandering in its streets to the Sisters of Charity Hospital or to the St. Vincent Insane Asylum, to be treated at city expense. But as the number increased, the board of health for reasons of economy began sending them to the city hospital, to the Quarantine Hospital and to the workhouse. These institutions provided little more than food, a bed and a minimum of general medical care.

On December 1, 1864, the cornerstone was laid for the St. Louis County Lunatic Asylum, at a site on the county farm in southwest St. Louis.[195] Four years later, the building was completed at a cost of $900,000, more than three times that of state mental institutions of comparable capacity.[196] The structure was impressive and unique architec-

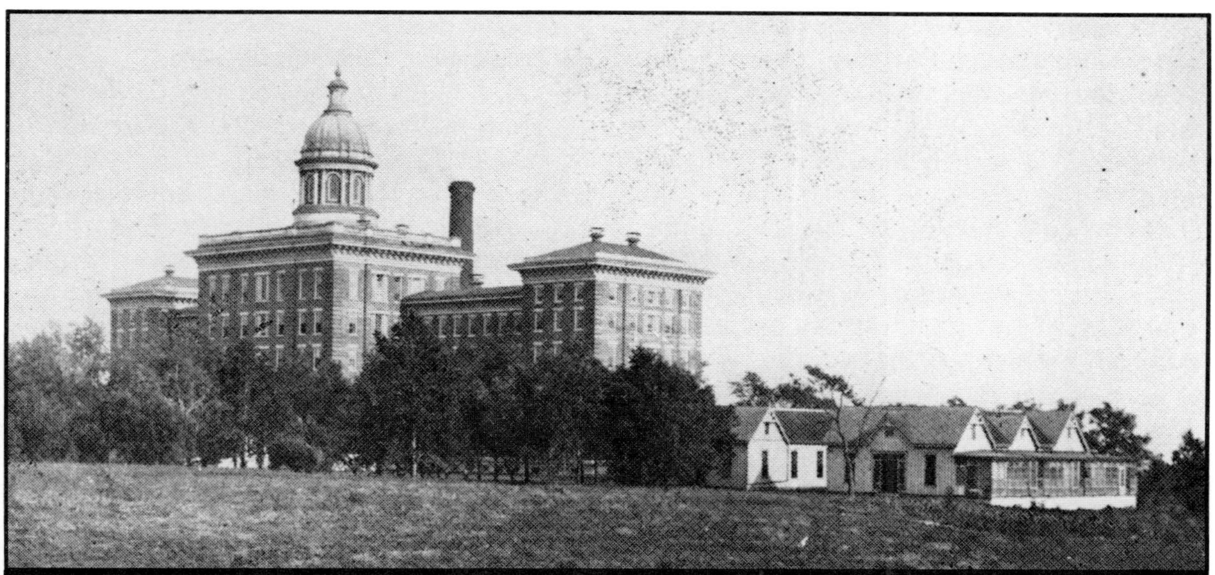

St. Louis mental hospital. Courtesy of the State Historical Society of Missouri.

turally, but poorly designed for a mental institution.

The main building, in which the administrative offices and service quarters were located, was five stories high. At each end of this central building was a four-story wing; adjoining each wing was a five-story structure. The wards for patients were in these five-story extensions.[197]

Since there were no elevators, hospital attendants spent much of their time and energy climbing stairs. The small rooms, eight by twelve feet, in each of which two persons lived, were difficult to cool in summer and heat properly in winter. The heating registers were located in the halls, not the individual rooms.[198]

In April 1870, 128 patients, comprising the entire group supported by the county at the Fulton mental institution, were transferred to the new St. Louis County Asylum.[199] Since the St. Louis asylum was caring for patients who otherwise would have gone to a state institution, the legislature in 1872 voted an annual appropriation of $15,000 for its support.[200]

A critical issue in mental hospital administration was the type of restraint to be used to keep patients quiet and to prevent their hurting themselves or others. A distressing incident involving this issue occurred on the night of August 14, 1875 at the county asylum, when four persons, three women and a man, died from apparent overdoses of a sedative mixture consisting of conium (hemlock), morphine and atropine (belladonna).[201]

At the inquiry held in connection with the death of the male patient, William Rocheford, William Dalton testified that on that occasion he was the night watchman or nurse in the hospital ward involved. Making his rounds through the darkened hospital with his lantern and bottle of conium mixture, his task was to administer the sedative to patients who were creating a disturbance by boisterous conduct. Since the hospital had acquired a new shipment of conium of stronger quality than that customarily used, the resident physician, Dr. N. DeVere Howard, instructed Dalton not to administer doses of the new mixture larger than one teaspoonful. But Dr. Howard failed to set a limit on the number of doses to be given during the night.[202]

Dalton gave Rocheford a teaspoonful at 12 P.M., another at 1:30 A.M.; then, contrary to order, two teaspoonfuls between 3:15 and 3:30 A.M. About 4:30 A.M. Rocheford went into convulsions and died.[203]

Shortly after this incident which shocked the city and raised concern regarding the conduct of the asylum, the Reverend W. G. Eliot and James E. Yeatman, former chairman of the Western Sanitary Commission, visited the institution and made a thorough investigation. Eliot publicized their observations and conclusions in a long letter in the St. Louis *Missouri Republican* of September 28, 1875.[204]

He reported that the asylum was kept in a clean and orderly condition, the patients were treated kindly, the food was of adequate quality and plentiful, and the patients enjoyed good physical health.[205]

Despite these favorable points, Eliot felt obliged to give the asylum an inferior overall rating. It was badly overcrowded. The atmosphere was depressing, with the patients spending their days sitting or walking in the halls. There was no planned entertainment or amusement, aside from an occasional dance. Lacking were books and magazines, outdoor exercise and religious services. There was no infirmary or hospital room in which to segregate sick patients. The compensation of the resident physician and his staff was low, making it impossible to get and keep professionally trained people. The treatment program relied upon dangerous sedatives, administered under conditions which made mistakes unavoidable.[206]

Eliot closed his critique with his concept of an ideal mental institution:[207]

Those who have studied the intricate subject of mental therapeutics, will not need to be told that moral, spiritual and aesthetic influences are those upon which the successful physician of the insane must chiefly rely. Give patients something to think about, something to do, in a word, treat them from beginning to end, just as you would treat other people, as far as you possibly can — appealing to common motives, awakening them to common interests, and thus, by bringing up the healthy side of their minds — if we may so speak — gradually giving a healthy tone to the whole. This, if any, is the road to their recovery, and, where care is hopeless, to their attainment of cheerfulness and peace. But all such methods imply the existence of agencies and opportunities very different from those now used, and unfortunately the best methods are not the easiest and not always the cheapest.

The only institution in the state which resembled Eliot's ideal hospital was the St. Vincent Insane Asylum, operated by the Sisters of Charity. The asylum occupied the building at the corner of Marion and Decatur streets, which previously housed the Convent of the Visitation. The clientele was mostly from the professional and business classes, not only of St. Louis but of Missouri and a number of Southern states. In July 1870, there were 149 inmates, of which twenty-eight were charity patients. Although operated by a Catholic order, members of all religious faiths were received.[208]

The asylum covered almost a whole city block. The edifice consisted of a central building and two wings. Shade trees and flower beds adorned the hospital grounds, through which the patients could stroll for exercise and enjoyment of nature. Occasional all-day outings were conducted to the farm the Sisters owned five or six miles out of the city.[209]

The walls of the hospital were decorated with paintings, and at the end of each ward was a display of flowers. Each floor had its separate dining room, where the patients and attendants could enjoy social relationships. To satisfy a variety of interests, the hospital had a library, billiard tables, an amusement room and a music conservatory.[210]

A major factor in the success of St. Vincent's was its nursing staff, the Sisters of Charity. Although not trained to meet today's standards, they were kind, dedicated and experienced practical nurses. In St. Louis's public institutions, the nurses were hospital attendants on the level with cooks, janitors and yard workers. They had not yet begun the climb to professional status. The treatment program at St. Vincent's was supervised by Dr. J. K. Bauduy, the leading psychiatrist in the city.[211]

In accordance with the terms of St. Louis's "Scheme and Charter," the municipal board of health, on April 21, 1877, took formal possession of the insane asylum and poorhouse, previously operated by the county. [212] Within a year the asylum, in the construction of which space for patients had been sacrificed to architectural pretentiousness, was badly overcrowded. In the section designed for 100 women, 183 female patients were being accommodated in June 1878.[213] To take care of the overflow, the upper stories of the nearby poorhouse were taken over for the insane. For the future, Commissioner Francis recommended the erection of several detached buildings, according to the "cottage plan." These were cheaper to build than large, multi-story structures and had advantages from the standpoint of light, ventilation, cleanliness and freedom from hospital infections.[214] The commissioner's suggestions were eventually carried out.

9. Medical Societies

Following the Civil War, the St. Louis Medical Society resumed its operations. An important feature of the meetings was the reading and discussion of papers on timely medical subjects. At the session of March 8, 1873, Dr. Edward Montgomery presented a paper on cerebro-spinal meningitis, a disease which was epidemic at the time. A discussion followed concerning the cause of the disease, in which barometric pressure, electrical conditions of the atmosphere and malarious influences were suggested as possible agents. The germ theory was not mentioned. Dr. T. F. Prewitt, resident physician at city hospital, explained the treatment he used, which comprised cupping, mercurial purgatives and quinine.[215] These were the old triad of medical remedies.

Internal squabbles occupied much of the time of the society. In November 1871, Dr. John T. Hodgen charged that Dr. Louis Bauer had attempted to solicit one of his patients. The charge was not sustained upon inquiry by the society.[216] Dr. Adam Hammer was expelled from the society because he had written a letter to the board of health alleging that a fellow member, Dr. A. P. Lankford, was an incompetent teacher and surgeon. The circuit court rescinded the expulsion, whereupon four members of the society resigned in protest. In both cases, the doctors charged were German-Americans, perhaps reflecting rivalry and hostility between Anglo-

Americans and German-American practitioners.[217]

The Missouri State Medical Association was reorganized at a meeting in St. Louis on December 10, 1867.[218] As a means of publicizing its activities and extending its membership, the association established the custom of meeting in different towns and cities throughout the state. In April 1871, the association appointed a committee of five members to promote the organization of county medical societies, affiliated with the state society.[219] This drive was quite successful. It was at this time that the Boone County Medical Society and also a district society in Central MIssouri were organized.[220] These local societies drew up constitutions and rules regarding ethical behavior of their members.

The American Medical Association began its annual meeting in St. Louis, May 6, 1873. Dr. Thomas M. Logan of Sacramento, California, in his presidential address dwelt on two subjects of great interest — the improvement of medical education and the establishment of a national system of health administration. Regarding the latter subject he declared:[221]

> The subject of public hygiene, or state medicine, is worthy of a more authorative recognition than has yet been awarded it, and should hold a place in their estimation upon the highest plane in medical education. Legislators are now turning their attention to the framing of laws bearing upon questions connected with medicine and boards of health for states and municipalities are rapidly multiplying everywhere. What seems to be, therefore, required in the premises is to effect a union of views as to the method of action, so as to bring every state into immediate communication by means of state boards of health, with a central office in Washington, to be presided over by a commissioner or secretary of public health, to be elected every four years or oftener by the association [American Medical Association], subject to the approval of the president of the United States and who shall have power to make all necessary subappointments.

10. Missouri State Board of Health

The State Medical Association at its annual meeting in 1880 petitioned the legislature to establish a state board of health.[222] Illinois already had taken this step. The Illinois Board of Health took a leading role in erecting quarantine stations along the Mississippi River to halt the yellow fever epidemic in 1879. In this action, the Illinois board cooperated with the St. Louis Board of Health and Health Commissioner, since there was no Missouri board of health.[223]

The delay in establishing a board of health was related to the chaotic situation in Missouri regarding medical practice. Originally there had been no control over the practice of medicine in the state. Legislation passed on February 16, 1847, conferred the status of physician on everyone who practiced medicine for a livelihood and paid a small license fee. In 1874 and 1877, laws were passed authorizing any person to practice if he had a diploma, even one from a bogus medical school.[224]

Under these permissive conditions, a wide variety of groups became part of the state medical profession. The largest consisted of the regular or allopathic physicians. They developed a strong organization in St. Louis and in 1850 perfected a state association.[225] They operated the Missouri Medical College and the St. Louis Medical College. These institutions graduated many of the doctors practicing in Missouri. The medical members of the St. Louis Board of Health, the doctors and interns at the municipal hospitals, and most of the doctors serving at the private hospitals in St. Louis belonged to the allopathic school.

Despite their dominant position, they did not command the full confidence of the public. Their diagnoses were largely guesswork, and their remedies the old stand-bys of calomel and quinine, and to some extent bleeding and blistering.

In reaction to the "heroic" remedies of the regular doctors, various reform schools had arisen. The most influential was homeopathy. Although its basic thesis that the doctor should prescribe medicines that duplicate the symptoms of the disease was probably mistaken, its emphasis on small doses was a step forward.

Occupying a position between the homeopaths and the regulars were the Eclectics. They, like the homeopaths, banned mercury, antimony, bleeding and blistering. They sought the best remedies from all sources, with a preference for vegetable products.[226]

The rural areas were served by doctors, many with only slight training. Often neighbors assisted each other in cases of sickness and childbirth.

The setting up of a board of health would be a move toward establishing a state-approved type and quality of medical practice.

This would curb folk medicine and reform movements such as homeopathy and Eclecticism. It would tend to limit the opportunity of persons to enter the medical profession and consequently make it an elitist calling.

The Eclectic Medical Society of Missouri, at its meeting in St. Louis, June 7-8, 1882, passed the following resolutions opposing a board of health that would be dominated by the allopathic practitioners:[227]

Resolved that we will protest against and oppose by all justifiable means any legislation that fails to guarantee equal rights to all legally qualified medical practitioners regardless of ethical considerations originating in differences which may exist in their medical theories or practice.

Resolved that believing such protection can only be thus assured we will insist upon definite provision by statute for the representation in equitable proportion of each branch of the medical profession in all executive, administrative or examining boards or offices which may be created by future enactment.

The general assembly, in an act of March 29, 1883, established the State Board of Health of Missouri, consisting of seven persons appointed by the governor, with the consent of the senate. They would serve terms of seven years. At least five members of the board were required to be "physicians in good standing, and of recognized professional and scientific knowledge, and graduates of reputable medical schools." The law provided that in appointments to the board "there shall be no discrimination made against the different systems of medicine that are recognized as reputable by the laws of this state."[228] The different systems from which members could be selected were not named, and no quota system for members was set up.

The board was given general supervision over the health and sanitary concerns of the people of the state. An important responsibility was to determine when any contagious disease existed in any part of Missouri or the United states to such an extent as to endanger the lives of citizens of Missouri. The board was authorized to establish and enforce quarantine regulations against such a city or district, using state and local officials to make the ban effective.[229]

Supervision of the registration of births and deaths was conferred on the board. The organization's secretary was made superintendent of this registration.[230]

The law made it mandatory that all physicians register their names with the clerk of the county where they resided. The practitioners were instructed to report to the county clerk all births and deaths occurring among their patients.[231]

An additional concern of the board was to investigate any fatal diseases prevalent among the domestic animals of the state and to publish the results of their inquiry.[232]

The board was required to meet in January and July of each year, with the January meeting to be held in Jefferson City. The only salaried official was the secretary. The members received reimbursement for travel and other expenses. The board was expected to issue an annual report giving health information and recommendations for legislative action.[233]

Following the establishment of the State Board of Health, the legislature, on April 2, 1883, enacted a law regulating the practice of medicine and surgery. The law provided two methods by which a person could obtain certification to practice in Missouri. The first was by presenting his diploma before the board, proving that it was genuine and that he was the rightful owner. The second method was by appearing before a meeting of the board and undergoing an examination covering his knowledge of medical science.[234]

The board was obligated to issue certificates "to all who shall furnish satisfactory proof of having received diplomas or licenses from legally chartered medical institutions in good standing" and also to those who successfully passed the board's examination.[235]

Every person holding a certificate signed by the board was required to have it recorded in the office of the county clerk of the district where he resided. The board was given discretion to refuse certificates to individuals guilty of unprofessional or dishonorable conduct and to revoke certificates for the same causes.[236]

A grandfather clause provided that the requirements of the law did not apply to persons who had been practicing medicine in Missouri for five years.[237]

Chapter V

Progress in Public Health Administration, 1866-1883

1   Max A. Goldstein, ed., *One Hundred Years of Medicine and Surgery in Missouri* (St. Louis, St. Louis Star, 1900), p. 155.

2   The political board of health in office during the 1866 cholera epidemic did not reveal to the press the extent of the city's losses. St. Louis *Missouri Republican,* Aug. 20, 1866, p. 3:6.

3   St. Louis *Missouri Republican,* Mar. 10, 1868, p. 2:5.

4   *Ibid.,* Aug. 13, 1866, p. 3:4. One hundred seventy-five noncommissioned officers and privates of the 56th U.S.C. Infantry, who died of cholera in 1866, were buried in the Quarantine Station Hospital cemetery. *Ibid.,* Aug. 3, 1878, p. 5:3-4.

5   Charles E. Rosenberg, *The Cholera Years* (Chicago, The University of Chicago Press, 1962) p. 193.

6   "Regular" is commonly interpreted to mean "allopathic."

7   *Laws of the State of Missouri, Passed at the First Session of the Twenty-fourth General Assembly, 1867,* (Jefferson City, Emory S. Foster, Public Printer, 1867), p. 180.

8   *Ibid.,* pp. 180-183.

9   *Ibid.,* pp. 181-182.

10   *Ibid.,* p. 182.

11   Goldstein, *opus cit.,* pp. 155, 334.

12   St. Louis *Missouri Republian,* Nov. 12, 1867, p. 3:4.

13   *Ibid.,* Aug. 28, 1867, p. 3:4.

14   *Ibid.,* July 20, 1869, p. 2:5.

15   *Idem.*

16   *Ibid.,* Mar. 10, 1868, p. 2:5.

17   *Idem.*

18   *Idem.* In the Fourth Ward the assigned physician visited all the houses in the ward and found 1931 families, with 4,070 children. He successfully vaccinated 3,319 of these. *Idem.*

19   Goldstein, *opus cit.,* p. 84.

20   St. Louis *Missouri Republican,* Sept. 8, 1869, p. 2:5.

21   *Idem.*

22   *Idem.*

23   *Ibid.,* Sept. 18, 1869, p. 2:7.

24   Rosenberg, *opus cit.,* pp. 195-196. The author of a letter published in the St. Louis *Missouri Republican* of June 21, 1871, was acquainted with the work of Drs. Snow and Pettenkofer, but disagreed with their conclusions. St. Louis *Missouri Republican,* June 21, 1871, p. 2:7.

25   Rosenberg, *opus cit.,* p. 193.

26   St. Louis *Missouri Republican,* July 22, 1868, p. 2:8.

27   *Idem.*

28   *Ibid.,* June 21, 1871, p. 2:7.

29   *Ibid.,* Nov. 12, 1867, p. 3:4.

30   *Idem.*

31   The retiring board, which served from 1867 to 1870, was highly praised by the St. Louis *Missouri Republican* in its issue of Apr. 26, 1870: "This board and assistants it must be said have proved a most efficient organization and they have the ruling sanitary system of the city in excellent working order. To those who recollect the confusion and inadequacy of the regime at the health office the present order of things appears as a complete and most important change of inestimable benfit to the city." St. Louis *Missouri Republican,* Apr. 26, 1870, p. 3:5.

32   The members of the new board were: Nathan Cole, mayor and ex-officio president; David Powers, vice president of the city council; Julius Hunicke from the board of police commissioners; Frank G. Porter, M.D.; and William S. Barker, M.D. *Edwards's St. Louis Directory 1871,* p. 34.

33   *The Revised Ordinances of the City of St. Louis, 1871* (St. Louis, George Knapp and Co., Book and Job Printers, 1871), pp. 104, 106.

34   *Ibid.,* pp. 107-108.

35   *Ibid.,* p. 104.

36   *Ibid.,* p. 398.

37   St. Louis *Missouri Republican,* Mar. 21, 1871, p. 2:6.

38   *Idem.*

39   *Idem.*

40   St. Louis *Missouri Republican,* Feb. 28, 1871, p. 2:5.

41   *Ibid.,* Sept. 13, 1870, p. 2:3.

42   Ibid., Aug. 26, 1870, p. 2:6.

43   Ibid., Feb. 27, 1868, p. 2:5.

44   *Idem.*

45   *Revised Ordinances, St. Louis, 1871,* p. 71.

46   St. Louis *Missouri Republican,* July 16, 1870, p. 2:5; *ibid.,* Aug. 26, 1870, p. 2:6.

47   *Ibid.,* Sept. 1, 1870, p. 2:4.

48   *Ibid.,* Aug. 23, 1870, p. 2:7.

49   George Worthington Adams, *Doctors in Blue: The Medical History of The Union Army in the Civil War* (New York, Henry Schuman, 1952), pp. 38-39.

50   St. Louis *Missouri Republican,* Aug. 23, 1870, p. 2:7.

51   *Ibid.,* May 18, 1871, p. 2:5.

52   *Ibid.,* June 21, 1871, p. 2:5.

53   *Ibid.,* Sept. 27, 1872, p. 2:4. *ibid.,* Sept. 20, 1872, p. 2:4.

54   *Ibid.,* Feb. 16, 1873, p. 8:1-2.

55   *Idem.* Dr. Eliot found the regulations deficient from the standpoint of protecting the public health. He warned that the superficial weekly examinations of the prostitutes did not guarantee that they were free from infection and could be patronized with immunity. He pointed out that the social evil regulation to be really effective should require the examination and registration of the men who visited the brothels as well as the inmates. Dr. Eliot believed that the only way to regulate prostitution was through the elevation of human nature by education and religion.

56   *Ibid.,* Aug. 17, 1873, p. 1:2.

57   *Ibid.,* Aug. 24, 1873, p. 10:1-2.

58   *Ibid.,* Apr. 1, 1874, p. 5:1-2.

59   *Idem.*

60   *Idem.*

61   *Idem.*

62   *Idem.*

63   *Ibid.,* June 24, 1875, p. 5:2.

64   *Idem.*

65   *Ibid.,* Nov. 26, 1871, p. 2:3.

66   *Ibid.,* Jan. 31, 1873, p. 8:1.

67   *Ibid.,* Dec. 11, 1874, p. 8:2.

68   *Ibid.,* Jan. 1, 1875, p. 8:3.

69   *Ibid.,* Sept. 29, 1871, p. 2:5.

70   *Ibid.,* Oct. 15, 1871, p. 4:3.

71 *Ibid.,* Nov. 14, 1873, p. 5:4.

72 *Ibid.,* Oct. 20, 1871, p. 2:5.

73 *Ibid.,* Mar. 15, 1872, p. 2:5.

74 *Ibid.,* June 6, 1873, p. 6:1.

75 *Laws of Missouri, Passed at the Adjourned Session of the Twenty-Seventh General Assembly, 1874,* (Jefferson City, Regan and Carter, State Printers, 1874), p. 111.

76 William Hyde and Howard L. Conard, *Encyclopedia of the History of St. Louis* (New York, The Southern History Co., 1899), Vol. II, p. 1010.

77 *Ibid.,* Vol. II, p. 821.

78 *Ibid.,* Vol. II, p. 1010.

79 *Ibid.,* Vol. II, p. 1008.

80 St. Louis *Missouri Republican,* Feb. 13, 1877, p. 3:3. Mr. Tolkacz was introduced as a defense witness, but much of his testimony was damaging to the pro-swill cause.

81 *Idem.*

82 *Ibid.,* Sept. 21, 1877, p. 5:3.

83 *Ibid.,* Mar. 7, 1879, p. 8:2.

84 *Ibid.,* June 25, 1875, p. 8:3.

85 *Ibid.,* Mar. 2, 1877, p. 7:1-2.

86 *Ibid.,* Mar. 16, 1877, p. 5:3.

87 *Ibid.,* Jan. 28, 1877, p. 6:3. This distrust of the medical practice of the day was expressed in the leading sentence of an editorial of the St. Louis *Missouri Republican* of January 28, 1877: "By slow degrees the civilized world is drifting to Macbeth's conclusion that there are times when it is best to throw physic to the dogs, although it is not at all likely that we shall ever come to that era of millennial perfection when physic will be entirely rejected."

88 *Laws of Missouri, Passed at the Adjourned Session of the Twenty-seventh General Assembly, 1874,* (Jefferson City, Regan and Carter, State Printers, 1874), p. 111.

89 St. Louis *Missouri Republican,* Feb. 15, 1878, p. 8:2-3.

90 *Ibid.,* Nov. 10, 1882, p. 5:3.

91 *Ibid.,* Dec. 22, 1882, p. 5:3.

92 *Ibid.,* July 26, 1879, p. 4:2.

93 Gerald M. Capers, Jr., *The Biography of a River Town. Memphis: Its Heroic Age* (Chapel Hill, The University of North Carolina Press, 1939), p. 194.

94 *Ibid.,* pp. 194-195.

95 *Ibid.,* p. 198.

96 Goldstein, *opus cit.,* pp. 82-84.

97 *Idem.*

98 *Idem.*

99 St. Louis *Missouri Republican,* July 26, 1879, p. 3:1.

100 *Idem.*

101 *Ibid.,* July 14, 1879, p. 1:3.

102 *Ibid.,* Aug. 8, 1879, p. 5:4.

103 *Ibid.,* Nov. 23, 1878, p. 2:3.

104 *Idem.*

105 *Ibid.,* July 6, 1874, p. 2:6.

106 *Ibid.,* July 17, 1870, p. 1:2-3.

107 *Ibid.,* Jan. 4, 1868, p. 3:7.

108 Former Mayor William Carr Lane, in a pamphlet with the title *Water for the City,* published in 1860, stated: "The Water which is at present supplied to us from hydrants, is pumped into the Reservoir from the Mississippi, near the shore, at Bates street. This source of supply is so far down the City, that the water suffers great deterioration from nuisances of every conceivable description, which are constantly and unavoidably cast into the River, above the Waterworks. The supply point is, moreover, below the mouths of Rocky Branch and Gingras Creek — each of which is the constant receptacle of a large and increasing mass of filth. In times past — before the extension of population above Bates street — Water taken from the River at this point, would remain sweet for more than a fortnight, in an earthern jar or a barrel; now it will spoil, more or less, in a single night." William Carr Lane, p2 *Water For the City* (St. Louis, n. p. 1860), p. 2.

109 St. Louis *Missouri Republican,* Feb. 22, 1863, p. 2:2.

110 *Laws of the State of Missouri, Passed at the Regular Session of the Twenty-second General Assembly, 1862-1863* (Jefferson City, J. P. Arent Public Printer, 1863), pp. 95-99.

111 St. Louis *Missouri Republican,* Feb. 22, 1864, p. 3:4.

112 *Ibid.,* Aug. 7, 1864, p. 2:2.

113 *Laws of the State of Missouri, Passed at the Regular Session of the Twenty-third General Assembly, 1864-1865* (Jefferson City, W. A. Curry, Public Printer, 1865), pp. 442-443; St. Louis *Missouri Republican,* Feb. 24, 1865, p. 3:1-3.

114 St. Louis *Missouri Republican,* Jan. 10, 1867, p. 1:2-3.

115 *Idem.*

116 *Ibid.,* Jan. 4, 1868, p. 3:7. If the dimensions given in the press were correct, the capacity of the basin should have been greater than 2,000,000 gallons. Possibly it was not filled to the top.

117 *Ibid.,* July 13, 1870, p. 3:4.

118 *Ibid.,* Apr. 19, 1871, p. 2:3.

119 *Ibid.,* Sept. 24, 1869, p. 2:6; St. Louis *Republic,* Nov. 11, 1896, 12:2.

120 *Ibid.,* Nov. 15, 1873, p. 8:1.

121 The move of the waterworks to Bissell's Point was apparently a major factor in reducing the number of typhoid deaths from 269 in 1870, to 174 in 1871, and 176 in 1872. Goldstein, *opus cit.,* p. 84.

122 William Hyde and Howard L. Conard, eds., *Encyclopedia of the History of St. Louis* (New York, The Southern History Co., 1899), Vol. IV, p. 2042.

123 *Idem.*

124 *Ibid.,* pp. 2042-2043.

125 *Ibid.,* p. 2044.

126 Goldstein, *opus cit.,* p. 84.

127 *Idem.*

128 St. Louis *Missouri Republican,* May 8, 1882, p. 4:2.

129 *Ibid.,* May 8, 1881, p. 11:1-2.

130 Owen H. Wangensteen and Sarah D. Wangensteen, *The Rise of Surgery: From Empiric Craft to Scientific Discipline* (Minneapolis, University of Minnesota Press, 1978), p. 439.

131 St. Louis *Missouri Republican,* June 3, 1877, p. 4:5.

132 *Ibid.,* Nov. 17, 1867, p. 3:3.

133 *Ibid.,* Oct. 20, 1871, p. 2:5.

134 *Ibid.,* Apr. 9, 1870, p. 2:5. A reporter from the St. Louis *Missouri Republican,* following a visit to city hospital, commented favorably on the skillful use of mechanical appliances to assist fractured limbs in the healing process, the reliance on chloroform in surgical

operations, the employment of carbolic acid and permanganate of potash as disinfectants, and the careful attention to diet in treating diarrhea, dysentery and feverish diseases. *Idem.*

135 *Ibid.,* Oct. 26, 1881, p. 5:2.

136 Dr. William Carr Lane died Jan. 6, 1863 (St. Louis *Missouri Republican,* Feb. 22, 1863, p. 2:2.); Dr. Charles A. Pope died July 5, 1870 (St. Louis *Missouri Republican* Aug. 7, 1870, p. 2:5; Joseph Nash McDowell died Sept. 25, 1868 (St. Louis *Missouri Republican,* Oct. 12, 1868, p. 2:3); Dr. John T. Hodgen died Apr. 28, 1882 (St. Louis *Missouri Republican,* Apr. 29, 1882, p. 4:3).

137 St. Louis *Missouri Republican,* Feb. 3, 1878, p. 6:6.

138 *Ibid.,* May 8, 1879, p. 8:2.

139 *Idem.*

140 *Ibid.,* June 12, 1881, p. 6:5. These were the American Medical College and the St. Louis Electic Medical College.

141 *Ibid.,* Mar. 8, 1883, p. 6:3.

142 *Idem.*

143 *Ibid.,* May 8, 1879, p. 8:2.

144 Walter B. Stevens, *St. Louis, The Fourth City 1764-1909* (St. Louis, The S. J. Clarke Publishing Co., 1909, Vol. I, p. 599.

145 Hyde and Conard, *Encyclopedia of the History of St. Louis, Vol. II,* p. 1052. The new building was not occupied by patients until July 1857. *Idem.*

146 St. Louis *Missouri Republican,* Sept. 10, 1871, p. 2:3.

147 *Ibid.,* Feb. 22, 1873, p. 8:1-2.

148 *Ibid.,* June 17, 1873, p. 5:1.

149 *Ibid.,* May 3, 1874, p. 4:2-3.

150 *Ibid.,* June 17, 1873, p. 5:1.

151 *Ibid.,* May 3, 1874, p. 4:2-3.

152 *Ibid.,* Jan. 16, 1875, p. 8:4.

153 *Ibid.,* July 6, 1872, p. 2:5.

154 Ibid., May 4, 1874, p. 8:2-3.

155 Hyde and Conard, *Encyclopedia of the History of St. Louis,* Vol. II, p. 1052.

156 "The treatment of a small-pox patient is simple in the extreme — pure air, proper ventilation, clean bedding, low diet, perfect quiet, and a thoroughly open system may be said to comprise the whole course. A person afflicetd with small-pox eats only when improving, for the preliminary stages are accompanied by intense pains and nausea. Morphine is judiciously administered when the mind is too active to admit of sleep and mind rest. Two thirds of the patients at one time or another during their illness become delirious...." Physical restraint was used in the later stages to prevent the patient from scratching. St. Louis *Missouri Republican,* Feb. 12, 1882, p. 7:1.

157 St. Louis *Missouri Republican,* Mar. 31, 1876, p. 2:5.

158 *Idem.*

159 *Ibid.,* Feb. 28, 1873, p. 8:4.

160 *Ibid.,* July 19, 1874, p. 8:4.

161 *Ibid.,* Aug. 13, 1871, p. 2:4; *ibid.,* Aug. 9, 1874, p. 5:1-2.

162 Hyde and Conard, *Encyclopedia of the History of St. Louis,* Vol. II, p. 1054; St. Louis *Missouri Republican,* May 30, 1873, p. 5:1; *ibid.,* Aug. 13, 1871, p. 2:4.

163 St. Louis *Missouri Republican,* Mar. 13, 1873, p. 8:1.

164 Hyde and Conard, *Encyclopedia of the History of St. Louis,* Vol. II, p. 1054.

165 Hyde and Conard, *opus cit.,* Vol. II, p. 1055.

166 *Idem.*

167 J. Thomas Scharf, *History of St. Louis City and County* (Philadelphia, Louis H. Everts and Co., 1883), Vol. II, p. 1534.

168 St. Louis *Missouri Republican,* May 27, 1882, p. 9:4; Hyde and Conard, *opus cit.,* Vol. III, p. 1392.

169 St. Louis *Missouri Republican,* Mar. 4, 1868, p. 1:3.

170 *Ibid.,* Mar. 4, 1868, p. 3:6.

171 *Ibid.,* Mar. 15, 1870, p. 2:5.

172 *Ibid.,* Apr. 5, 1872, p. 2:5; Stevens, *St. Louis: the Fourth City,* Vol. I, p. 605.

173 St. Louis *Missouri Republican,* May 17, 1878, p. 8:2-3; *ibid.,* Feb. 28, 1879, p. 8:5.

174 *Ibid.,* Aug. 22, 1875, p. 2:5-6.

175 *Ibid.,* Mar. 6, 1879, p. 8:4.

176 *Ibid.,* Mar. 7, 1877, p. 8:4.

177 *Ibid.,* Mar. 3, 1877, p. 8:2.

178 *Ibid.,* Dec. 18, 1874, p. 5:4.

179 *Laws of Missouri, General and Local Laws Passed at the Adjourned Session of the Twenty-seventh General Assembly, 1874* (Jefferson City, Regan and Carter, State Printers, 1874), p. 111; *Missouri Revised Statutes, Myers' Supplement to Wagner's Missouri Statutes* (St. Louis, Mo., W. J. Gilbert Publisher, 1877), pp. 270-271.

180 *The Revised Ordinances of the City of St. Louis, 1881* (St. Louis, Times Printing House, 1881), pp. 509-511.

181 St. Louis *Missouri Republican,* Dec. 18, 1874, p. 5:4; *ibid.,* June 20, 1876, p. 8:4.

182 *Ibid.,* Jan. 15, 1875, p. 8:3.

183 *Ibid.,* Feb. 20, 1879, p. 3:1.

184 *Ibid.,* Nov. 23, 1880, p. 8:2.

185 *Ibid.,* Nov. 28, 1880, p. 11:4.

186 *Ibid.,* Sept. 30, 1881, p. 4:5.

187 *Ibid.,* Apr. 12, 1863, p. 1:2.

188 *Ibid.,* Jan. 16, 1864, p. 2:1.

189 *Ibid.,* Dec. 4, 1868, p. 2:3; Goldstein, *opus cit.,* p. 271.

190 St. Louis *Missouri Republican,* Dec. 4, 1808, p. 2:3.

191 *The Statutes of the State of Missouri, Compiled by David Wagner,* Second edition, 1870 (St. Louis, W. J. Gilbert, Publisher, 1870), Vol. I, pp. 712, 718.

192 *Laws of the State of Missouri, Passed at the Adjourned Session of the Twenty-sixth General Assembly, 1871-1872* (Jefferson City, Mo., Began and Edwards, Public Printers, 1872), pp. 160-161.

193 St. Louis *Missouri Republican,* Nov. 10, 1874, p. 5:1-2.

194 *Ibid.,* June 4, 1874, p. 4:3.

195 *Ibid.,* Dec. 2, 1864, p. 2:3-4.

196 *Ibid.,* Aug. 12, 1869, p. 2:4; *ibid.,* Nov. 10, 1874, p. 5:1-2.

197 *Ibid.,* Nov. 6, 1867, p. 2:4, *ibid.,* Aug. 12, 1869, p. 2:4.

198 *Ibid.,* Sept. 28, 1875, p. 6:1-3.

199 *Ibid.,* May 4, 1870, p. 2-3.

200 *Laws of Missouri, 1871-1872,* p. 11.

201 St. Louis *Missouri Republican,* Aug. 15, 1875, p. 10:3-4.

202 *Ibid.,* Aug. 22, 1875, p. 10:2-4.

203 *Idem.*

204 *Ibid.,* Sept. 28, 1875, p. 6:1-3.

205 *Idem.*

206 *Idem.*

207 *Idem.*

208 *Ibid.,* July 17, 1870, p. 4:1-2.

209 *Idem.*

210 *Idem.*

211 *Idem.*

212 *Ibid.,* Apr. 22, 1877, p. 7:2.

213 *Ibid.,* June 2, 1878, p. 4:2.

214 *Idem.*

215 *Ibid.,* Mar. 9, 1873, p. 8:3.

216 *Ibid.,* Nov. 19, 1871, p. 2:6.

217 *Ibid.,* Mar. 18, 1873, p. 2:5. *ibid,* Mar. 30, 1873, p. 4:2.

218 Robert Ernest Schlueter, *History of the Missouri State Medical Association* (Fulton, Mo., Ovid Bell Press, 1950), p. 5.

219 St. Louis *Missouri Republican,* Apr. 27, 1871, p. 3:5.

220 *Ibid.,* Mar. 13, 1873, p. 5:3.

221 *Ibid.,* May 7, 1873, p. 8:2.

222 Schlueter, *opus cit.,* p. 9. The State Medical Association at its 1876 and 1877 meetings had made the same request. St. Louis *Missouri Republican,* Apr. 20, 1876, p. 5:1; *ibid,* Apr. 19, 1877, p. 2:3.

223 St. Louis *Missouri Republican,* Aug. 8, 1879, p. 5:4.

224 Health Commissioner Francis, in an interview on Jan. 6, 1883 with a reporter from the St. Louis *Missouri Republican,* argued strongly for a state board of health with power to regulate medical practice: "You see it is possible under the state law for any set of men, however, ignorant and unscrupulous, to charter a 'medical college'. Having taken out such a charter they can issue diplomas utterly regardless of the attainments or qualifications of the men to whom they are issued, there being no standard or regulation fixed by law. A man holding a diploma from a regular chartered medical college can call upon our city register, present his diploma and demand that he be registered as a regular practicing physician. The register has no right to even require proof of the identity of the applicant with the person whose name is given in the certificate...." Apparently St. Louis's ordinance No. 10,386, which under the authority of the city's new "Scheme and Charter" had placed restrictions on the practice of medicine, had been invalidated by the courts. St. Louis *Missouri Republican,* Jan. 7, 1883, p. 2:1-2.

225 Schlueter, *opus cit.,* p. 3.

226 St. Louis *Missouri Republican,* June 9, 1882, p. 5:3.

227 *The Revised Statutes of the State of Missouri, Revised and Promulgated by the Thirty-fifth General Assembly, 1889* (Jefferson City, Mo., Tribune Printing Co., 1889), pp. 1298-1299.

228 *Ibid.,* p. 1299.

229 *Ibid.,* pp. 1299-1300.

230 *Ibid.,* p. 1300.

231 *Ibid.,* p. 1301.

232 *Ibid.,* pp. 1300-1301.

233 *Laws of Missouri, Passed at the Session of the Thirty-Second General Assembly Begun and Held at the City of Jefferson, January 3, 1883* (Jefferson City, State Journal Printing Co., State Printers, 1883) p. 115.

234 *Idem.*

235 *Ibid.,* p. 116.

236 *Ibid.,* p. 117.

Chapter 6

State Involvement in Health Services, 1883-1900

1. St. Louis Near the End of the Century

ST. LOUIS during the last quarter of the nineteenth century, experienced a period of vigorous growth. From 350,518 in 1880, its population increased by twenty-nine percent to 451,770 in 1890, and by twenty-seven percent to 575,238 in 1900. In that year it ranked fourth in the country behind New York, Chicago and Philadelphia. By 1890, St. Louis was fourth in the value of its manufactured products and fifth in funds devoted to manufacturing.[1] St. Louis's trade territory embraced much of the lower Mississippi Valley and the Southwest, access to which was available through excellent water and rail connections.

The prosperity enjoyed by manufacturers, merchants and bankers was not shared by the workers.[2] Competition kept wages close to the level of mere subsistence.[3] Efforts of laborers to improve their incomes and working conditions by unionization were generally ineffective. Government, dedicated to the principles of laissez-faire economics, provided no assistance.

In St. Louis the homes of the workers were located mainly in an area about a mile wide and several miles long, bounded by Franklin and Cass avenues, the Mississippi River and Fifteenth Street.[4] This was the location of the original French and American city. Older homes and stores had been cut up into rental apartments. In the spacious backyards of the old town, tenements were erected, facing the alleys. Since this area was adjacent to the railroad stations and boat landings, it became the first home of newcomers, and for some, particularly the blacks, their permanent abode.

Many immigrants arrived in St. Louis with their funds exhausted and had to share quarters with relatives, friends or acquaintances. Overcrowding was the rule. Some three hundred families inhabited the Ashley tenement stretching along the block between Ashley and O'Fallon streets.[5] Water for washing and cooking had to be secured from wells or outside hydrants. Meat and vegetables, too far decayed to be disposed of in middle-class markets, were sold to the poor at reduced prices. Since there was no regular collection service, trash and garbage were thrown into the streets and alleys to rot and emit foul odors. During the hot summer nights, many of the inhabitants slept shoulder to shoulder on the wide stone sidewalks outside their suffocating homes.[6] In these ghettos, cholera infantum, typhoid fever, diphtheria, scarlet fever, consumption and other diseases took a heavy toll.

Sweatshops, particularly in the clothing industry, flourished. Child labor of young girls twelve years old and up was employed in many of the shops. The pay for the younger children was as low as $.75 a week for six twelve-hour days.[7]

Scattered among the tenements were gambling dens, saloons and houses of prostitution. Violence and murder were frequent in such notorious neighborhoods as Fort Sumter, Castle Thunder and Clabber Alley.[8]

Charitable organizations worked to provide some relief for the destitution and suffering of the poor. The St. Louis Provident Association was organized in 1860. It operated two depots for the reception of gifts in kind, such as food and clothes. At one of its stations, ovens were installed so that it could provide bread to the poor. A preliminary visit was made upon families seeking assistance, in order to establish the fact of need. For the year ending in October 1873, $20,000 was collected and disbursed, and a total of 5,580 persons assisted.[9]

The order of St. Vincent de Paul was established in St. Louis in 1845. The work of the society was carried on by twenty-two local conferences or committees. The local committees collected and distributed to the poor the supplies of which they were most in need. The expenditures and the number of persons aided during the 1873 period were slightly below those reported by the provident society.[10]

By his will filed in 1851, Bryan Mullanphy established a fund for the relief of immigrants and travelers. The trustees, in addition to making money grants to assist stranded immigrants, operated the Mullanphy Emigrant Home on Fourteenth and Mullanphy streets. The estimated value of the assets of the trust in 1874 was $676,493.98.[11]

St. Louis, in the last decades of the century, came under the control of a corrupt political machine. The city's prosperity may have had the side effect of causing St. Louisans to neglect their civic responsibilities. The prospect of making a fortune in business or banking exercised more attraction than any honest rewards politics could offer.

Politicians had a bad image. When Theodore Roosevelt, in 1880, expressed his intention to enter politics, his friends tried to dissuade him by remarking that political organizations were not controlled by gentlemen but by saloon-keepers, horse-car conductors and other such working-class characters.[12] The scandals of the Grant administration, including the operation in St. Louis of the Whiskey Ring, certainly contributed to this unattractive reputation.

The St. Louis charter of 1876, designed to give the city an honest and efficient government, had the opposite effect. By diffusing responsibility among a mayor, a bicameral legislature and a number of semi-independent boards, the charter created confusion, frustration and stalemate.[13] Citizens, who had no qualms about working with saloonkeepers and street car conductors, must still have hesitated to spend endless hours in serving a political process so futile and unproductive.

For these and other reasons, the potential governing class of St. Louis, instead of enlisting in the campaign to cope with the problems of an emerging metropolis, moved westward to quiet suburban communities, leaving city management in less worthy and capable hands.

This situation created the opportunity for an extra-legal organization to assume control of city affairs. The boss of the local Democratic machine was Edward Butler, who emigrated from Ireland to America about

1850. Following his move from New York to St. Louis, he worked his way through the apprenticeship system to the rank of master blacksmith and the owner of his own successful shop.[14] He later branched out into the collection and disposal of the city's garbage — a very lucrative enterprise.

An early failure to get a contract to shoe the mules that pulled the city's streetcars taught him that political influence was an important factor in the award of city contracts and franchises. Throughout the last quarter of the century he was active in municipal politics, working to secure the election of councilmen, regardless of political labels, who would follow his orders. Through his control of a majority in the council, he was able to dictate the granting of contracts and franchises to private corporations at prices which involved a substantial bribe to the corrupt legislators who had approved the sales.[15] His influence extended also to the state legislature.

2. *The Battle for Wholesome Food and Drink*

In the final quarter of the nineteenth century, a change occurred in the focus of the efforts of the St. Louis Board of Health. Previously its attention had been directed mainly toward the abatement of nuisances, such as filthy streets and alleys, overcrowded housing, stagnant pools of water, insanitary stables and industries that polluted the water and atmosphere in their vicinity. As the St. Louis municipal bureaucracy expanded, the board of health was able to relinquish some of these concerns to other city agencies, e.g., the board of public improvements.

The change of emphasis did not mean that the board of health, by the application of sanitary science, had eliminated all nuisances. A letter to the editor, by F. Mansfield, published in the St. Louis *Republican* of April 15, 1885, complained of the vast cesspool along the Iron Mountain Railway between Anna and Miller streets into which hundreds of scavenger wagons were dumping the city's garbage and also the refuse from dairies, breweries and sausage factories.[16] In the industrial town of Lowell, on the northern edge of the city, a dozen or more fertilizer factories and rendering establishments were processing carloads of dead cattle shipped in from the states of the West and Far West. The drainage from these factories entered the river in the vicinity of the waterworks intake tower.[17]

With the downgrading of nuisance abatement, the board accorded top priority to the provision for the citizens of St. Louis of wholesome supplies of food and drink. To achieve this goal, the board would have to overcome the opposition of certain well-entrenched special interest groups.

A start toward assuring St. Louis a safe milk supply was made when the council, in 1871, authorized the board of health to exercise broad control of the production and distribution of this important food item. The board drew up stringent rules that empowered the health officer to inspect all milk sold in the city, and to seize for condemnation any found impure or adulterated.[18] This legislation proved ineffective because of the inability of the board to prove to the satisfaction of the council and the courts that milk produced by swill-fed cows was impure and unhealthful.

The council returned to the issue of dairy regulation sixteen years later when it passed the following ordinance: [19]

The maintenance of cow stables or other conveniences for the purpose of carrying on a dairy business within the city limits shall be exercised only under the supervision of the board of health, who may condemn such stable or convenience as a nuisance, if not kept in a cleanly manner; and upon such condemnation, said stable, or convenience shall be vacated forthwith, and shall not again be used for dairy purposes, without permission of the board of health; provided, that no such stable or convenience shall be maintained in any block of the city without the written consent of the majority of the property owners of such block; provided, further, that any person or persons maintaining such stable or convenience within the city limits shall comply strictly with all regulations framed by the board of health and shall not feed to his or their animals any swill or other deleterious food.

This law proved to be unenforceable for reasons explained by Charles W. Francis, the chief sanitary officer, in an interview with a reporter from the St. Louis *Republican* on January 23, 1887:[20]

The ordinance is inoperative for the simple reason that the municipal assembly cannot delegate to any person or persons the power given to them by charter. The charter gives them, among other things, the power to regulate dairies, but they cannot turn their power in this case over to the board of health.

The resulting situation was thus described in a leading article of the St. Louis *Republican* of February 1, 1887:[21]

The unearthing of the filthy dairies and offensive cowsheds of St. Louis has concentrated public attention upon the horrible concoctions sold to consumers in the city under the guise of milk. In the absence of a milk inspector the very heart of the city has become honeycombed with the vilest of sheds, in which cows are immured, deprived of light, pure air and exercise, and fed on the refuse of the distilleries — where offal is thrown in heaps, where steaming odors arise day and night, and where besotted cows give forth poisoned milk, teeming with the germs of consumption and fevers, and where the air is filled with a nauseating stench that breeds pestilence and contagion. All over the city these dens of filth and hotbeds of disease send their pestilential vapors day and night, winter and summer — all the more dangerous because they are invisible. In the center of population, where their evil influences can be most felt, there they increase and multiply, as if glorying in their power to spread contamination, unseen and unsuspected. For years these so-called dairies — a libel on legitimate institutions of this character — have existed and flourished in St. Louis, and their number has increased until now there are over 400 within the city limits. Their influence is great, not only because it is unseen and has been, to a great extent, unknown, but because it is subject to no control. The few ordinances now existing concerning them are inoperative and there is no officer to put the ordinances into execution if they were otherwise; and so the concoction is sold, thousands and thousands of gallons daily, and children sicken and die and these vile holes continue to exist, without restraint.

The political power of the milkmen was exercised through the "St. Louis Dairymen's

Benevolent and Protective Union," which maintained a full-time legal staff. Counsel was available to defend any member summoned before the board of health or the courts on charges involving the operation of his dairy. Union representatives monitored the activities of the board of health, the St. Louis City Council and the state legislature, in order to defeat, or at least weaken by amendments, any legislation hostile to the dairy enterprise.[22] The union had powerful allies in the brewery and distillery industries, the waste products of which were sold as cattle feed. The political clout of the dairymen and their allies, and the venality of the city councils, dominated by the Ed Butler machine, assured the milkmen wide freedom from supervision.

The dairy lobby gave striking evidence that its power was strong in Jefferson City as well as in city hall in St. Louis. The state legislature, on June 14, 1889, passed a comprehensive milk inspection bill, applicable to cities having a population of 300,000 or more.[23] St. Louis was the only city that qualified.

The act permitted the board of health of St. Louis to appoint one chief milk inspector and such assistants as might be needed. The law made it illegal for any dairymen to market "milk to which water or any foreign substance has been added, or milk produced from cows fed in whole or in part on the refuse or residue from distilleries, vinegar, glucose or starch factories, whether designated as swill, distillery slop, grains, feed for livestock, or by any other name . . . ."[24]

Two years later, under pressure from the dairy and distillery lobby, the state legislature repealed the milk inspection law and substituted for it the following provision:[25]

All cities and towns in the state shall have power, by ordinance, to license and regulate milk dairies, and the sale of milk, and provide for the inspection thereof.

The repeal of the state law was a setback for the St. Louis Board of Health, forcing it to renew efforts to persuade the local government to pass adequate legislation.

Two developments gave promise that St. Louis would eventually enjoy a wholesome milk supply. The first was the progress that had been made in dairy science. By the 1890s, the major features of modern dairying, including refrigeration, chemical analysis to determine solid content of milk, bacteriological inspection for disease germs, and pasteurization, had been developed. An increasing volume of "railroad milk" was being shipped into St. Louis from large dairy farms in nearby counties of Missouri and Illinois. Some of this milk was produced under the sanitary conditions of the new dairy science. Because of its greater cost, it was purchased mostly by the wealthy families. The poor continued to use the milk from the city dairies.

The second development was the appointment, in 1895, by Mayor Cyrus P. Walbridge of a vigorous new health commissioner, Dr. Maximilian C. Starkloff. Starkloff was born in Quincy, Illinois, December 30, 1859, and was educated in the St. Louis public schools. He read medicine for four years under the preceptorship of St. Louis's distinguished physician, Dr. John T. Hodgen. He also attended a broad program of lectures at the St. Louis Medical College, from which he received his doctor's degree in 1882.[26]

Dr. Starkloff was an excellent administrator as well as doctor. He had a strong political following and ran on the Republican ticket as a candidate for mayor in the 1897 election. He was an effective public speaker and debater, talents which he frequently exercised in appearances before hostile council commit-

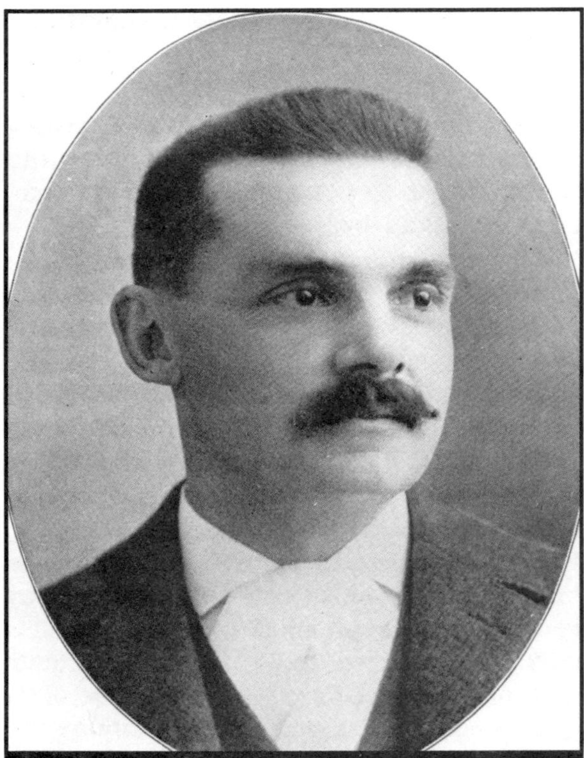

Missouri Historical Society, Max C. Starkloff, M. D., from Notable St. Louisians, 1900.

Dr. Max C. Starkloff

tees in advocating board of health measures. He brought to his new job immense energy, determination and knowledge. Dr. Starkloff retained his post for almost thirty years. During this period, he was twice elected president of the international society of public health officials.[27]

Dr. Starkloff successfully guided through the council, on March 31, 1896, a strong dairy inspection bill, which contained the following requirements: (1) clean, well-ventilated stables; (2) sewer connections to the city's mains; (3) discontinuance of the pollution of public water courses and streams by dairy wastes; (4) sufficient breathing room for the cows and an open lot for exercise; (5) the maintenance of rigid precautions whenever disease showed itself at any dairy.[28]

The inspection of meat supplies posed another difficult problem for the board of health. The city was slow in establishing inspection procedures, with the result that it became a dumping place for injured and diseased animals that were barred from sale in adjoining states.[29]

Under the provisions of city ordinance No. 13,068, a meat inspection force consisting of a chief inspector and six assistants was organized on January 19, 1885. In a two-weeks period at the St. Louis and East St. Louis stockyards, the inspectors examined 10,790 cattle, 38,010 hogs and 9,729 sheep. Of these, 109 cattle, 990 hogs and 30 sheep were condemned.[30]

This inspection program proved unsatisfactory. The magnitude of the job and the cost involved were greater than a single city could handle. Federal or state assistance was needed. Further, the program failed to provide inspection of the hundreds of small slaughterhouses and butcher shops scattered over the city.

In July 1885, the council adopted a different approach to the inspection problem. Instead of trying to examine all animals passing through the local stockyards, the council determined to concentrate on improving the quality of food sold to consumers in stores and markets. The office of inspector of meat, fish, game and poultry was established, with a staff of four officials. They were empowered to enter all markets and to condemn any meat, fish, game or poultry found to be tainted, diseased or unwholesome. Food thus condemned had to be destroyed. The offering for sale of unwholesome meat, fish, game or poultry was made a misdemeanor. The names of offending dealers were to be published in the local papers.[31]

In the middle 1880s, the board of health made another effort to close the thousands of city wells, which were suspected of spreading cholera, typhoid fever and other diseases. An attempt in 1868 to force homeowners whose wells had been condemned as unwholesome to use city water had failed.[32]

Asiatic cholera in the summer of 1884 had launched a major invasion of Europe. The cities of the Mediterranean coast were particularly plagued. In France, two-thirds of those attacked had died.[33] The experience of St. Louis in 1849 and 1866 foretold that European epidemics eventually would reach the United States and Missouri.

Fortunately, the scientific knowledge was available that would enable St. Louis to protect itself. John Snow of London had demonstrated in 1849 that the disease is communicated by contaminated water supplies. Robert Koch, in 1884, discovered the bacillus, which causes the disease.[34] The transformation of this knowledge into effective sanitary measures in St. Louis, however, would require a massive mobilization of public opinion.

On the evening of March 6, 1885, President W. B. Potter of Washington University delivered a lecture on "Water" before almost 1,000 people at the Pickwick Theater auditorium. The talk was part of a course on public health presented by Alpha Council of the Legion of Honor. Professor Potter showed pictures of sidewalk hydrants located within several feet of sewers, also of wells sandwiched in between rows of privies.[35] He pointed out that the limestone rock underlying St. Louis was fractured by weathering, facilitating the seepage of sewage from vaults and sewers into water supplies.

Summarizing the situation in St. Louis regarding its wells, he declared:[36]

Already the question has been repeatedly asked by those concerned for the welfare of the city, is St. Louis prepared for a visitation of the cholera? With the knowledge that there are 6,000 to 8,000 surface wells of the character shown tonight, and surrounding them 25,000 to 30,000 privy vaults, saturating the soil with corruption and making sewers of the wells, and there are besides several thousand private cisterns more or less polluted, how is it possible to believe that the city is prepared to face an epidemic? May we not with reason go further and most emphatically declare that the city is in a dangerous as well as disgraceful condition? The danger, unfortunately, is not alone in the public wells and cisterns and overflowing vaults, it is also to a large extent in the ignorance and apathy concerning these matters that prevail to such an alarming extent among all classes of citizens and even the city authorities themselves.

Spurred by the threat of an epidemic, the municipal assembly, on March 24, 1885, passed a general well-closing law. The measure, as summarized in the *St. Louis Globe-Democrat* of that date, closed "all the wells in the city, except those used for manufacturing purposes, or stables or for watering stock, or those proven to contain pure water." The law embodied an amendment from the house to the effect "that all wells containing water with more than six grains of chlorine to the gallon shall be declared nuisances and abolished."[37] It was weakened by the three major categories of exemptions from forced closure. However, the house amendment put some teeth in the measure by providing a rule by which the city chemist could distinguish between wells that were allowable and those which must be condemned as nuisances.

On the evening of March 31st, a large number of citizens met at the Central Turner Hall and formed the "Well-Owners Protective Association." They elected officers and collected funds to hire chemists to analyze the water in the wells and to engage legal talent to fight any injustice in the carrying out of the law.[38]

To the city council on June 9, 1885, a petition signed by 1,500 persons was presented. The main point of the remonstrance was that the presence of chlorine — an ingredient of table salt — did not prove that well water was impure. At this meeting, the city counselor was instructed to represent the municipality in a suit brought by the well-owners' organization in the Missouri Supreme Court challenging the constitutionality of the well-closing law.[39]

The case was argued before the Missouri Supreme Court, June 15, 1885, with Leverett Bell representing the city and Judge Gottschalk and Colonel F. T. Ledergerber speaking for the well owners. Bell asserted that the city, in licensing the wells on the public streets, retained the right to abolish them without notice or compensation. He argued that no property right existed in the wells so situated and that the private convenience must give way to the public welfare.[40]

The lawyers for the appellants contended that their clients, with the consent of the city, had dug and erected wells on the sidewalks adjoining their real estate and that the water of the wells was healthy and wholesome. They protested the filling up of the wells and threatened to bring suits against the city for their destruction.[41]

Before the supreme court rendered its decision, the city council repealed the well-closing ordinance.[42] Several considerations account for the retreat. The threatened cholera epidemic failed to materialize. The

closure of the wells aroused the wrath of a powerful special interest group, whose displeasure could be anticipated at the next election. Enforcement of the law would have involved the city in endless litigation and possible damage judgments. Finally, the failure of the council to provide an abundant and wholesome supply of water from its municipal works certainly contributed to the reprieve which the well owners gained.

Short-sighted planning was responsible for this failure. In 1865, a board of water commissioners had been named to draft plans for a new waterworks to replace the Bates Street pumping station and the Benton Street reservoir. The board's chief engineer, James P. Kirkwood, visited a number of successful systems in England, France and Germany in preparation for designing the St. Louis plant.[43]

Kirkwood's plan called for moving the pumping site to the Chain of Rocks, almost ten miles above the Bates Street inlet. It provided for three reservoirs, each 400 by 700 feet, in which the initial deposit of sediment would take place. From these basins, the water would be fed into a series of eight filter beds, each 200 by 280 feet, with an individual capacity of 4,500,00 gallons of water daily.[44]

The council, for reasons of economy, rejected the Kirkwood plan, which had the support of the water commissioners, and decided to build the works at Bissell's Point, only three miles above Bates Street. They eliminated the filter beds completely and reduced the capacity of the settling basins to 16,000,000 gallons daily.[45] The first water was pumped from Bissell's Point in 1871.

By the end of the decade, St. Louisans were again complaining that their water was muddy and frequently in short supply. The water scarcity was aggravated by the enormous wastage that was occurring. Meters were not in general use. Customers paid charges based on the number of rooms in their houses or the type of business involved. Many consumers left their hydrants and water closets running constantly. In winter, the practice was justified as necessary to keep the pipes from freezing. Many housewives considered that a continuing flow of water was required to flush the sewer drains and thus prevent disease.[46] It was estimated in 1879 that from fifty to sixty percent of the water pumped from the river was wasted.[47]

The city faced a water famine in the summer of 1881. In July, consumers were using each day 1,500,000 gallons more than the waterworks were providing. The high-service engines were pumping 31,000,000 gallons daily into the Compton Hill reservoir, but the city was using 32,500,000 gallons. The exhaustion of the Compton Hill store would have left many parts of the city entirely without water. In this emergency, Thomas Whitman, water commissioner, urged the mayor to enforce the ordinance restricting sprinkling by homeowners and also to limit the use of water on public parks and buildings.[48]

The water shortage demonstrated the pressing need for an expansion of the municipal works. But the issue of where the enlargement should be made had not been settled. The board of public improvements, in its 1881 annual report, recommended that the pumping station be moved approximately seven miles up river from Bissell's Point to the Chain of Rocks. There the intake would be above the city's sewer drainage and the contamination from industries in north St. Louis. At the Chain, the foundations of the waterworks buildings and their heavy machinery could be installed on solid rock, instead of upon the unstable river bank at

Bissell's Point. Also the settling basins could be constructed on an elevation which would permit their draining and cleaning at all stages of the river.[49]

Minor improvements continued to be made at the waterworks pending the decision regarding its relocation. A second stand-pipe or water tower was erected at Twelfth and Bissell streets in 1885, in connection with the extension of the high service works at Bissell's Point. The tower was situated about 3,200 feet from the pumping station at the point. It had a capacity to move 70,000,000 gallons daily. Its function was to maintain the pressure in the distribution system.[50]

The high-service engines at Bissell's Point were divided into two groups. The new water tower would permit each group of high service pumps to have its own water tower. The two water towers were interconnected. Ordinarily they functioned separately, but in an emergency one system could take over the entire job of providing the city with water.[51]

While the city teetered on the brink of disaster, the municipal assembly continued its policy of procrastination. To keep the hydrants flowing, water was pumped into the distribution mains with hardly a pause in the settling basins. It is possible that the boodling assembly was deliberately discrediting the public ownership and operation of the waterworks in order to sell it to a private corporation, as the St. Louis *Republican* of August 1, 1887 suggested:

The assembly has recently acquired a bad habit of devoting nearly its whole time to the pleasing and alluring arguments of lobbyists for corporations that want the city to grant them valuable franchises without compensation. The question of waterworks extension is pressing and vital. The funds with which to carry out the work are available. There is not a single obstacle in the way of a prompt and straightforward settlement of the whole policy to be pursued, and the policy once settled, work could be carried on in sections each year until completed. The necessity for action is so urgent that the assembly has been guilty of little less than criminal negligence in omitting to consider the matter.

In a special session of the municipal assembly held on September 7, 1887, a bill for the enlargement of the waterworks narrowly passed after surviving a series of parliamentary moves by its opponents to delay or defeat it. It mandated that the "pumping station, inlet tower and settling basins of the extension of the low-service division of the St. Louis waterworks are hereby established at or near Chain of Rocks."[53]

A new danger, from an unexpected quarter, threatened to nullify the hard-won victory. The St. Louis *Republican,* in its issue of October 18, 1887, pointed out that the city of Chicago was developing plans to divert its sewage from its existing destination in Lake Michigan into a drainage canal which would join the Illinois River at Peru. If this project were completed, the sewage would progress down the slow-moving Illinois River to the Mississippi and threaten the water supply of St. Louis at the Chain of Rocks. The writer suggested that this disastrous possibility could be avoided if the St. Louis waterworks inlet were built on the Missouri River at some location above St. Charles.[54]

Colonel Henry Flad, president of the St. Louis Board of Public Improvements, hastened to the defense of the Chain of Rocks site. He strongly opposed a proposal by Mayor David R. Francis to appoint a commission to investigate the effect of the Chicago drainage canal on the St. Louis water supply. Colonel Flad cited two main reasons why he foresaw no future health hazard from the Chicago plan. He was confident that the Chicago sewage would be decomposed by oxidation by the time it reached St. Louis. He argued further that the waters of the Missouri and Mississippi rivers continue as separate streams for scores of miles after their merger. Since St. Louis would be using water which hugs the western shore, there would be slight possibility of contamination of its supply.[55]

On January 31, 1888, it was announced that engineers had begun surveying the route of the major conduit to connect the new works at the Chain of Rocks with the existing plant at Bissell's Point. The new works were scheduled to go into operation in four years, at a cost of $3,000,000. The low-service pumps and the settling basins of the enlarged works would have the capability of handling 100,000,000 gallons daily. Consumption in 1888 averaged 34,000,000 every twenty-four hours.[56]

The new Chain of Rocks plant was officially put into operation, April 6, 1895, and was completed four years later. Water entered the system through an intake tower in the river 1,500 feet from shore and flowed through a tunnel carved out of solid rock to the pumping pits of the low-service engines. These consisted of two E. P. Allis Company engines, each with a daily capacity of 30,000,000 gallons of water, and two Worthington pumps with a capability of 20,000,000 gallons each twenty-four hours.[57] The engines moved the water into six settling basins, with dimensions of 670 feet by 400 feet. From the settling basins, the water was pumped into the clear wells.

From the clear wells 40,000,000 gallons each day went through the mains to a new substation at Baden, in northwest St. Louis, about five miles from the Chain. There high-service engines distributed it to areas about Compton Heights and west of Kingshighway that were too high to be serviced by the Compton Hill reservoir. The other 60,000,000 gallons of the Chain of Rocks daily output was sent to Bissell's Point and distributed by the high-service station there.[58] The water from both the Baden and Bissell's Point stations passed through one of the two water towers en route to consumers. Any surplus of water not drawn by users was diverted into the Compton Hill reservoir. Daily consumption had increased to 55,000,000 in 1894.[59]

With the completion of the pumping station and settling basins at the Chain of Rocks, the city had taken an important step toward providing an adequate supply of pure, wholesome water. But more remained to be done. On June 13, 1896, an ordinance was introduced in the St. Louis House of Delegates providing for the construction of an experimental filtration plant. The plant would introduce into river water pumped into a settling basin a coagulant, i.e., alum, for the purpose of precipitating the suspended inorganic matter as well as the coloring matter and bacteria. The plan was indorsed by Water Commissioner M. L. Holman and the board of public improvements. If the experiment were successful, the coagulation process would be adopted as the first stage of the city's pure water program.[60] The second stage would pass the water through sand and rock filters.

A rival filtration ordinance was pending in the assembly. This provided for private construction and ownership of the filtration plant, with the city guaranteed the option of purchasing it.[61]

Opposition to Commissioner Holman's filtration plan was expressed by the St. Louis *Republic* of March 25, 1897, because of the scientific method proposed:[62]

It is not sufficient to say that the use of alum is only slightly harmful. No substance deleterious to health, however slight the effect, should be added to the water supply by the filtering process. Before resorting to any such device it should first be determined that there is no other process that will give as good a result in the matter of filtration.

The lack of action in the municipal assembly on the earlier filtration ordinance prompted the board of health, in the fall of 1899, to intervene in the matter. Health Commissioner Starkloff instructed the city chemist and city bacteriologist to make analyses of the Mississippi River water in the vicinity of the Chain of Rocks. Their findings established the fact that the city's water supply was polluted by sewage from upstream towns.[63]

In a meeting on October 23, 1899, the board of health unanimously adopted the following resolution:[64]

Be it resolved, that the Board of Health strongly recommend and urge that for the protection of the public health of this city, the Board of Public Improvements, as speedily as possible, prepare an ordinance to be submitted to the Municipal Assembly, which ordinance shall provide for the clarification and purification of the water supply of this city.

The ordinance, drafted by the board of public improvements, provided for the appropriation of $75,000 for conducting experiments to determine the best method of filtration. It was killed in the city council by a vote of seven to six; the adverse majority was constituted by Colonel Ed Butler's political combine.[65] The experiments would have led to the establishment of an operational filtration plant to provide the city with wholesome water.

The St. Louis *Republic* labeled the defeat of the measure a classic example of corrupt politics:[66]

> The combine was not voting against the ordinance as it pretended, but against the communication from the Board of Public Improvements, which made plain the board's intention to recommend finally that the city filter its own water, as the most practicable and economical which can be effected. The combine will consent to no ordinance which does not provide for the letting of a filtering contract to a private corporation, and for the use of the patented device which a certain company exclusively controls, thus guaranteeing the contract to the company at whatever price it demands.

The defeat of the pure water ordinance came at the time when St. Louis was in the midst of a typhoid epidemic. Forty-six new cases were reported on November 17, 1899. The focus of the outbreak was in the wealthy western suburbs, which were supplied with water from the Chain of Rocks pumping station that was distributed by the Compton Hill reservoir. Contrary to previous experience with epidemics, very few members of the working class were affected. The wealthy patients went to private hospitals or were treated at home. To meet the demand for nurses, hospital attendants were brought in from Chicago, Cincinnati and other points.[67]

Stirred by the threat to the health of the city from its contaminated water supply, fifty representatives from twenty-one leading organizations met at the Mercantile Club on the evening of January 26, 1900, and formed a permanent association. They adopted resolutions calling on the board of public improvements and the municipal assembly to determine as quickly as possible the best system of filtration and to apply this system in securing clear and pure water for St. Louis.[68]

3. Medical Progress

The editor of the St. Louis *Republic,* in surveying the contributions to science of Louis Pasteur, Robert Koch and their contemporaries, asserted in the issue of March 24, 1896:[69]

> There is not a single science in the whole range of human knowledge, perhaps, unless it be that of electricity, which has made more marvelous progress in the way of development during the last two decades than that of bacteriology — by which is meant the study of "bacteria," "microbes," "disease germs" and their allied microorganisms . . . .

> Learned biologists are now studying the best mode of killing them when they once find lodgment in animal tissue without killing the man or animal so afflicted. The microscope is the great instrument in this study, and within a few years the doctor who starts out without a tested instrument of that class will be as much an object of ridicule as a hunter without a dog and gun.

St. Louis doctors were quick to adapt the germ theory and the microscope to their practice. An excellent example was Dr. Herman Tuholske, who had received his medical education at the Missouri Medical College and at the leading medical centers in Vienna, Berlin, London and Paris. He served as physician at the St. Louis dispensary and other municipal hospitals. In 1890, he established the St. Louis Surgical and Gynecological Hospital at Locust Street and Jefferson Avenue, where he catered to a large private practice.[70] Dr. Tuholske personally examined each patient and determined the necessary treatment. Two assistants worked with him, one doing the surgical dressing, the other conducting chemical and bacteriological tests.[71]

Other important advances in medical practice occurred in the closing decades of the nineteenth century. One was the conquest of diphtheria, a disease endemic to St. Louis, which from time to time claimed hundreds of young lives in the city. In 1883, Theodor Albrecht Klebs and Friedrich Loeffler identified the *bacillus diphtheriae* and successfully cultivated it on an artificial medium. Seven years later, Emil Adolph von Behring and Shibasaburo Kitazato discovered the curative and immunizing power of diphtheria antitoxin.[72] The antitoxin is the blood serum of an animal, usually a horse, which has been immunized against the disease.

Local doctors were involved in the early use of the X-ray for locating foreign objects in the human body. In March 1896, Dr. Tuholske attended a young man who had suffered a gunshot wound in the left side of his chest. Instead of attempting to find the bullet by exploratory surgery, Dr. Tuholske decided to use an X-ray machine. For the construction of the machine Dr. Tuholske enlisted the help of Dr. Charles O. Curtman, professor of chem-

istry at the Missouri Medical College. Dr. Curtman directed the manufacture of a large Crookes tube at the Columbia Incandescent Lamp Company. He also secured a powerful coil to generate an electric spark and a sensitized plate to record the image of the patient's chest area.[73] It is not clear whether the attempt was successful.

A year later, Dr. Waldo Briggs at the Baptist Hospital in St. Louis, by the use of the X-ray, located and removed a bullet lodged against the spinal column of fifty-one year old Marcellus Sullivan. It was anticipated that the removal of the bullet would end the paralysis that had affected Sullivan since he was shot seven years   previously.[74]

An important change in the pattern of disease in St. Louis took place in the final decades of the nineteenth century. From 1883 to 1900 not a single case of cholera or yellow fever was reported in St. Louis.[75] Influenza made an occasional visit, as in 1889-1890, though not in an epidemic form.[76]

A major reason why these diseases from foreign lands failed to appear was the establishment in the United States of an effective national health agency with strong quarantine powers. In this expansion of the responsibility of the federal government for public health, St. Louis-born Dr. Walter Wyman played a significant role.

After graduating from St. Louis Medical College in 1873, Dr. Wyman served for two years as an assistant physician in the St. Louis municipal hospital system. In 1876 he was placed in charge of the United States Marine Hospital in South St. Louis. His efficient administration won for him rapid advancement to the superintendency of the nation's largest marine hospital, located on Staten Island. In 1891 he was commissioned as supervising surgeon general of the entire United States Marine Hospital Service.[77]

In the fall of 1892, when passenger vessels were sailing from cholera-infected Hamburg without adequate medical inspections, Dr. Wyman directed American port authorities to detain incoming ships up to twenty days. This policy discouraged passenger boats from embarking for the United States. The next year, Congress passed the national quarantine law, which extended the powers of the Marine Hospital Service and gave to the surgeon general the responsibility of executing the quarantine laws.[78] Previously the states, and often individual cities on the coast or inland waterways, had imposed quarantines.

Under Dr. Wyman's supervision, medical officers were detailed to foreign ports to serve in the consular offices and to enforce sanitary requirements on outbound ships. Uniform sanitary regulations for all ports of the United States were established. His office had charge of the medical inspections of all immigrants arriving in the United States.[79]

The most fatal diseases of the late nineteenth century were those affecting children. Of those, diphtheria topped the list. In 1886, 3,504 cases occurred in St. Louis, with 889 deaths. The following year there were 2,964 cases and 961 fatalities.[80] The ratio of deaths to cases was approximately one to three. The cause of death in many instances was the formation in the throat of a membrane which obstructed swallowing and breathing. Before the use of antitoxin, the patient was treated by passing a tube down his throat through which air could be delivered to his lungs; in other cases an incision was made in the child's neck.[81]

In the epidemic of 1886-1887, the board of health found that the diphtheria cases clustered around the city dairies and were probably caused by contaminated milk. The cases increased with the opening in the fall of the schools, where children were crowded fifty to sixty in a room, with poor ventilation and insanitary toilet accommodations.[82]

In mid-December 1894, the board of health established at quarantine station, on the river south of the city, a laboratory for the production of diphtheria antitoxin. Dr. George Homan, health commissioner, Dr. Amand Ravold, city chemist and Dr. Thomas A. Buckland, assistant city chemist, were in charge of the project.[83]

Five worn-out horses, most of them retired from the city ambulance service, were chosen for the experiment. Two of them suffered from serious diseases. Three or four times a week the horses were injected with diphtheria toxin in increasing amounts, in order to induce them to produce antitoxin or antibodies. As the inoculations proceeded, the physicians recorded each day the temperature and other vital signs of the animals. When the horses had developed immunity to the toxin, their blood was ready for using. Thereafter, the animals were tapped from time to time and a quart of blood taken, the serum of which would be employed in treating human patients.[84]

A month later Captain Charles B. Ewing, assistant surgeon at Jefferson Barracks, received authorization from Surgeon General Sternberg of the United States Army, to produce diphtheria antitoxin at his station. With the resources of the army at his command, the captain was able to avoid certain mistakes made by the St. Louis Board of Health in their diphtheria laboratory. For his experimental animals, he secured healthy young horses. Before beginning his work, he immunized them against the most common diseases, including glanders and tuberculosis. He tested daily the increase in the germicidal power of their blood until he was certain the animals were completely immunized and ready to produce an effective quality of diphtheria serum.[85]

During 1895, another diphtheria epidemic struck St. Louis causing 3,196 cases and 526 deaths. The widespread use of antitoxin by the doctors that year was credited with helping reduce the ratio of deaths to one out of six cases, instead of the previous ratio of one of three.[86]

The destructiveness of even the minor childhood diseases before the advent of immunization programs is illustrated by the statistics on croup. Of the 2,177 cases of croup recorded for St. Louis for the period between 1887 and 1898, 1,303 of the patients died.[87] In interpreting these figures, it must be kept in mind that many doctors diagnosed diphtheria as croup.[88]

Scarlet fever rivaled diphtheria in the number of cases that occurred, although the death rate was considerably below that of diphtheria.[89]

Typhoid fever occurred with such frequency that many doctors did not bother to report it.[90] A major outbreak occurred in 1892, with 3,624 cases and 514 deaths.[91] This epidemic was attributed to the drainage of the Prairie Street sewer into the river above the Bissell's Point waterworks inlet. Three North St. Louis creeks, which carried much of the sewage of the Lowell area, dumped their contents into the city's water source.[92]

At a meeting of the St. Louis Medical Society on the evening of December 4, 1892, a committee appointed to look into the nuisances in the Lowell area and to test the city water supply made its report. The group testified that on the basis of their careful investigation, they were unwilling to use for cooking or drinking purposes the water as it came from the hydrants. Chief Sanitary Officer Francis strengthened this indictment of the

municipal supply by stating that in 2,110 of the 2,217 houses where typhoid fever had broken out city water was used.[93]

The most lethal disease among adults was tuberculosis, which accounted for approximately ten percent of the annual deaths in St. Louis, numbering from 800 to 1,000 a year.[94] Crowded housing, poor ventilation and malnutrition were factors in its prevalence. The doctors had no medicines to halt its ravages. Tuberculosis, for a variety of reasons, was not classified as a contagious disease.[95] Consequently, persons suffering from it could not be compulsorily quarantined as were victims of smallpox or cholera.[96] Alarmed by the growing rate of tuberculosis both locally and nationally, a group of St. Louis doctors considered sponsoring a bill in the 1898 session of the general assembly for the regulation of the treatment of consumptives, perhaps after the plan used successfully in the state of New York.[97] An ordinance to accomplish the same purpose, introduced in the municipal assembly, died in committee.[98]

4. The Effect of Scientific Progress on Medical Education

The expansion of scientific knowledge produced by the researches of Pasteur, Koch and their associates had important repercussions upon medical education in St. Louis. Traditionally, the typical medical course had begun with a short period of apprenticeship under an established physician. Then, the student entered a medical college and listened to two years of lectures on anatomy, physiology, surgery and materia medica. The college year began in November and ended in March. This gave farm boys an opportunity to put in and harvest a crop in the long summer break. The medical course was not graded, the second program of lectures being merely a repetition of the first. The old medical science dealt with the gross features of the human body — organs, bones, nerves and blood vessels.

The new medicine embraced the world of microbiology — germs, cells and molecules. Its study required a knowledge of biology, zoology, organic chemistry and physics. Since the high schools of the times provided little or no scientific training, these new subjects had to be grafted upon the medical college's training program. This required a lengthening of the program, either by extending the school year or by adding another year of study. By the 1890s, the school year had been extended from four to seven months. The Missouri Medical College and the St. Louis Medical College, the two oldest colleges, had moved up to a three-year program.[99] This move was in line with the recommendations of the American Medical Association, the American Medical College Association and a majority of the practicing physicians of the state.[100]

The colleges that had lengthened their programs had to pay a price for the privilege of being pioneers. Enterprising groups of doctors, confident that there was still a demand for the two-year school, opened new institutions. The Marion-Sims Medical School, organized in 1890, reported 275 students in attendance during the term which ended in April 1892.[101] The newly established Barnes Medical College conferred 177 medical diplomas in the spring of 1898.[102] St. Louis Medical College, however, had only sixteen graduates at its 1894 commencement.[103]

The various sectarian systems — Thomsonianism, homeopathy, hydropathy, electicism and others — were threatened by the new European medicine. These minor medical cults had played an important role in the early nineteenth century in combatting the excesses of the prevailing "heroic" medicine, such as bleeding, purging and blistering. But by the latter part of the century, regular medicine had largely abandoned these practices. The result was that homeopathy and eclecticism, two of the sectarian systems which had survived, were forced to compete with a reformed, scientific system of regular medicine.

In this confrontation Samuel Hahnemann's two healing principles, the law of similars and the law of infinitesimals,[104] appeared more as articles of dogmatic faith than as proved therapeutic practice.[105] For the treatment of diphtheria, for example, his minute doses of medicine could not compare in effectiveness with the immunizing and curative antitoxins of regular medicine. By the end of the century, homeopathic doctors in St. Louis were appropriating much of the therapy of the regular school.[106] With homeopathy declining in popularity, the St. Louis college of the system closed its doors in 1910. The American Eclectic Medical College continued in operation, freely adopting the successful practices of the new scientific medicine.

From their organization in the 1840s until the end of the century, St. Louis's medical colleges were proprietary institutions, owned by small groups of doctors. At first all a college needed was a building with space for classrooms, library and a surgical laboratory. The professors were unpaid and depended on the sale of tickets to their lectures for compensation. With the new scientific medicine and its demand for more laboratory space and equipment, the operation of a private college became unprofitable. In 1899, the St. Louis Medical College and the Missouri Medical College united to form the medical department of Washington University.[107] Shortly afterwards Marion-Sims Medical College and

Beaumont Medical College joined to establish the medical branch of St. Louis University. The trend of the future, set by Johns Hopkins University, was for medical schools to be part of university-hospital complexes.

5. St. Louis's Municipal Hospitals Beset With Problems

The increase in population and the growing tendency of sick persons to prefer institutional to home care, created a demand for additional hospitals in St. Louis. The Alexian Brothers, in 1890, added a five-story wing to their hospital on Jefferson Avenue at Osage Street. During two visits to hospitals in Europe, Dr. F. J. Lutz, chief surgeon, gathered ideas which were advantageously applied to the St. Louis institution. The new structure had a number of private rooms, also wards with from five to twenty beds. It was equipped with elevators, electric lighting and steam heating.[108]

Dr. William Henderson Mayfield founded the Missouri Baptist Sanitarium in 1884 and served as superintendent and chief surgeon until 1896, when he withdrew and established a private hospital.[109] The St. Louis Baptist Hospital was organized in 1893. It accepted all classes of patients, except those with contagious diseases. The hospital had a capacity of fifty beds. It operated a training school for nurses. In 1899, it established a bacteriological and pathological laboratory.[110]

To take care of the needs of the large population of young, unmarried and homeless men and women in the city, the Protestant Hospital was established. This was supported by the Evangelical Alliance, made up of a number of small Protestant denominations, which were unable individually to operate a hospital.[111] These three hospitals, as well as the older private sanitaria in the city, were founded and supported by religious organizations and were charitable institutions.

Two new hospitals of a different nature made their appearance. Jay Gould's western line sponsored the Missouri Pacific Railway Hospital, which offered a whole range of medical and surgical services for its employees. It was financed by an assessment of fifty cents a month on each worker earning $60 or more a month, and twenty-five cents on workers drawing less than $60. The railroad's hospital in St. Louis was located in a four-story brick building at California Avenue and Henrietta Street.[112]

The Barnes Hospital, still in the planning stage in 1897, was a privately endowed institution. Robert A. Barnes, a wealthy businessman, had established a trust fund of $950,000 for the erection and maintenance of the hospital. The benefactor did not intend his institution should be a competitor of the free city hospital. Patients, who were able, would be expected to pay for their treatment.[113]

While these modern private hospitals were developing, St. Louis's municipal institutions were plagued with problems of overcrowding and mediocre service. City hospital, the main part of which had been built in 1867, needed major repairs. It was poorly ventilated; the upper floor reached 103 degrees in summer. Aside from the resident superintendent, the doctors were fresh internes, just out of medical school. The young practitioners were expected to diagnose and treat every sort of disease. Patients complained of long delays and even failure to receive urgently needed treatment.[114] One patient, who was suffering from pneumonia, was diagnosed as an alcoholic case by an interne; he died several days after he was dismissed without treatment.[115]

The Female Hospital, opened in 1872, was also in disrepair. In some rooms, blankets were nailed to the ceiling to prevent the plaster from falling. To accommodate patients for whom there was no room in the building, tents were set up in the yard. Several patients in cold weather died from the resulting exposure. There was no classification of patients by disease. The lack of a detached lying-in ward exposed mothers and infants to infections of various kinds.[116]

Conditions in the St. Louis Insane Asylum and the poorhouse were even more demoralizing. The insane asylum, with a capacity of 250, housed approximately 500 patients. Two or three persons were crowded into single rooms. In the wards, beds and mattresses at night were closely packed from wall to wall. During the early days of the asylum, nurses administered sedatives to noisy patients. But when the hospital became overcrowded, that practice was abandoned, so that both day and night rest was disturbed by maniacal yelling and screaming. For a majority of patients, there was no treatment program, the attendants limiting their attention to preventing the inmates from hurting themselves or each other. Whereas in the best operated asylums, a cure rate of eighty percent was achieved, in the St. Louis hospital, only ten percent left in sound mental condition.[117]

A reporter for the *St. Louis Republic* made a tour of the asylum in late June 1888 and wrote this indictment of the conditions he observed:[118]

Unfortunate are they who are so burdened with affliction that they must be consigned to the walls of an asylum, but their misery is multiplied when they must go, not to an asylum, but to this insane jail where what degree of intelligence is left must be sacrificed . . . . When they enter there they do leave hope behind, and truly may they cry: "I am not mad, but soon will be."

The poorhouse, adjacent to the insane asylum, by 1888, had been taken over largely by hopelessly insane patients. In the remaining space of the poorhouse and in several outhouses and a nearby barn, indigents and epileptics of both sexes and all ages were miserably housed. During the winter of 1888, there were 902 inmates in the different accommodations of the poorhouse.[119]

The city comptroller, in an interview with a representative of the St. Louis *Republic* on June 26, 1888, attempted to justify the municipal assembly's miserly care of its unfortunate citizens. He stated that if better accommodations and treatment were provided, more patients would flock to St. Louis to take advantage of them. He considered that the care of the insane and indigent was a state responsibility, not a local obligation. If the state wanted St. Louis to operate an asylum and a poorhouse, he declared, it should provide the funds for carrying on this work.[120]

A tornado, which cut a wide swath of destruction through the Mill Creek valley during the evening of May 27, 1896, demolished the city hospital. Patients from the wrecked building were moved to the vacant House of the Good Shepherd at Pine and Seventeenth streets.[121] Fortunately, the municipal assembly the previous month had passed a law establishing a hospital commission to draw up plans for a modern health care system. The legislation provided that one percent of the city's annual revenue, amounting to about $50,000, should go into a hospital construction fund.[122]

The hospital commission consisted of Mayor Cyrus P. Walbridge, Professor Halsey C. Ives of the city council, Edward Mepham of the house of delegates, Health Commissioner

Maximilian C. Starkloff, Dr. Albert Merrell, and Dr. Charles H. Hughes of the board of health, and Louis J. Singer of the board of charity commissioners. The commission, after studying hospitals in a number of Eastern cities, submitted a report recommending the erection of a central or emergency hospital on the site of the old city hospital. This structure would also house the city dispensary. The report proposed the construction of the city's main hospital in the vicinity of the old poorhouse.[123]

Mayor Henry Ziegenhein, who succeeded Cyrus Walbridge, rejected a plan to build the new emergency hospital in stages as money became available. He favored diverting the approximately $800,000 in the Mullanphy Fund to that purpose. The fund had been established in 1851 to assist emigrants from the Eastern states and Europe who were passing through St. Louis en route to homes in the West. Many, in the flood of emigration during 1849 and 1850, reached St. Louis sick, hungry and without resources. By the end of the century, however, the number of emigrants coming through St. Louis had dwindled, and the fund had ceased to render the charitable service its founder had contemplated.[124]

The city of St. Louis, as trustee of the fund, with the support of a majority of the fund directors, entered a suit in Circuit Court Number 4, asking for authorization to divert the assets of the Bryan Mullanphy Emigrant Fund to a new use. The petition was based on the rule of law that permits a charitable fund, when the purpose for which it was established no longer exists, to be redirected to another similar goal.[125]

Judge Daniel D. Fisher, in an opinion rendered July 12, 1899, denied the city's request. To allow the fund to be diverted to the building of a hospital, to be called the Bryan

Mullanphy City Hospital, would be a violation of the original trust, he ruled. Such a hospital, he declared, would be a city hospital, built on city land and, in effect, city owned. He suggested that the nearest charity to the one for which the fund was created would be "a hospital for the use of indigent nonresidents who might be found in the city sick and helpless and with no one to care for them."[126]

Shortly before the announcement of Judge Fisher's decision in the Mullanphy Fund case, the city hospital commission forwarded four ordinances governing the proposed new city hospital to the council for approval. The first provided for the erection of a public emergency hospital, designed according to the pavilion plan, at the site of the old city hospital at Lafayette Avenue and Linn Street.[127]

The second ordinance specified that the institution should be under the administration of a superintendent, who would direct all the affairs of the institution except the treatment of patients. This aspect of the hospital was to be controlled by a board of hospital administration, consisting of members of the faculties of the city's medical colleges, who would be chosen by the health commissioner. Each of these attending physicians or "clinicians" would have charge of a particular clinic and would be obligated to attend those cases in which he performed a clinical demonstration until the patient was discharged or died. The board of hospital administration would have absolute control of the internes and would direct all the medical and surgical activities of the hospital.[128]

The third ordinance mandated the addition of a professionally trained bacteriologist to the hospital staff. The fourth proposed law amended the existing rule, which required that all nurses employed in the city hospital must be recruited from the St. Louis Training School for Nurses. The new ordinance provided that the graduates of any accredited nursing school would be eligible for hiring.[129]

6. Nursing as a Profession

The nurses to which the hospital commission looked to staff the hospital were a new professional group, consisting mainly of young women. It was not until the Civil War that women in considerable numbers entered the nursing field. An exception was the Catholic nursing orders. However, the nuns looked upon nursing as a religious calling rather than as a professional career. During the war, most of the nurses, except in the general hospitals, were convalescent soldiers. Even after the conflict, men continued to play a prominent role in the care of the sick. Nursing was a menial task, involving scrubbing floors, making beds, emptying bed pans and administering medicines according to doctors' orders. There was nothing about the work that defined it as particularly fitting for feminine hands.

The organization, on December 7, 1883, of the St. Louis Training School for Nurses marked the inauguration locally of the new profession. The sponsors of the school were leaders of the Western Sanitary Commission, the Ladies Union Aid Society, the Fremont Relief Society and the Young Men's Christian Association.[130] These organizations had been active during the Civil War and the postwar period in recruiting nurses for Union hospitals and in providing charitable relief.

The meeting, at which the school was founded, was held on the Washington University campus and was chaired by Chancellor William G. Eliot, St. Louis's most distinguished civic leader. The aims of the group were to train young women for new career opportunities; also to furnish to the city's many hospitals nurses capable of apply-

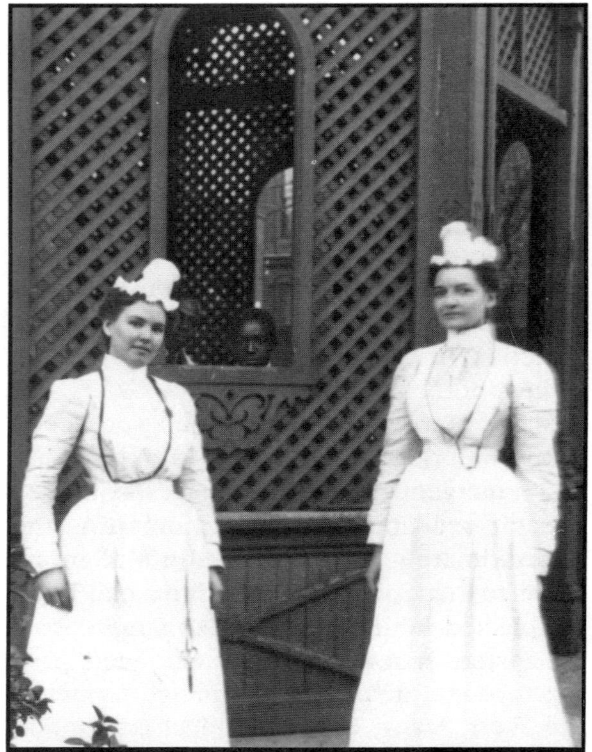

Nurses of the 1890's. Courtesy of the State Historical Society of Missouri.

ing the latest medical knowledge. The first class of students, three in number, enrolled April 7, 1884.[131]

The city made an arrangement with the school by which the students received on-the-job training at city hospital under a superintendent from the faculty of the training school; the other nurses were directed by a different supervisor. The student nurses were paid by the city while they worked and learned; the first-year students received $20 a month, the second-year nurses $25. Both classes got board, lodging and laundry service.[132] As a token of their new profession, the nurses adopted a uniform of spotless white dress and shoes, an apron and a jaunty little cap perched on the top of their heads.

The routine of a nurse in city hospital involved procuring and distributing medicines, bandaging wounds, changing beds, giving out clean garments to patients and making reports. It is not clear when they were given responsibility for checking patients' vital signs — temperature, pulse and blood pressure. The nurses in public hospitals assigned convalescent patients to perform various housekeeping duties.[133] The fact that the patients were charitable cases made them liable to exploitation.

Many private hospitals established and operated training programs for nurses.[134] These consisted at first of apprentice training ranging from simple housekeeping duties to service in the surgical department.[135] Later these programs developed into two- or three-year sequences of lectures and demonstrations combined with on-the-job experience in hospital wards.[136]

The prospects of implementing the hospital commission's four-fold plan were bleak. Judge Fisher's ruling had put the Mullanphy Fund off limits for this purpose. In addition, a financial crisis raised the threat that the $200,000 accumulated in the hospital construction fund might have to be used to keep the city government running. [137]

As the cost of hospital construction and operation increased, the issue of how far the city should go in providing free hospital care was discussed. Shortly after he became health commissioner, Dr. Starkloff had established the rule that persons able to pay for private medical treatment should not be admitted to city hospitals and dispensaries except in emergency situations. The board of health, at its meeting of January 31, 1897, adopted a resolution advocating the investigation of the financial status of patients admitted in emergencies and the collection of the costs of their treatment from those who were solvent.[138]

In a move designed to reduce hospital admissions, the board of health established three additional dispensaries, one in the western suburbs, another in the southern sector of the city and a third in the northern portion. The new dispensaries would be staffed by a physician and an ambulance. The existing central dispensary had its staff increased to a chief physician, four assistants and a sixth physician to attend sick and indigent persons in their homes. This expanded outpatient service would reach persons who found it difficult to get to the central dispensary.[139]

7. *The Influence of Medical Societies*

The American Medical Association and its state and local chapters exerted a powerful influence during the late nineteenth century upon the way that medical services would be delivered. The gradual decline of the sectarian systems, such as homeopathy and Eclecticism, removed a major opposition to the association's plans. The success of the new scientific medicine practiced by the allopathic doctors won for them a degree of popular support not previously enjoyed.

Doctors generally had not gained the prestige and financial compensation received by other professions, such as law, banking and engineering. A study, made by the American Medical Association, revealed that well into the twentieth century only ten percent of the nation's doctors were earning a decent living.[140] There were too many doctors, most poorly prepared for their profession.

The situation in St. Louis confirmed this analysis. With a population in 1892 of 542,922 persons, the city had 737 doctors and 249 midwives.[141] There were eleven medical schools, graduating from 300 to 400 doctors each year. Many of these new physicians received their diplomas from two-year colleges. The Missouri State Board of Health was required by law to grant certificates to all graduates of medical colleges "in good standing."

Besides competition from fellow doctors in private practice, St. Louis practitioners lost business to local medical institutions. The city maintained free hospitals and dispensaries. The various medical schools,   in order to give their students practical training, operated clinics and dispensaries. The denominational hospitals, as part of their charitable work, provided dispensary service.

The American Medical Association, dating back to 1847, maintained a code of ethics covering relations of doctors to each other, to patients and to the public.[142] The provisions of the code reflected a mixture of altruism and professional self interest. The code encouraged high standards of medical practice. But it was monopolistic, since it recognized the claims of no form of practice except the regular or allopathic.[143]

This exclusiveness of the code brought the regular establishment in St. Louis into conflict with the sectarians over appointment to city jobs. The homeopaths unsuccessfully sought one ward in each of the city hospitals where their own practitioners could treat patients who preferred the milder therapy.[144] They also applied for appointments in the state's mental institutions. Under Governor Lon V. Stephens, they got an opportunity. Governor Stephens, who personally preferred homeopathic treatment, in March 1897 appointed Dr. James T. Coombs of Kansas City as superintendent of State Lunatic Asylum No. 1 at Fulton. The regular doctors protested the appointment and predicted that the patients at Fulton would suffer under the new system of treatment. Instead, Dr.

Coombs's administration brought a definite improvement at the institution.[145] The   hospital was restored to control by doctors of the regular school in 1902.[146]

The code barred consultation between members of the national association and homeopaths. The New York State Medical Society broke with the national organization and adopted a new set of rules permitting consultation with homeopaths and other schools recognized by state law.[147]

The act, of March 29, 1883, establishing the State Board of Health of Missouri, provided that in appointments to the board "there shall be no discrimination made against the different systems of medicine that are recognized as reputable by the laws of this state."[148]

Governor Thomas T. Crittenden, who was largely responsible for the creation of the state board, addressed the Missouri Medical Association at its meeting on May 15, 1883. He urged the association to follow the example of the New York state society and "to preserve to each physician perfect liberty to decide with whom he shall act."[149]

Dr. A. E. Gore, president of the Missouri society, replied to the governor's address with a scathing attack on homeopathy:[150]

We believe homeopathy an imposition from beginning to end; conceived in the brain of a visionary fanatic, who had failed as a regular practitioner of medicine, and adopted this deception for the purpose of imposing upon and fleecing a credulous public.

Dr. Gore rejected unconditionally any cooperation or consultation between regular physicians and homeopaths.[151]

A provision of the code that caused much trouble was the ban on advertising by physicians. It was aimed at a favorite means used by quacks for attracting business. In December 1894, Dr. Heine Marks, one of St. Louis's leading physicians and the superintendent of the city hospital, was charged with violating the code by giving information to the press regarding operations he performed at the hospital.[152] He was found guilty and was asked to resign from the society, but chose to ignore the request.[153]

A major issue was created by the emergence of contract plans for medical and hospital care. An example of the new service was the system established by the Missouri Pacific Railway for its employees. Also, several joint stock companies had been formed to provide care on a prepaid basis. The companies collected monthly premiums and hired doctors to provide the stipulated services.[154] The new plan was opposed by the local medical society because it would interpose a third party between doctor and patient. It would also reduce the doctor's income by the amount of the company's operating costs and profits. A campaign was waged to force the resignation from the local society of all physicians connected with contract medical plans.[155]

8. Treatment of the Insane

The report of a legislative committee, appointed by the governor to inspect the various state institutions, revealed that in 1889 there were 3,501 cases of insanity in Missouri. The figure did not include the population of several private asylums, which would likely bring the total to approximately 4,000 persons.[156]

The numbers of these patients confined in St. Louis and state hospitals were as follows: St. Louis Insane Asylum, 530; St. Louis Poorhouse, 449; Missouri State Asylum No. 1 (Fulton), 548; Asylum No. 2 (St. Joseph), 482; Asylum No. 3 (Nevada), 206; State Penitentiary, 50. The total in these institutions was 2,265. Twelve hundred and thirty-six insane persons were kept in the counties, the majority in poorhouses and in private accommodations.[157]

The quality of treatment in these hospitals varied greatly. The St. Louis Insane Asylum and poorhouse, because of overcrowding, offered little more than custodial care. A major reason for this was that many patients were brought to St. Louis from other communities and abandoned. They were picked up wandering about the streets and, after a superficial examination, sent to the asylum or poorhouse. Since most of these patients were incurable cases, they had to be confined until death released them.

The state's three asylums could be more selective. They were permitted to refuse admission to persons they considered would not profit from treatment; and they could send back to the counties patients they judged could not benefit from additional care.[158]

The origin of this dual system of state and local care for the insane dated back to 1868 when St. Louis County, because of the difficulty of getting its patients over poor roads and the unbridged Missouri River to the Fulton asylum, opened its own mental hospital.[159] This was transferred to the city of St. Louis in 1877. Shortly afterwards, St. Louis asked the legislature for an appropriation to assist in caring for patients from outside its limits. Governor John S. Phelps vetoed a $70,000 legislative grant on the grounds that the St. Louis asylum was not a state institution. The issue was appealed to the Missouri Supreme Court, which rendered an opinion in behalf of the city. But the court attached a condition that any funds appropriated must be used exclusively for the treatment of patients for which the state was responsible.[160] This barred St. Louis citizens from any benefits from the state appropriation.

In accordance with the court's decision, the legislature made appropriations for the use of the St. Louis institution, beginning with a $70,000 grant for 1877-1878. The subsidy was reduced to $50,000 for the biennial periods starting in 1883 and 1885, but was raised to $70,000 in 1887 and 1889, and to $85,000 in 1891. For the rest of the decade, the biennial subsidies were as follows: 1893, $50,000; 1895, $40,000; 1897, $30,000; 1899, $40,000.[161]

The subsidy for the asylum was the source of continuing friction and ill feeling between the legislature and the city of St. Louis. Despite the fact that the city of St. Louis contributed one third of the state's taxes, its citizens were deprived of any benefits from state appropriations for treatment of the mentally ill.[162] The grants that were made to St. Louis for the treatment of outsiders were less generous than those given to the state's three asylums.[163] Further, St. Louis was given no credit for the fact that its mental hospital was constructed with local rather than state funds.[164]

The state legislature had valid complaints against St. Louis. The annual payments made to St. Louis were placed in the city's general revenue fund and no accounting was made of how the asylum subsidy was used. The city was never able to give accurate figures regarding how many outsiders it was taking care of in its asylum. The homeless, destitute and mentally deranged persons involved were often unable or unwilling to tell where they formerly resided.[165]

The legislature, in order to get more satisfactory information on how its grants were used, attached the following restriction on its

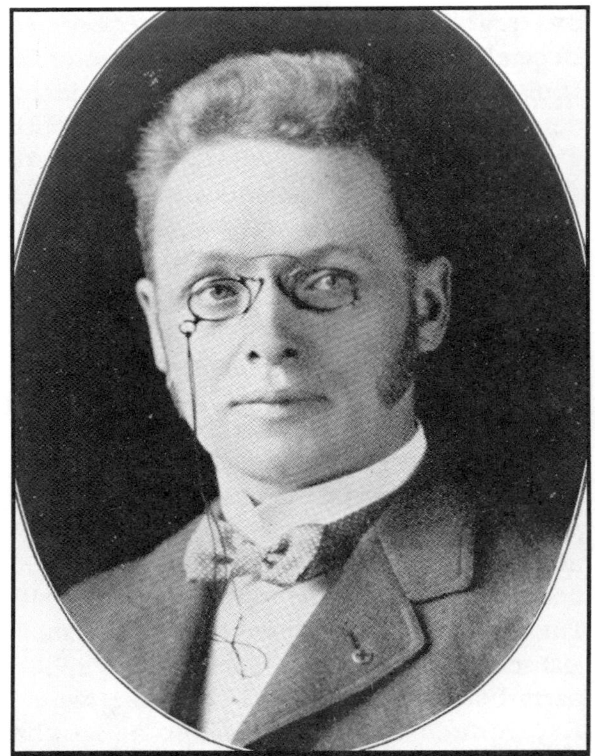

Missouri Historical Society, Edward C. Runge, M. D. Notable St. Louisians, 1990, p. 131.
Dr. Edward C. Runge

1899 subsidy of $40,000 to the St. Louis asylum:[166]

The officers of said asylum shall make under oath a detailed and itemized statement to the state auditor of the manner in which and the purposes for which said appropriation was expended, and shall keep a separate account under the head of "state appropriation for the support of the St. Louis Insane Asylum," showing how said appropriation was expended, and no part thereof shall be expended except for the support of the inmates of said asylum.

An enlightening account of the state of the art for the treatment of insanity is found in the 1898 report of Dr. Edward C. Runge, superintendent of the St. Louis Insane Asylum. Dr. Runge, a native of St. Petersburg, Russia, emigrated to the United States and settled in St. Louis. From St. Louis Medical College, he received his M.D. degree in 1891. He was appointed superintendent of the St. Louis Insane Asylum in 1895.[167]

Dr. Runge began his report with a short discussion of the nature of insanity. He stated that there is a narrow dividing line between sanity and insanity, and that a healthy body is the key to sound mental health. According to Dr. Runge, "Any condition of the brain that affects the psychic centers, no matter how induced, should bear the label 'insanity'." He cited acute alcoholic intoxication as an example of insanity.[168]

Dr. Runge's program of therapy followed naturally from his definition of insanity:[169]

The medical treatment of the patients has not differed to any extent from the one previously reported. Plenty of fresh air and good nourishing food, exercise in some cases, rest in others, have filled and will fill for all time to come the most important place under this caption. Prolonged and oft-repeated baths have been again employed with a great deal of success, especially in cases of unadulterated mania simplex, one young man recovering under the hydropathic regimen without ever having taken a single dose of medicine, and another patient, a girl aged 17, did as well, but for five small doses of trional. The opium treatment fulfilled its promises only in a few instances. In the light of our present knowledge our chief aim must be to improve the general nutrition, and thus to affect favorably the special nutrition of the brain; besides, our efforts are to

be directed toward reaching the psychic cerebral centers with measures of a psychic nature. With regard to the use and results of hypnotics and other means of combatting insomnia, I state again that we have employed the former to but a small extent.

During 1898, 196 patients received hypnotics. For women, potassium bromide was most frequently used; for male patients, choral hydrate was favored. Morphine, duboisine and hyoscyamine were administered in cases of patients passing through the maniacal phase of dementia paralytical. Trional was found to be a safe and effective depressant.[170]

To relieve overcrowding in existing facilities, two new asylums were constructed. The first stage of Missouri's third mental hospital, located at Nevada, Missouri, was completed in the fall of 1887. This consisted of the center building and three wings. Three additional wings were planned to provide a maximum capacity of 600 patients.[171]

The Sisters of Saint Vincent's Order in 1896 moved their asylum from a downtown location to a ninety-three acre site on the Wabash Railway close to Normandy, about a mile beyond the city limits. The new site combined the quiet of the country with the beauty of nature. A four-story brick building, consisting of a central section and two extensive wings, was erected; the overall frontage was 700 feet. The main section was devoted to administrative functions. The two wings contained private and ward rooms for patients. The designed capacity was 500 inmates. The structure was the largest — and possibly the finest — private asylum in the United States.[172]

St. Vincent's differed in several ways from the usual public institutions. The Sisters had a strict rule against overcrowding, so that each patient was guaranteed the space and privacy needed for his restoration to normalcy. The architectural model of the building was that of a home rather than a prison. Locks and bars were used only in extreme cases. A complete separation of violent patients from the harmless unfortunates was enforced. Extensive gardens and a modern dairy provided much of the food for the staff and patients.[173]

9. State Board of Health

The first state board of health consisted of Dr. E. H. Gregory, president; Dr. G. M. Cox of Springfield, vice president; Dr. J. C. Hearne of Hannibal, secretary; Dr. P. D. Yost and Dr. W. B. Conery of St. Louis; Dr. G. T. Barrett of Poplar Bluff and Dr. H. E. Hereford of Kansas City.[174] Drs. Gregory, Hearne, Conery, Barrett and Hereford were allopathic physicians. Dr. Yost belonged to the Eclectic school.[175] Dr. Cox practiced according to homeopathic principles, although he had a diploma also in allopathic medicine.[176] Dr. Gregory was a prominent physician of St. Louis and was elected president of the American Medical Association when it met in St. Louis in 1886.[177]

The legislature gave the board an initial appropriation of $6,000.[178] One of the committee's first acts was the publication of a circular treating the control of contagious diseases. The circular established the procedure for the reporting by doctors of cases of contagious diseases under their care. The reports were to be filed with the county clerks for forwarding to the state board. The circular provided for the quarantining in their homes of persons suffering from contagious diseases, the removal where necessary of serious cases to county or city hospitals, and the fumigation of dwellings following occupation by persons suffering from communicable infections.[179]

The circular, which duplicated the system of disease control in St. Louis, aroused a mixed reaction. It laid the burden of collecting and forwarding disease reports on the county clerks, who were also made responsible for posting quarantine signs and for arranging the transfer of serious cases to hospitals.[180] The extra duties, which would involve constant risk from disease infection, were imposed on the clerks without any provision for compensation or assistance.[181] It is probable that this circular turned the clerks, the most powerful people in the county courthouses, against the new organization.

The board, at its meeting in Jefferson City, January 9, 1884, refused to recognize the St. Louis Eclectic Medical College, the Kansas City Hospital College of Medicine and the American Eclectic Medical College of Cincinnati as institutions in good standing.[182]

In exercising its control over the accrediting of physicians, the board revoked the licenses of a number of doctors and turned down many applications for permission to practice. The total number of practitioners thus eliminated approached 100 during the first year of the committee's operation.[183] Although the doctors eliminated were probably inefficient, in many cases they were all that certain rural communities had or could afford.

Meanwhile, the legislature and many citizens, especially in the rural areas, were having second thoughts about the state organization. They questioned whether it would work successfully in Missouri where local boards of health were practically nonexistent and where public revenues were   minimal.

The St. Louis *Republican,* in an editorial of May 7, 1884, expressed these misgivings:[184]

A law is passed and a state board of health created. The members are appointed, usually without salary. Then it is found that to render the work of the board effective a somewhat cumbrous machinery is necessary. There must be chemists, analysts, veterinarians, inspectors and a system of records with clerks to keep them. It is found that in order to enforce penalties in the courts a somewhat expensive process is required in securing evidence. Naturally the board wants its special attorney to look after its prosecutions. Thus the number of officers and employees increases rapidly. The field is limitless. Abuses everywhere seem to call for investigation and correction. Legislators become sensible that the public views with distrust a great increase in the number of paid employees, and the result generally is a scant appropriation, which necessarily curtails the work and often renders the board almost powerless.

A movement in the legislature, in February 1885, to terminate the board drew strong opposition from the Missouri State Medical Association and other medical organizations.[185] Responding to this show of support, Governor John S. Marmaduke proceeded to fill the existing vacancies on the board. The composition of the new panel was as follows: Dr. Albert Merrell, St. Louis, Eclectic; Dr. George Homan, St. Louis, allopathist; Dr. Jefferson D. Griffith, Kansas City, allopathist; Dr. G. A. Goben, Kirksville, allopathist; Dr. George M. Cox, Springfield, homeopathist; Major William Gentry, Sedalia, farmer and stockman; and James B. Prather, Maryville, farmer and stockman. The board organized by appointing Major Gentry president and Dr. Homan secretary.[186]

The governor called attention to the fact that the law creating the board gave it responsibility for diseases among livestock. To emphasize this part of the board's responsibility, he had added to it two farmers and stockmen.[187]

The new board was designed to elicit statewide support for its work. The dominant role of St. Louis was eliminated; the city's representation was reduced from three to two members. While the original board had consisted entirely of doctors, the new panel had two nonprofessional members.

The legislature, indifferent or even hostile, ceased making appropriations for the board. From 1885 to 1889, the members and the secretary paid the costs of operation out of their own pockets.[188]

The board avoided the mistake of its predecessor in trying to do too much too quickly. An important achievement was the establishment at the state university in Columbia of a laboratory for preparing fresh vaccine virus.[189]

The board continued the registration of qualified physicians. The work was facilitated by the decision of the Missouri Supreme Court in the case of *E. G. Granville vs. the State Board of Health*, decided in December 1884, in which the court ruled that the board of health had the authority to draft reasonable criteria for judging whether the diploma of a candidate for registration was from "a legally chartered medical institution in good standing." In performing this function, the decisions of the board were not subject to overrule by writ of mandamus. The graduates of schools found not "in good standing" could be denied certification for practice in Missouri.[190]

The registry of physicians, as of December 31, 1886, showed a total of 4,105 practitioners. Of these 3,104 were graduates of medical colleges, 977 were certified on the basis of five years of service in Missouri before the medical practice act went into effect and 24 were granted certificates following examinations before the board.[191]

In its report covering the period July 2, 1885, to December 31, 1886, the board recommended the following measures:[192]

a local board of health in every county and large town in the state; compensation of county clerks for making reports; the extension of the board's quarantine authority to communicable diseases among animals; the enlargement of the vaccine laboratory so as to embrace experimental researches into biology and bacteriology; the appropriation of an emergency health fund, to be drawn on when pestilential diseases threaten to become epidemic; and the subjection of accoucheurs and midwives to the practice act.

Dr. George Homan, secretary of the board, in June 1888, sent inquiries to the clerks of every county in the state seeking information regarding the existence of county health boards and county health officers, and also concerning town or city boards. The replies indicated there were county health officers in six counties, i.e., St. Charles, Clay, Pettis, Moniteau, Buchanan and Schuyler. In Pettis and Schuyler, there were also county boards of health. Twenty cities had local boards of health. Regarding the question whether public opinion favored the organization and maintenance of county boards of health, there were eight unqualified "Yes" replies from counties, and eight unqualified "Nos." There were also twelve qualified favorable replies and twenty-two qualified negative responses.[193]

The opposition to the establishment of local boards of health is understandable. The major mission of a board of health would be to make war on nuisances, such as unpenned hogs, contaminated water supplies, insanitary privies, filthy stables and foul-smelling industries like slaughterhouses. All of these were customary features of small towns and rural communities. People change old ways slowly, particularly when improvement has a price tag.

The report of Dr. Homan at the organization's meeting in Jefferson City, January 29, 1891, expressed frustration over the board's inability to awaken concern over public health:[194]

If any spirit of sanitary progress, or desire to excel in that form of wisdom which aims to prevent rather than cure, ever pervaded the state, it seems dead or dying — the only evidence to the contrary being the efforts of medical men, individually and through their local and State societies, to arouse the public to a sense of the necessities of the situation.

Only two counties, the report indicated, had made the returns of births and deaths for 1890, as required by law. The obligation of doctors to give early notification of the occurrence of contagious diseases in their practice was being generally disregarded.[195]

On the positive side, the report called attention to the growing interest on the part of doctors throughout the state in extending the required medical course from two to three years. Already nine of the state's medical colleges, located in St. Louis, Kansas City and St. Joseph, were requiring three years of attendance as a condition of graduation. Advances in medical science were mentioned as the cause of the extension:[196]

Medicine to-day is not the same art and science as that of a few years ago. To-day the clinic, the laboratory, the demonstration constitute the medical school — not a set of text-books or their rehearsal in the classroom.

Another hopeful sign was that in 1889, after a four-year lapse in payments, the legislature appropriated $3,000 for the salary of the secretary of the board of health and $1,000 for the expenses of the board for 1889 and 1890. In addition, $1,070.60 was provided for reimbursing members for personal funds they had expended during the past two years in carrying out their duties.[197]

The legislature, in 1891, appropriated $5,000 for the support of the board of health, including the salary of the secretary, the recording of vital and mortuary statistics and the expenses of the office. The grant covered a two-year period.[198] Two years later, the basic appropriation was raised to $5,500. In addition, the legislature established a credit of $10,000, which the board could use for the preservation of public health in case an epidemic of Asiatic cholera attacked the state.[199]

By a law approved April 18, 1893, the general assembly reduced the terms of the seven members of the board to four years. Members, at the time the law was passed, however, were permitted to serve the full terms for which they were appointed.[200]

The two-year appropriation for the board was reduced to $5,000 in 1895. The legislature that year authorized the board to request the services of the state veterinarian to aid in the investigation of diseases of livestock, which were transmissible to human beings, and in the examination of meats, milk and other foods for wholesomeness.[201] Laws of 1897 and 1899 made appropriations of $5,000 for the salary of the secretary and other expenses of the board.

In January 1895, a bill was introduced in the legislature providing for the creation of local boards of health in every county of the state. It passed the house but was defeated in the senate.[202]

The existence of smallpox in a number of communities induced the state board of health to place the penitentiary in Jefferson City under quarantine. The board, in order to force the counties to establish local health organizations, on May 10, 1895, passed a resolution to the effect that no prisoner would be received at the penitentiary unless he was accompanied by a health certificate signed by the board of health of the county from which he was sent.[203]

The board of health, also at the May meeting, established the policy that a medical school must have a graded course of study in order to be considered "in good standing." In many medical institutions, the second year was merely a repetition of the first.[204]

In its continuing campaign to improve medical education, the board inaugurated the rule that matriculates of all state medical colleges must be graduates of high schools or colleges, or if not graduates, at least qualified to pass examinations for first grade teaching certificates. The board sent notices to the various medical schools in the state asking for information regarding the basis on which each of its students had been matriculated. From an examination of the replies, the board determined that 185 students enrolled in St. Louis medical schools did not meet the preliminary educational requirements and would have to withdraw. The numbers of students enrolled and the totals of deficient students were distributed as follows: Barnes Medical College, 275 students, number who failed to pass, 97; St. Louis Medical College, 70 students, number who failed to pass, 15; Missouri Medical College, 260 students, number who failed to pass, 30; Marion-Sims, 200 students, number who failed to pass, 7; Beaumont, 75 students, number who failed to pass, 6; Physicians and Surgeons, 230 students, number who failed to pass, 30. The American Eclectic Medical College, the Homeopathic Medical College and the Woman's Medical College were fortunate that all their students met the matriculation requirements.[205]

Since the passage of the medical practice act of March 27, 1874, the possession of a diploma from a legally chartered medical school "in good standing" had entitled a candidate to certification in Missouri. Profiting from the experience of the state of Illinois, the Missouri Board of Health had developed certain criteria for determining the good standing of a medical school. The school must have a complete faculty of qualified professors; it must offer a three-year course of study; the students enrolled must have the equivalent of a high school or college education.

The board of health, in its 1893 report, proposed a more efficient method of screening candidates than the current one of trying to evaluate the colleges from which they received their degrees:[206]

> The duty of pronouncing upon the standing of medical colleges in all parts of the world is one that, from the circumstances of the case, cannot be satisfactorily performed by any State Board of Health; and this duty has been largely imposed upon this Board during the past by the immigration into this State of physicians from all quarters of the globe.

As other States become more stringent in their requirements, their refuse material crowds into Missouri. An examining board that would accept no diplomas, but require the only evidence of knowledge, i.e., the passing of a thorough examination as to the acquirements and qualifications of the applicants — would protect the people of the State against ignorant practitioners, and relieve the Board of a difficult, delicate and disagreeable duty, as well as stimulate all medical educational institutions to the establishment of a higher standard for graduation, and more thorough methods of instruction.

The board of health prepared and sent to the legislature a bill calling for the creation of a state board of medical examiners.[207] The proposal failed to win the approval of the general assembly.

Chapter VI
State Involvement in Health Services, 1883-1900

1 James Neal Primm, *Lion of the Valley: St. Louis, Missouri* (Boulder, Colorado, Pruett Publishing Co., 1981), p. 345.

2 Primm dramatically describes this contrast: "The great commerical emporium had not served the poor well. The squalor of 'Castle Thunder,' 'Wildcat Chute,' and 'Clabbor Alley' and other degraded tenements and hovels, wage-cuts, chronic hunger and unemployment, and municipal soup kitchens stood in stark contrast to the lordly mansions which loomed behind the market, the elegant ladies who descended daintily from their glittering carriages, and the rich merchants and land-lords who dined on lobster and champagne at Tony Faust's Oyster House, one of the nation's finest restaurants." Primm, *opus cit.*, p. 328.

3 St. Louis *Republic*, Jan. 18, 1899, p. 9:2-4.

4 *Ibid.*, June 18, 1890, p. 4:5-6.

5 *Idem.*

6 *Ibid.*, Aug. 9, 1896, p. 32.

7 *Ibid.*, Jan. 18, 1899, p. 9:2-4.

8 *Ibid.*, Nov. 22, 1896, p. 24.

9 St. Louis *Missouri Republican*, Nov. 23, 1873, p. 4:6.

10 *Idem.*

11 *Ibid.*, Mar. 7, 1874, p. 4:3.

12 John A. Garraty, *The American Nation: A History of the United States* (New York, Harper and Row Publishers, 1966), p. 535.

13 David D. March, *The History of Missouri* (New York, Lewis Historical Publishing Co., 1967), Vol. II, p. 1225.

14 *Ibid.*, Vol. II, p. 1226.

15 St. Louisans had a special title for this type of political corruption: "Boodle was the local term for the practice of bribing city officials or legislators to win utilities franchises, licenses, low tax assessments, garbage cotracts, or other special privileges." Primm, *opus cit.*, pp. 374-375.

16 St. Louis *Republican*, Apr. 15, 1885, p. 10:5.

17 St. Louis *Republic*, Nov. 30, 1892, p. 4:3.

18 St. Louis *Missouri Republican*, Mar. 21, 1871, p. 2:6.

19 *The Revised Ordinances of the City of St. Louis 1887* (St. Louis, Nixon, Jones Printing Co., 1887, p. 591.

20 St. Louis *Republican*, Jan. 23, 1887, p. 16:3.

21 *Ibid.*, Feb. 1, 1887, p. 5:1.

22 *Ibid.*, Jan. 19, 1887, p. 5:3-4.

23 *Laws of Missouri, Passed at the Session of the Thirty-Fifth General Assembly, Begun and Held at the City of Jefferson, January 2, 1889.* Regular Session (Jefferson City, Mo., Tribune Printing Co., 1889) p. 92.

24 *Ibid.*, p. 93.

25 *Laws of Missouri, Passed at the Session of the Thirty-Sixth General Assembly, Begun and Held at the City of Jefferson, January 7, 1891.* Regular Session (Jefferson City, Mo., Tribune Printing Co., 1891) p. 163.

26 William Hyde and Howard L. Conard, eds., *Encyclopedia of the History of St. Louis* (New York, The Southern History Co., 1899) Vol. IV, pp. 2127-2128.

27 "Historical Notes and Comments," *Missouri Historical Review*, Vol. XXXVI (Oct. 1941), No. 1, p. 389.

28 St. Louis *Republic*, Mar. 28. 1896, p. 11:6.

29 St. Louis *Republican*, Jan. 27, 1885, p. 9:6. *Ibid.*, June 30, 1885, p. 5:3.

30 *Ibid.*, May 20, 1885, p. 9:1-3.

31 *The Revised Ordinances of the City of St. Louis 1887* (St. Louis, Nixon-Jones Printing Co., 1887) pp. 575-576.

32 St. Louis *Missouri Republican*, July 22, 1868, p. 2:8.

33 St. Louis *Republican*, Aug. 10, 1884, p. 9:3.

34 *Ibid.*, Nov. 6, 1883, p. 3:6, *ibid.*, Sept. 9, 1884, p. 10:3.

35 *Ibid.*, Mar. 7, 1885, p. 5:4; *ibid.*, Mar. 29, 1885, p. 18:1-2.

36 *Ibid.*, Mar. 7, 1885, p. 5:4.

37 St. Louis *Globe-Democrat*, Mar. 24, 1885, p. 8:1.

38 St. Louis *Republican*, Apr. 1, 1885, p. 8:3.

39 *Ibid.*, June 10, 1885, p. 7:1.

40 *Ibid.*, June 16, 1885, p. 9:2.

41 *Idem.*

42 *Ibid.*, July 8, 1885, p. 5:1-2. The well-closing law was repealed July 7, 1885.

43 *Ibid.*, Mar. 20, 1878, p. 2:4-5.

44 *Idem.*

45 *Idem.*

46 *Ibid.*, Mar. 1, 1879, p. 4:6.

47 *Idem.*

48 *Ibid.*, July 9, 1881, p. 5:1.

49 *Ibid.*, July 23, 1881, p. 7:1-4. At Bissell's Point the drain pipe for sluicing out the settling basins was below the level of the river at its high stages.

50 *Ibid.*, Oct. 13, 1885, p. 6:6.

51 *Idem.*

52 *Ibid.*, Aug. 1, 1887, p. 4:2-3.

53 *Ibid.*, Sept. 8, 1887, p. 7:3.

54 *Ibid.*, Oct. 18, 1887, p. 4:7.

55 *Ibid.*, Nov. 6, 1887, p. 3:3.

56 *Ibid.*, Jan. 31, 1888, p. 9:5.

57 St. Louis *Republic*, Nov. 20, 1894, p. 6:4.

58 *Idem.*

59 *Ibid.*, Apr. 7, 1895, p. 6:3.

60 *Ibid.*, June 14, 1896, p. 9:1.

61 *Ibid.*, Aug. 18, 1896, p. 1:5.

62 *Ibid.*, Mar. 25, 1897, p. 8:1.

63 *Ibid.*, Oct. 24, 1899, p. 14:3.

64 *Idem.*

65 *Ibid.*, Nov. 18, 1899, part II, p. 1:6.

66 *Idem.*

67 *Ibid.*, Nov. 18, 1899, Part II, p. 1:1-3.

68 *Ibid.*, Jan. 27, 1900, p. 8:2.

69 *Ibid.*, Mar. 24, 1895, p. 12:3-4.

70 Hyde and Conard, *opus cit.*, Vol. IV, pp. 2311-2312.

71 St. Louis *Republic*, Mar. 22, 1896, p. 26:1-3.

72 *Encyclopedia Americana* (New York, Americana Corporation, 1953) Vol. IX, pp. 139-140.

73 St. Louis *Republic*, Mar. 25, 1896, p. 1:2-3.

74 *Ibid.*, Mar. 20, 1897, part II, p. 1:6.

75 Max A. Goldstein, ed., *One Hundred Years of Medicine and Surgery in Missouri* (St. Louis, St. Louis Star, 1900) p. 84.

76 St. Louis *Republic*, Dec. 28, 1889, p. 1:2; *ibid.*, Sept. 21, 1890, p. 21:3.

77 Hyde and Conard, *opus cit.*, Vol. IV, pp. 2559-2560.

78 *Ibid.*, p. 2560.

79 *Ibid.*, p. 2561.

80 Goldstein, *opus cit.*, p. 84.

81 St. Louis *Republic*, Dec. 24, 1894, p. 8:4.

82 *Ibid.*, May 19, 1887, p. 10:3; *ibid.*, Jan. 21, 1889, p. 8:2-3.

83 *Ibid.,* Dec. 8, 1894, p. 3:5.

84 *Ibid.,* Dec. 17, 1894, p. 1:5-6.

85 *Ibid.,* Jan. 6, 1895, p. 14:3.

86 Goldstein, *opus cit.,* p. 84.

87 *Idem.*

88 St. Louis *Republic,* Nov. 23, 1894, p. 8:2.

89 Goldstein, *opus cit.,* p. 84.

90 *Idem.*

91 *Idem.*

92 St. Louis *Republic,* Dec. 5, 1892, p. 2:5.

93 *Idem.*

94 Goldstein, *opus cit.,* p. 84.

95 Tuberculosis, at least until the germ theory, was considered a hereditary affliction. Besides, its onset was usually so slow and with so few visible signs of suffering and decay that little effort was made to guard against its transmission. St. Louis *Republic,* Dec. 23, 1894, p. 24:3-4.

96 St. Louis *Republic,* Mar. 11, 1898, p. 8:7.

97 *Ibid.,* Jan. 22, 1898, part II, p. 1:1.

98 *Ibid.,* Mar. 11, 1898, p. 8:7.

99 Ibid., Jan. 4, 1891, p., 5:7.

100 Robert P. Hudson, "Abraham Flexner in Perspective: American Medicine Education 1865-1910." Judith W. Leavitt and Ronald L. Numbers, eds., *Sickness and Health in America: Readings in the History of Medicine and Public Health* (Madison, Wisc., The University of Wisconsin Press, 1978), p. 109; St. Louis *Republic,* Jan. 29, 1891, p. 5:3.

101 St. Louis *Republic,* Apr. 26, 1892, p. 7:2-3.

102 *Ibid.,* Apr. 14, 1898, p. 7:4.

103 *Ibid.,* Mar. 17, 1894, p. 7:4.

104 Ronald Numbers, "Do-It-Yourself the Sectarian Way," Leavitt and Numbers, *opus cit.,* p. 89.

105 Robert P. Hudson, "Abraham Flexner in Perspective: American Medical Education 1865-1910," Leavitt and Numbers, *opus cit.,* p. 110.

106 *Idem.*

107 St. Louis *Republic,* Apr. 19, 1899, p. 5:5.

108 *Ibid.,* Oct. 5, 1890, p. 21:3.

109 Hyde and Conard, eds., *opus cit.,* Vol. III, p. 1382.

110 Goldstein, ed., *One Hundred Years of Medicine and Surgery in Missouri,* p. 169.

111 St. Louis *Republican,* Dec. 7, 1886, p. 7:3.

112 St. Louis *Republic,* Jan. 1, 1893, p. 25:1-2.

113 *Ibid.,* Jan. 24, 1897, p. 18:4.

114 *Ibid.,* Aug. 12, 1888, p. 21:3-4. Under Health Commissioner Starkloff, who took office in 1895, steps were taken to improve the city hospital staff. Under his administration, it comprised the superintendent, an assistant superintendent, two senior physicians and eighteen internes. St. Louis *Republic,* Sept. 10, 1897, p. 9:5-6.

115 St. Louis *Republican,* Jan. 28, 1885, p. 8:3.

116 St. Louis *Republic,* June 24, 1888, p. 17:7.

117 *Ibid.,* p. 17:1-5.

118 *Ibid.,* p. 17:5.

119 *Ibid.,* p. 17:4-5.

120 *Ibid.,* June 27, 1888, p. 4:6.

121 *Ibid.,* May 28, 1896, p. 1.

122 *Ibid.,* July 10, 1896, p. 11:3, *ibid.,* Jan. 13, 1899, p. 6:4-5.

123 *Ibid.,* Mar. 25, 1897, p. 3:5; *ibid.,* Mar. 23, 1897, p. 11:4.

124 *Ibid.,* Aug. 11, 1898, p. 12:2.

125 *Idem.*

126 *Ibid.,* July 13, 1899, p. 11:3.

127 *Ibid.,* June 28, 1899, p. 6:4.

128 *Idem.* The ordinance providing for the nonpolitical management of the new city hospital was killed by Ed Butler's combine by a vote of ten to three in the upper house of the municipal assembly on Nov. 7, 1899. St. Louis *Republic,* Nov. 8, 1899, p. 5:4.

129 St. Louis *Republic,* June 28, 1899, p. 6:4.

130 Edwin A. Christ, *Missouri's Nurses: The Development of the Profession, Its Associations, and Its Institutions* (Jefferson City, The Missouri State Nurses' Association, 1957), p. 63.

131 *Idem.*

132 *Idem.*

133 St. Louis *Republic,* Aug. 12, 1888, p. 21:3-4.

134 Christ, *opus cit.,* pp. 65-77. The following St. Louis hospitals established training programs: St. Luke's Hospital Training School, 1889; Evangelical Deaconess Hospital and Training School for Nurses, 1889; Protestant Hospital Training School for Nurses, 1890; Rebekah Hospital Training School for Nurses, 1893; St. Louis Baptist Hospital Training School for Nurses, 1893; Mullanphy Hospital Training School for Nurses, 1894; Missouri Baptist Sanitarium Training School for Nurses, 1895; Mayfield Sanitarium Training School for Nurses, 1896.

135 St. Louis *Republic,* May 7, 1899, part IV, p. 12:1-4.

136 Christ, *opus cit.,* p. 70.

137 St. Louis *Republic,* Mar. 14, 1900, p. 7:1-2.

138 *Ibid.,* Feb. 1, 1897, p. 7:2.

139 *Ibid.,* June 7, 1895, p. 14:2.

140 "Image and Income," Leavitt and Numbers, *opus cit.,* p. 129.

141 Gould's *Directory of St. Louis, 1892, passim.*

142 St. Louis *Republic,* Jan. 21, 1894, p. 13:3-4.

143 St. Louis *Missouri Republican,* June 5, 1885, p. 5:3.

144 *Ibid.,* June 20, 1876, p. 8:4.

145 Donald H. Ewalt, Jr., "Patients, Politics and Physicians: The Struggle for Control of State Lunatic Asylum No. 1, Fulton, Missouri," *Missouri Historical Review,* Vol. LXXVII, No. 2(January 1983), pp. 172-174, 183-184.

146 *Ibid.,* p. 187.

147 St. Louis *Republican,* June 23, 1887, p. 9:5.

148 *The Revised Statutes of the State of Missouri, Revised and Promulgated by the Thirty-Fifth General Assembly, 1889* (Jefferson City, Mo., Tribune Printing Co., 1889), pp. 1298-1299.

149 St. Louis *Republican,* May 16, 1883, p. 3:3-4.

150 *Idem.*

151 *Idem.* This hard line attitude was reflected in the action of the American Medical Association in 1885 expelling from its membership those doctors owing allegiance to the New York State Medical Society. *Ibid.,* June 23, 1887, p. 9:5.

152 St. Louis *Republic,* Dec. 11, 1894, p. 1:4-6.

153 *Ibid.,* Mar. 25, 1895, p. 5:4.

154 *Ibid.,* Mar. 28, 1897, p. 3:4.

155 *Idem.*

156 *Report of the Committee Appointed by the Governor to Visit the Various State Institutions.* Thirty-Fifth General Assembly (Jefferson City, Mo., Tribune Printing Co.,

1889), p. 29. Published in *Appendix to Senate and House Journals of the Thirty-Fifth General Assembly of the State of Missouri, 1889* (Jefferson City, Mo., Tribune Printing Co., 1889)

157 *Idem.*

158 *General Statutes of the State of Missouri, Revised by Committee Appointed by the Twenty-Third General Assembly* (Jefferson City, Emory S. Foster, Public Printer, 1866), pp. 304-307.

159 St. Louis *Republic*, June 27, 1888, p. 4:6; St. Louis *Missouri Republican*, Aug. 12, 1869, p. 2:4.

160 *Appendix to Senate and House Journals of the Fortieth General Assembly of the State of Missouri 1899* (Jefferson City, Mo., Tribune Printing Co., 1899), p. 137.

161 *Laws of Missouri, 1883-1899, passim.*

162 St. Louis *Republic*, Feb. 18, 1895, p. 4:2-3.

163 *Ibid*, Mar. 9, 1895, p. 11:1. St. Louis's comptroller in a report to the mayor, estimated that during 1893 and 1894 the state appropriated $92.55 per capita biennially for insane patients in its three asylums, but only $46.73 per capita for indigent insane in the St. Louis Insane Asylum.

164 *Idem.*

165 *Appendix to Senate and House Journals, 1899,* p. 138.

166 *Laws of Missouri, Passed at the Session of the Fortieth General Assembly, Begun and Held at the City of Jefferson, January 4, 1899* (Jefferson City, Mo., Tribune Printing Co., 1899), p. 20.

167 Goldstein, ed., *opus cit.,* pp. 326-327.

168 St. Louis *Republic*, Aug. 6, 1898, part II, p. 1:1.

169 *Ibid*, Aug. 6, 1898, part II, p. 1:4.

170 *Idem.*

171 *Ibid*, June 10, 1887, p. 9:5.

172 *Ibid*, Aug. 20, 1893, p. 20:2-5.

173 *Idem.*

174 St. Louis *Republican*, July 24, 1883, p. 5:5.

175 *Ibid*, Aug. 17, 1883, p. 5:5.

176 *Ibid*, July 11, 1884, p. 8:2.

177 *Ibid*, May 7, 1886, p. 3.

178 *Ibid*, Dec. 10, 1887, p. 3:6.

179 *Ibid*, Nov. 18, 1883, p. 2:5.

180 *Idem.*

181 *Idem.*

182 *Ibid*, Jan. 10, 1884, p. 4:7.

183 *Ibid*, July 10, 1884, p. 8:2.

184 *Ibid*, May 7, 1884, p. 4:3.

185 *Ibid*, May 25, 1885, p. 4:4; *ibid*, Feb. 3, 1885, p. 7:2.

186 *Ibid*, June 27, 1885, p. 2:2.

187 *Idem.*

188 *Ibid*, Dec. 10, 1887, p. 3:6.

189 *Ibid*, Jan. 27, 1886, p. 10:5.

190 *Ibid*, Dec. 4, 1884, p. 10:3-5.

191 *Ibid*, Jan. 16, 1887, p. 4:2.

192 *Idem.*

193 St. Louis *Republic*, Aug. 14, 1888, p. 12:5.

194 *Ibid*, Jan. 29, 1891, p. 5:3.

195 *Idem.*

196 *Idem.*

197 *Laws of Missouri, Passed at the Session of the Thirty-Fifth General Assembly, Begun and Held at the City of Jefferson, January 2, 1889* (Jefferson City, Mo., Tribune Printing Co., 1889), p. 7.

198 *Laws of Missouri, Passed at the Session of the Thirty-Sixth General Assembly, Begun and Held at the City of Jefferson, January 7, 1891* (Jefferson City, Mo., Tribune Printing Co., 1891), p. 5.

199 *Laws of Missouri, Passed at the Session of the Thirty-Seventh General Assembly Begun and Held at the City of Jefferson, January 4, 1893* (Jefferson City, Mo., Tribune Printing Co., 1893) p. 5.

200 *Ibid*, p. 177.

201 *Laws of Missouri, Passed at the Session of the Thirty-Eighth General Assembly, Begun and Held at the City of Jefferson, January 2, 1895* (Jefferson City, Mo., Tribune Printing Co., 1895), pp. 6, 37.

202 St. Louis *Republic*, Mar. 23, 1895, p. 11:4.

203 *Ibid*, May 11, 1895, p. 5:1.

204 *Idem.*

205 *Ibid*, Jan. 15, 1896, p. 2:4-5.

206 "*Report of the State Board of Health of the State of Missouri,*" *Thirty-Seventh General Assembly, 1893* (Jefferson City, Mo., Tribine Printing Co., 1893), pp. 9-10. Printed in the *Appendix to Senate and House Journals of the Thirty-Seventh General Assembly of the State of Missouri,* 1893 (Jefferson City, Mo., Tribune Printing Co., 1893) Report No. 20, pp. 9-10.

Chapter 7

An Era of Progress and Reform, 1900-1920

1. A New St. Louis

THE ELECTION OF ROLLA WELLS,[1] on April 2, 1901, marked the emergence of the "New St. Louis." The landslide vote for the Democratic candidate indicated the desire of the citizens of St. Louis for a change from the inefficient and corrupt administration, which had made the government of the city a national disgrace.

The term "boodling" had been coined to describe the bribery of officials in order to secure franchises and contracts. The intellectual as well as moral level of lawmakers was low.[2] The needs of a growing city had been badly neglected. After almost seventy years of the operation of a municipal plant, the water from the faucets was still muddy and contaminated by sewage. The city hospital was conducted in a former convent which was ill-adapted to medical requirements. Mentally ill patients, packed to overflowing in the St. Louis Insane Asylum and the poorhouse, were provided little more than custodial care. The city's business leaders made deals with the corrupt officials, instead of eliminating them and assuming the responsibility of running the city.

The first decade of the twentieth century was a period of reform in the United States.

Theodore Roosevelt carried the banner of Progressivism on the national scene. In major cities, old political machines were overthrown and power returned to the people. Young college-trained men were entering politics and providing honest and efficient leadership. The teachings of the Social Gospel made citizens more conscious of the needs of the sick, the insane and the poor.

The choice of St. Louis as the site for the 1904 World's Fair strengthened the local reform forces. The fair would bring to the city millions of visitors from all over the world. Pride demanded that St. Louis have an abundant supply of clear and wholesome water, adequate sewers, clean streets and first-quality medical and hospital services. Preparation for and operation of the fair united all groups in the magnificent civic enterprise.

The task of destroying the Butler political machine was accomplished by Joseph Folk, a young lawyer elected as circuit attorney in 1900. Folk inaugurated a series of investigations which led to the trial and conviction of key members of the combine. Ed Butler, in a case moved to Columbia on a change of venue, was found guilty of attempting to bribe a member of the St. Louis Board of Health in connection with the award of a contract for the collection and disposal of the city's garbage.[3] Although some members of the combine escaped prison on the basis of legal technicalities, Folk's crusade had the practical effect of putting the Butler coalition out of business.

2. Hospitals and Dispensaries

In becoming acquainted with his new responsibilities, Mayor Wells made a tour of inspection of the city hospital, insane asylum, poorhouse and female hospital. Following his visits, he announced the priorities for his administration:[4]

> Our first duty . . . is towards the poor and infirm who occupy the eleemosynary institutions. If the people of St. Louis could witness the decay of the city's asylum and hospital buildings, and the consequent deplorable conditions existing therein, I have no doubt that they would agree with me.

Realizing the impossibility of satisfactorily repairing the older hospitals, he favored new construction. Since the city had only approximately $250,000 in its building fund, Mayor Wells advocated the issuance of bonds to provide the needed capital. Such a step would require changes in the city charter.[5]

A start had already been made to replace some of the older structures. The municipal assembly, on August 14, 1900, approved a bill appropriating $258,000 from the building fund for the erection of the first units of a new city hospital, to be located on the site of the original hospital destroyed by the 1896 tornado.[6] The initial appropriation was designed to cover the cost of an isolation ward, an octagonal ward, connecting corridors, a laundry, a kitchen and a boiler house. These buildings would constitute an operational hospital with a capacity of 300 patients.[7]

Strikes, shortages of materials, and a scarcity of funds slowed the completion of the total hospital.[8] Small appropriations from the city's general revenue were made from time to time to supplement the one percent earmarked for the building fund.

To secure space for an emergency hospital pending the availability of the new city hospital, the council purchased, for $50,000, the building at the northeast corner of Fourteenth and O'Fallon streets. This edifice, which had been occupied formerly as the Pius Hospital by the Sisters of St. Anthony, was equipped with elevators, laundry, baths and a powerhouse.[9]

Five years after the ground breaking, the new city hospital received its inmates. The move of 400 patients from the old hospital at Seventeenth and Pine streets to the new institution on Carroll, Grattan and Fourteenth streets took place on August 10, 1905. Since there were no elevators in the old building, bedridden patients were strapped to stretchers and carried by orderlies down the narrow stairways to waiting ambulances. Patients, who could sit up, were transported in buses. Ambulatory cases boarded cars for the ride to their new home.[10]

The new hospital consisted of five interconnected buildings. The administrative building provided space for the hospital offices and quarters for the physicians and male employees. Two five-story buildings, designated as Division B, West Octagonal and Division C, East Octagonal, were devoted to hospital wards. Division D had operating rooms on the second floor and reception offices on the ground level. The fifth building housed the kitchen and other service functions.[11]

The building was pronounced by experts to be "as perfect and complete as the present state of medicine, sanitation or building is capable of."[12] In its new home, the city hospital had the facilities to provide the quality of service available in the finest private medical centers, so that it could begin to make the transition from a strictly charitable institution to a fee-based hospital. The city's bacteriological laboratory was established in the hospital and performed laboratory work for the institution's staff and for the local medical fraternity. The separation of male and female patients, which began in 1875, was abandoned in the new quarters.[13]

In an election held June 12, 1906, the Wells administration submitted nine propositions, totaling $11,200,000, for voter approval. In a rare display of public unity and support, all proposals received the required two-thirds vote. Proposition Two provided for the spending of $800,000 for the construction and expansion of hospitals. Proposition Three called for the utilization of $1,000,000 for repairing and enlarging the St. Louis Insane Asylum.[14]

A new four-story addition to city hospital was opened during June 1911. The new wing, costing $1,000,000, completed the occupation of the whole block bounded by Lafayette Avenue, Carroll, Sixteenth and Grattan streets. With the transfer to the enlarged city hospital of the remaining inmates of the female hospital, the building, thus vacated, could be used as an infirmary for old people from the poorhouse. The new wing became the administrative center for the hospital and also served as a home for the nurses.[15]

A major change in the administration of health services in St. Louis was made in April 1910. The change involved the establishment of a separate and independent hospital board and a hospital commissioner. Previously, the board of health and the health commissioner had complete control of all health matters. Following the division of responsibility, the board of health was charged with issues involving sanitation and the prevention of disease, the hospital board with the care and treatment of the sick in public institutions.[16] The hospital board consisted of seven members, with the mayor as presiding officer. No two members of the board could be from the same medical college.[17]

The new law provided for the appointment of a superintendent at each municipal hospital who would conduct business matters. He was to be assisted by a staff of resident physicians. The resident physicians would be directed and supervised by a board of visiting specialists who would have charge of all phases of medical and surgical treatment.[18]

The reasons for the change were persuasive. The growth of the city's population and the expansion of its health services placed an excessive burden upon a single administrative board and commissioner. The hospital superintendent under the old system had to handle business affairs as well as medical and surgical services. He had an assistant superintendent and a staff of senior physicians, junior physicians and internes to assist him. The superintendent and his subordinates were unable to provide the wide spectrum of specialized knowledge and skill needed for treating a hospital population of 500-800 patients, as in city hospital. Politics had played an important role in the choice of members of hospital staffs.[19] It was hoped that this factor would be eliminated under the new system.

Controversy erupted over the method of selecting the visiting specialists. The ordinance governing the issue stated that the "visiting staff shall be appointed by the hospital board and all selections shall be made after investigations of such character as will determine, to the satisfaction of the hospital board, the fitness of the candidate for the position to which he aspires, and in no case shall political reasons govern the appointments."[20] The hospital board divided on the question whether the investigation should include competitive examinations of candidates.[21] Doctors generally opposed having to take examinations.[22] If they did poorly they would suffer damage to their self-image and possibly to their private medical practice. Another controversy was over the formula for the distribution of the visiting positions among the various medical schools.

At a lively meeting on June 10, 1910, the hospital board by a tally of four to three decided to require candidates for the visiting staff to take examinations. However, the board proceeded to select a temporary visiting staff of thirty-six members without formal examinations. To satisfy the principle of fairness, twelve of the visiting doctors were from Washington University, twelve from St. Louis University, and twelve from other medical schools. The distribution by specialties was as follows: general surgery, 7; general medicine, 7; genito-urinary diseases, 4; gynecologists, 3; neurologists, 5; oculists, 5; ear, nose and throat, 4; dermatologists, 2.[23]

A chaotic period, during which incoming patients at city hospital were "simply stored in the institution, awaiting diagnosis," occurred between the passage of the new hospital ordinance and the organization of the first panel of visiting doctors. Dr. Walter C. G. Kirchner, superintendent, and Dr. Cleveland H. Shutt, assistant superintendent, had resigned in protest to the new hospital arrangement.Many of the hospital's staff of internes had quit and the new class of

internes were taking their examinations. The organization of the panel of visiting doctors had been delayed by controversies in the hospital board. Finally on June 14, the visiting staff assembled at city hospital and began the preliminary task of examining the patients on hand and placing them into the categories of medical, surgical and insane cases.[24]

A new hospital bill covering the resident staffs at the municipal hospitals was passed in the summer of 1911. It established the rule that the resident physician, assistant physicians and internes should not serve more than a year, except when reappointed following competitive examination. The request of hospital internes for a small salary was turned down; their compensation consisted of room, board and laundry.[25]

The law authorized the hospital commissioner to appoint pupil nurses at the ratio of one for each six patients. The pupil nurses were of two classes. Junior nurses were those who had not received a year's training and education in nursing in a training school. Senior nurses had been trained for one year or longer in a training school or had been employed for at least a year as junior nurses in the municipal hospital department. The junior nurses received a salary of ten dollars a month, the senior nurses fifteen dollars a month. Both classes got free board, lodging and laundry at the hospital where they were employed.[26]

Although the new city hospital, with its 1911 addition, had a capacity of 700 or more patients, the number of beds available in public institutions had not greatly increased. With the completion of the new building, the old institution at Seventeenth and Pine streets and the female hospital on Arsenal Street had been withdrawn from general hospital use. Thus, the increased capacity at city hospital did little more than balance the number of beds, which had been lost at the emergency hospital and the female hospital. The result was that the municipal hospitals were generally short on space to accommodate the increasing demand.

Several procedures were instituted to reduce hospital overcrowding. Dr. John Young Brown, while superintendent, established outpatient clinics at city hospital. Patients with minor wounds or dislocations were treated and discharged instead of being put into a hospital ward for convalescence. However, they were given an identification card entitling them to return for any follow-up treatment that might be needed. Persons suffering from disease were diagnosed and provided with medicine and counsel. They too were entitled to continued care from the hospital's staff.[27]

A rule was established at city hospital in 1908 limiting its services to those who had been residents of St. Louis for six months. Applicants from outstate, thus rejected, could seek charitable help in one of St. Louis's many private hospitals or clinics.[28]

In times of serious overcrowding at city hospital, the superintendent got in contact with private institutions in the city. Where a private hospital would accept patients and charge only what it would cost to keep them in city hospital, the superintendent would transfer part of the excess of patients to private care.[29]

In addition to its general hospitals, St. Louis had two specialized medical centers. In the city bacteriologist's office in the city hospital, five rooms were set aside for the operation of a Pasteur Institute for the free treatment of hydrophobia. Each summer St. Louis usually had two or three cases a day of this disease. Treatment required injections for upward of fifteen days. The St. Louis clinic was the first in the United States west of the Mississippi.[30]

The high incidence of tuberculosis prompted the hospital board to transform the quarantine station south of Jefferson Barracks into a sanatorium. The station was away from the city's industrial contamination, with plenty of fresh air, sunshine and space for recreation. These were the requisites for the type of treatment then popular in the American Southwest. The institution was named the Robert Koch Hospital, in honor of the German scientist who had discovered the tuberculosis bacillus. Most of the patients sent to quarantine were in the advanced stages of the disease. The emphasis consequently was less on their treatment and cure than on preventing them from spreading the disease in the crowded wards of the city's general hospitals.[31]

The early twentieth century witnessed the organization of new private hospitals and the enlargement of old established ones. The cornerstone of the St. Louis Jewish Hospital at Delmar Avenue, just west of Union Avenue, was laid May 16, 1901. The completed building was dedicated May 18, 1902.[32] It had a capacity of thirty-five patients.

To meet a pressing need, the Sisters of St. Mary built, at Carondelet Heights just south of the River des Peres, the Mount St. Rose Hospital for Consumptives. The building had a frontage of 210 feet and a depth of 50 feet. Two wings extended westward, each with a length of 65 feet. The hospital was the largest of its kind in the Middle West.[33]

In July 1905, the St. Louis Skin and Cancer Hospital on North Jefferson Avenue was founded. It was the second such infirmary in the United States, the other being in New York City. Its initial funds were raised by popular subscription. The rationale for its establishment was that many hospitals refused to admit cancer patients. Dr. Guthrie McConnell, state bacteriologist, served as pathologist for the hospital, and Dr. Washington E. Fischel as president of the medical staff. During its first eighteen months, 522 persons entered the institution for examination and treatment.[34]

The hospital engaged in research as well as treatment of patients. In its first report, the staff announced the following tentative conclusions: (1) that cancer is not caused by a parasitic agent and is not contagious; (2) that treatment by X-rays, radium and other light rays was only slightly successful; (3) that the only safe method of treatment is early recognition and extensive removal of the diseased tissue.[35]

On June 1, 1908, it was announced that George D. Barnard, a wealthy St. Louis businessman, had given $100,000 to the association. The gift was made on the following conditions: that a cancer hospital be built on a tract of land on the north side of Forest Park Boulevard, between Newstead and Taylor avenues; that it be forever a free institution; and that it be renamed the Barnard Free Skin and Cancer Hospital.[36]

The Masonic Home Board of Missouri voted, on December 13, 1910, to invite bids for a $100,000 hospital to be erected on Delmar Avenue slightly west of Union Avenue. The site selected was known as "Hospital Row," being the neighborhood in which the Jewish Hospital and St. Luke's Hospital were located. The building would be of brick construction, three-stories high, with accommodations for 142 patients. The sanitarium was designed as a private institution, for the free use of Masons and their families.[37]

The managers of the Mayfield Memorial Hospital enterprise announced, in May 1912, that they were ready to proceed with the construction of their planned building to be located on a five-acre tract bounded by Oakland, Tamm and Berthold avenues. The

hospital was to be three stories high, with a large dome in which the operating room would be located. A number of wards, in which the patient would pay only five dollars a week, were planned. Control of the institution was to be vested in the Baptist churches of the entire United States rather than in the local or state church organizations.[38]

In the fall of 1914, the Barnes Hospital at Euclid Avenue and Kingshighway received its first patients. The institution owed its existence to the generosity of Robert A. Barnes, a wealthy businessman and civic leader, who twenty-two years previously had left $950,000 for the building and endowment of a hospital. Smith P. Galt, Richard M. Scruggs and Samuel M. Kennard were appointed trustees to carry out the benefactor's wishes. The will provided that only $100,000 could be used for building and equipping the hospital, the rest being retained as a permanent endowment.[39]

It quickly became apparent that $100,000 would not be sufficient to build an outstanding hospital, since construction costs were going up and hospital design and equipment were changing. So the trustees prudently invested the fund and adopted a policy of "watchful waiting." Meanwhile, they made a study of the finest hospitals in Europe and America. In 1908, they hired the well-known architect Theodore Link, with instructions to design a hospital on the pavilion plan, using the Johns Hopkins Hospital as a general model. In 1912, the fund having grown to $1,500,000, they ordered construction to begin.[40]

The Barnes Hospital, as delivered by the contractor in 1914, was an extensive complex of buildings, the property of different corporate owners, but with all units bound together by contracts of mutual aid and cooperation.[42] East of Euclid Avenue stood two four-story buildings; these were the north and south laboratories of the Washington University Medical School. In the space between them was the medical school's administration building.[43]

The administration building of Barnes Hospital was on the west side of Euclid Avenue and faced Kingshighway. It was a massive four-story structure, with east and west wings in the shape of the letter "T". The second and third floors of the central portion of the building provided housing for the resident medical staff. A large medical lecture hall occupied the fourth floor. In the east and west wings were the medical and surgical wards. Adjoining the west wing rose a three-story addition containing private wards. Behind the administration building was the service center, in which were found the kitchens, dining rooms, bakery, laundry and sleeping quarters for employees. In the northwest corner of the hospital grounds was the children's hospital; and at the northeast corner, facing Euclid Avenue, stood the four-story clinical and pathological building.[44]

Barnes Hospital was completed for a total cost of $1,250,000. Its endowment fund not only remained intact but increased from $850,000 to $950,000.[45]

To the two traditional functions of a hospital, i.e., the care of the sick and the training of doctors and nurses, Barnes Hospital added a third — the advancement of medical knowledge.[46] It thus provided a model for other Missouri hospitals, such as the medical center of the University of Missouri at Columbia, to follow.

A number of older, well-established hospitals transferred their operations to more spacious quarters, usually in the western part of the city. St. Luke's in 1903 moved into a four-story structure, consisting of three connected pavilions, located at Delmar Boulevard and Holt Avenue.[47] The Evangelical Deaconess Home and Hospital Society, in 1905, announced plans to build a $77,000 hospital at 4117 West Belle Place.[48] The St. Louis Mothers' Hospital opened its obstetric dispensary at 711 Carr Street in December 1905.[49]

Archbishop John Glennon, on May 7, 1911, laid the cornerstone of the new St. John's Hospital at Park View, Euclid and Audubon avenues. The hospital was under the auspices of the Sisters of Mercy. The Reverend Christopher Byrne, pastor of the Holy Name Parish, in a tribute to the work done in St. Louis by this religious order, explained the motivation behind the building of most of St. Louis's private hospitals:[50]

It is fitting that the corner stone of this institution is laid amidst religious ceremonies, for religion has always fostered the science of medicine. The work of healing was born of the spirit of the Savior, who said to the leper: "I will that thou be made clean."

From the very beginning of Christianity religion has had pity and compassion for the ills to which human nature is subject, and has always sought to alleviate them. We find after the master himself Christian men and women devoting their lives, their abilities and their talents to the alleviation of suffering."

There were other hospital changes. The Good Samaritan, the city's homeopathic sanitarium, abandoned its historic affiliation and installed an allopathic staff of doctors in August 1902.[51] Because of the decline of shipping on the inland waterways, the St. Louis Marine Hospital closed its doors in 1906.[52] The Martha Parsons Free Hospital for

Children and the St. Louis Children's Hospital merged in 1910.[53] They later built a new hospital on Kingshighway that became a part of the Barnes Hospital group. Beaumont Hospital, which had been associated with Beaumont Medical College, went out of business in 1912.[54]

A survey, conducted by the St. Louis *Republic* in December 1906, indicated that the city had thirty-two major hospitals[55] and possibly twenty-five minor ones, with a total capacity of 3,455 patients. The average daily occupancy rate was 2,712 patients; of these 1,231 were charity cases.[56]

The years from 1890 to 1910 were a transition period for St. Louis hospitals. Earlier hospitals had been charitable institutions — asylums for the sick, disabled and homeless citizens. They were supported by public funds and by the benefactions of wealthy citizens and church organizations. Visiting staffs of doctors provided the medical and surgical care free of charge. Middle-class persons preferred to be treated at home by their family physicians.

Beginning in the 1890s and increasingly in the following decades, as the *Republic*'s 1906 survey revealed, the middle class was choosing hospital treatment rather than home care. The extended family was breaking down; the smaller family often lacked the space and the helpers to provide family nursing. The newer hospitals were becoming more comfortable, rivaling hotels in their accommodations. They were staffed by professional nurses. They were learning to cope with the hospital infections, which previously had given them a bad reputation. Only a hospital could provide the diagnostic and therapeutic equipment required by the practice of the new scientific medicine.[57]

Some of the features of the older practice of medicine persisted. The visiting staffs of unpaid doctors continued to serve in many hospitals. However, the new Barnes Hospital had its own salaried staff of practitioners. Many women still preferred to have their babies delivered at home. A large part of the patronage of denominational hospitals, as well as the city institutions, continued to be charitable cases. But as the costs of the new hospitals rose, they were forced to pass more of the financial burden to their customers.

3. *The Board of Health*

Mayor Wells took a keen interest in, and exercised close supervision over, the operations of the board of health. A tragic accident involving the board occurred in the fall of 1901. Thirteen children treated with diphtheria antitoxin prepared in the city's bacteriological laboratory contracted tetanus and died. Mayor Wells personally presided over the court of inquiry set up to discover how the serum had become contaminated with tetanus toxin. Weeks of testimony were taken from officials and employees of the board of health in order to establish the facts.[58]

On September 30, 1901, an employee of the board had bled "Jim," a broken-down horse used for the production of antitoxin. About six quarts of blood were secured and processed by extracting the serum. Several days after he was bled "Jim" developed tetanus and had to be killed. Although Dr. Amand Ravold, city bacteriologist, was informed of the death of the horse, he failed to order the destruction of the contaminated serum. During Dr. Ravold's absence in Chicago in connection with the Chicago Drainage Canal case, the laboratory exhausted its supply of diphtheria antitoxin. Henry Taylor, the janitor, issued to doctors with diphtheria cases a number of doses of the poisonous serum which had been poured into individual vials and labeled.[59]

The investigation revealed the careless fashion in which the laboratory operated. The horses used for the antitoxin were old, retired animals. They were kept at the poorhouse in a yard the soil of which had become contaminated by tetanus. The poisoned blood drawn from "Jim" was not immediately destroyed but was put into the refrigerator with the good serum. It was not tested on a guinea pig before being issued. In the absence of Dr. Ravold, the janitor who lacked professional training was left for days in charge of the laboratory.

Because of his failure to safeguard the quality of the antitoxin produced under his supervision, Dr. Ravold was dismissed from his position in the health department. Henry Taylor was fired for making under oath conflicting and misleading statements regarding his role in the tragedy. The board of inquiry recommended that the ban on the manufacture of serum by the Health Department, which had been imposed immediately following the first deaths, should be made permanent.[61]

Perhaps stimulated by the antitoxin matter, a thorough reorganization of the Health Department began to be publicly discussed.[62] Under the existing system, the mayor appointed the health commissioner and the superintendents of the municipal hospitals. The health commissioner chose the physicians, nurses and clerks who served under the superintendents. The procedure denied the superintendents the opportunity of selecting their own subordinates and laid the basis for friction between the health commissioner and the hospital chiefs. This system placed a heavy administrative burden upon the commissioner. The staff at city hospital alone consisted of thirty-two physicians, forty-six nurses and one hundred and eighty other employees. The arrangement gave the health commissioner a tempting opportunity to distribute the hospital jobs to members of his political party or to his personal friends.[63]

A coalition of representatives of St. Louis's various medical societies, in February 1907, proposed a scheme for the restructuring of the Health Department. The plan was designed to curb the excessive power of the health commissioner and also to provide a more efficient administration of health services. The proposal, with some amendments, was approved by the municipal assembly in 1911. It established a Hospital Department separate from the Health Department. Visiting staffs of unpaid specialists were given a major role in providing medical and surgical treatment in the hospitals. The change brought St. Louis's municipal hospitals in line with the practice prevailing in similar institutions in major Eastern cities.[64]

Tuberculosis and pneumonia were the two most fatal diseases with which the health organization of St. Louis had to contend. Tuberculosis attacked all classes of society. The blacks were particularly susceptible. Crowded insanitary housing, lack of fresh air and sunshine, and inadequate diets were partial causes of their vulnerability. Stuffy, tightly closed houses and lack of outdoor exercise brought the disease into middle-income families. Dr. William H. Mayfield's only son died of the "White Plague."[65]

There were 11,521 deaths from consumption in St. Louis in the decade 1900 to 1910. The population of the city was 575,238 in 1900 and 687,029 in 1910.[66]

Dr. Starkloff, the health commissioner, in November 1901, introduced a bill in the municipal assembly for curbing tuberculosis. The measure declared tuberculosis a communicable disease. The ordinance further provided that:[67]

> physicians shall report every case of tuberculosis to the Health Commissioner, that the Health Commissioner shall cause an examination of the premises to be made, including all details about their sanitary condition and the number of persons living in the house; that he may order an examination of the sputa of every suspected case; and that the room occupied by the invalid shall be fumigated.

The St. Louis Medical Society, meeting on November 9, 1901 with representatives of the homeopathic and Eclectic schools, voted unanimously to ask the municipal assembly to defeat the bill.[68]

The main objections to the legislation were: that the sputum test was inconclusive to establish the presence of the disease; that the compulsory testing of sputa was an invasion of the patients' privacy; that the procedure established by the bill would displace the family physician and set up a program of public treatment of consumptives;[69] and that the periodic fumigation of quarters would be ineffective and excessively expensive.[70] The doctors were of the opinion that only education by the medical profession would safeguard the public against infection.[71] Their opposition was effective in defeating the bill.

To promote greater public awareness of the disease, its cause and cure, the municipal commission on Tuberculosis was formed in 1909. The commission held neighborhood mass meetings at which doctors lectured and showed a series of stereopticon slides.[72]

In 1910, the quarantine station below Jefferson Barracks was converted into a tuberculosis sanatorium. The Mount St. Rose Hospital for Consumptives had opened its doors as a private sanatorium some years earlier.

St. Louisans took a leading role in the establishment at Las Vegas, New Mexico, of a national tuberculosis sanatorium. This development was an outgrowth of the popular reception accorded the Temple of Fraternity, which had been contributed to the St. Louis World's Fair by the Associated Fraternities of America. When the fair ended, the fraternal association, in a spirit of idealism and service, decided to transport the temple building to New Mexico as the headquarters for an open-air hospital for consumptives. Offers of land and buildings were solicited. The following committee was chosen to go to New Mexico to select the exact site: W. R. Eldson, president of the Associated Fraternities of America; August Schlafly, president of the Missouri-Lincoln Trust Company; Dr. H. A. Warner of Topeka, Kansas; M. P. Moody, manager of the American Baptist Publication Society; and Dr. W. H. Mayfield, president of the Mayfield Sanitarium.[73]

The town of Las Vegas, by its offer of 10,000 acres of fertile farm land, won the approval of the committee. The Atchison, Topeka and Santa Fe Railroad, which served Las Vegas, gave 1,000 acres and the Montezuma Hotel. The two land grants formed a tract fifteen miles square adjoining the town. This site met the committee's specifications in regard to altitude, precipitation, temperature, healthfulness and available transportation.[74]

The plan was to build a city for consumptives with a maximum population of 25,000. Patients from fraternal organizations, which contributed to the support of the project, would be entitled to free care. Others would be admitted at a minimum charge. As the health of the patients improved, they would be provided work on the farm or at house-keeping duties.[75] It was anticipated that St. Louis, with its yearly average of nearly 2,000 consumptives and its excellent rail service to the Southwest would send a large contingent of patients to this new health spa.[76]

It was not until July 28, 1916, that Dr. Starkloff's ordinance declaring consumption contagious brought the malady under the supervision of the Health Department and gave the commissioner the same control over it that he exercised over smallpox, diphtheria and scarlet fever, including the authority to placard the residence of tuberculosis patients.[77]

The second most deadly disease in St. Louis was pneumonia, dreaded as "The King of Death." During the decade 1900-1910, a total of 9,971 persons succumbed to this malady.[78] While consumption worked slowly in destroying its victims, pneumonia moved swiftly. No specific remedies to halt its progress were available. About one fourth of the cases ended fatally. Pneumonia often followed another disease, such as a cold or a case of influenza.[79]

Typhoid fever claimed 1,615 lives in St. Louis in the first decade of the twentieth century.[80] Contaminated supplies of milk and water were the main causes of this death toll. Much of the city's milk was produced by small neighborhood dairies, operated under insanitary conditions. St. Louis's water supply, pumped from the Mississippi River at the Chain of Rocks, was polluted by sewage from upstream cities as well as by discharges from St. Louis's own sewer system.

A major offender among the upstream cities was Chicago. In 1900, the Chicago Drainage Canal began discharging the city's sewage into the Illinois River which emptied into the Mississippi. Previously, these wastes had been pumped into Lake Michigan. St.

Louis sought an injunction to halt this diversion. The state of Missouri intervened in behalf of St. Louis, and the case came before the United States Supreme Court as the *State of Missouri* vs. *the State of Illinois and the Sanitary District of Chicago.*[81]

On February 19, 1906, the Supreme Court published its judgment unanimously rejecting Missouri's charge that its water supply was being polluted by its neighbor. The tribunal affirmed that Missouri did not come into court with clean hands. Although the state had the authority to do so, it had made no effort to prevent St. Louis and other Missouri cities from fouling the Mississippi River by discharging their sewage into it.[82] The court pointed out that a more accurate classification of diseases in the early twentieth century might have contributed to the mistakenly reported increase in typhoid fever in St. Louis. Previous censuses frequently classified typhoid cases as intermittent, remittent, typho-malarial and typhus fever. The court considered it significant that, contrary to St. Louis's experience, there had been no increase of typhoid in cities along the banks of the Illinois River since the opening of the canal.[83]

The loss of the case in the Supreme Court was more a blow to St. Louis's pride than to its public health. In 1904, two years before the announcement of the court's decision, the St. Louis waterworks had perfected a method utilizing filtration and a coagulating agent to assure the city a clear, pure and plentiful supply of water.[84]

Influenza dominated the health situation in St. Louis and Missouri during the second decade of the twentieth century.[85] The first news St. Louisans received of the outbreak of the disease in the fall of 1918 was a report of October 2 out of Washington announcing the spread of the epidemic in army camps and civilian centers along the Atlantic and Gulf coasts.[86] In response to this alarm, Health Commissioner Starkloff, on October 4, introduced in the board of aldermen a bill requiring St. Louis doctors to report to the Health Department all cases of influenza coming to their attention. The ordinance declared influenza a contagious disease and empowered the health commissioner to utilize the broad powers provided in the charter for fighting epidemic infections.[87] The same day the St. Louis chapter of the American Red Cross notified its local chapters to register all available nurses, nurses' aides and other persons who had completed elementary training in home care of the sick. This mobilization involved home defense groups and nurses who were not under orders for military service.[88] To supplement the work of the Red Cross, all public health and visiting nurses' organizations were instructed to assemble their forces to combat the disease. Nurses in service were required to wear gauze masks.[89]

The first death reported in St. Louis from influenza was that of A. A Jest, twenty-five years old, who died on October 3 at his home. Jest was enrolled in the naval training program and was given a furlough and sent home when he was stricken with the disease.[90] The practice of sending home from army and navy training centers recruits who showed signs of influenza was one of the means by which the ailment was spread from service camps to civilian centers.

At a meeting held in the office of the health commissioner on October 7 and attended by representatives of the city's business, educational and health agencies, the mayor, after listening to status reports, proclaimed that influenza was fast becoming epidemic in the city. This proclamation gave the health commissioner authority to order the immediate closing of theaters, motion picture shows, schools, Sunday Schools, billiard halls, cabarets, lodges and societies, public funerals, open-air meetings, dance halls and conventions. The order applied also to military parades and Liberty Loan mass meetings.[91] All requests for exemptions were turned down by the health commissioner. Although streetcars were permitted to continue running, they were required to provide adequate ventilation.[92]

In addition to forbidding formal meetings, Dr. Starkloff instructed the police to disperse groups of more than six persons, gathered in saloons or idling on the streets and in public buildings.[93]

Beginning October 21, retail stores (excluding groceries and drug shops) in the downtown business district east of Twelfth Street were ordered to delay opening until 9:30 A.M. and to close by 4:30 P.M. The plan was designed to prevent shoppers from overcrowding the streetcars on which the employees of banks, insurance companies and government offices were going to work.[94]

On Saturday, November 9, Commissioner Starkloff imposed a four-day ban on business operations in the city. However some thirty-six categories of exemptions were established. In justifying this drastic move, Dr. Starkloff cited the increase in new cases during the previous week and also the massive popular celebration in downtown St. Louis on the evening of November 7, which had greeted the premature announcement that an armistice had been signed ending World War I. The four-day ban was generally opposed by the St. Louis business leaders.[95]

In addition to the measures taken to prevent the spread of influenza, Dr. Starkloff established a comprehensive system of care for those who had contracted the disease. Following the closing of the schools, the superintendent of public instruction tendered the services of the system's hygiene division and the entire teaching staff, numbering 2,500 teachers, nurses and doctors, to help combat the epidemic. The teachers were employed in visiting the homes in their school districts and working with the children of their classes, under the guidance of Dr. James Stewart, supervisor of school hygiene.[96] City patrolmen were instructed to make sickness surveys of their districts and report cases of disease where the patients had no medical care. Doctors from the Health Department were stationed in the different police stations to answer calls from families reported by the police.[97]

On October 15, it was announced that a general visiting nurse and home assistance plan for the city had been set up. Under Red Cross management nurses and nurses' aides would be sent to any address in the city to be helpful in any way necessary as the result of members of the family being incapacitated by illness. Physicians were notified to give wide publicity to the program, but to use their judgment in selecting the most urgent cases for this free service so as not to exceed the available nursing staff.[98]

By the end of October, the Health Department's nursing program was staffed and operated as follows:[99]

There are now available 40 graduate visiting nurses, 10 Red Cross aids, 25 elementary hygiene workers and nine practical nurses. Transportation is being furnished for the workers by the Red Cross Motor Corps, which has made available for their use seven automobiles each day

. . . .

Not only are nurses being furnished, but bedding and linen is being provided

where the family is too poor to buy it, milk is being given by the tuberculosis society and the Health Department is furnishing free medical aid.

The progress of the war on influenza was charted by the weekly mortality statistics: week ending October 12, 86 deaths; week ending October 19, 186 deaths; week ending October 26, 233 deaths; week ending November 2, 257 deaths; week ending November 9, 229 deaths; week ending November 16, 228 deaths; week ending November 23, 190 deaths; week ending November 30, 235 deaths.[100]

The 1918 influenza outbreak differed from previous epidemics which St. Louis had suffered. The cholera epidemic of 1849 had been introduced locally by tides of immigration proceeding up the Mississippi River. It was spread by the use of contaminated water supplies and could have been halted by the boiling of drinking water. Epidemics of malaria and yellow fever were propagated by mosquitoes. These three diseases were selective in their targets; many communities, particularly those away from main waterways, escaped.

The 1918 influenza, being air-borne, advanced with great rapidity until it blanketed the entire nation. In St. Louis, it ravaged the wealthy suburbs as well as the downtown slums. No public measure existed that could effectively halt it, aside from the impossible step of forbidding all human contacts. The prevailing strain, known as "Spanish influenza," was the most virulent on record. For many patients, influenza was followed by pneumonia, which produced almost certain death. On autopsy, the lungs of these patients were found to be filled with a frothy, bloody fluid.[101] There were no specific medicines to cure influenza. Rest, fresh air, adequate food and warm bed covers were generally advised.[102]

St. Louis utilized its own local agencies — the board of health and the health commissioner — to conduct the war against the invading enemy.[103] As soon as the mayor proclaimed the existence of an influenza epidemic, the health commissioner was clothed with all the powers, which were ordinarily exercised by the municipal assembly. Dr. Starkloff was no newcomer to responsibility. He had served as health commissioner for most of the previous twenty years and had demonstrated marked efficiency and success in the office. He enjoyed the confidence and support of St. Louis citizens and could afford to stand firm against special interests. His administration of the anti-influenza campaign was facilitated by the willingness of people on the home front during World War I to accept restrictions and make sacrifices for the common good.

With the signing of the armistice with Germany on November 11, 1918, the popular mood changed. Disregarding the ban against gatherings of more than six persons, the citizens of St. Louis on the evening of the good news jammed the downtown district in a joyous celebration. Then they turned their attention to immediate peace time concerns. Merchants were anxious to begin advertising their Christmas goods and hoped to attract crowds of customers. Parents wanted the schools to reopen so their children would not lose a whole year of academic credit. Theater owners looked forward to resuming the showing of their films. With a guilty conscience for staying away from religious services for a month or more, church goers were ready to renew their regular pattern of worship.

These were some of the considerations that caused Dr. Starkloff, on November 12,

despite the fact that more than 200 persons per week were dying in the city from influenza and pneumonia, to order the lifting of the meetings ban.[104] His action appears to have been based on two assumptions: (1) that the declining trend of new cases and deaths would continue; (2) that the citizenry would follow the rules of good health without being forced to do so by government.

On November 27, new cases unexpectedly jumped to 659, an increase of 141 from the previous day. Fifty-three percent of the new patients were children, including 100 from a single orphan asylum. The following day, Dr. Starkloff ordered the closing of all schools. In addition, children under sixteen years of age were forbidden to attend theaters and stores. All large public meetings, except with a special permit, were banned.[105] Consideration was given to a plan to keep all schools closed until after the Christmas holidays.

Instead, Dr. Starkloff issued an order permitting third and fourth year high school students, who were over sixteen years old, to return to classes on Monday, December 9.[106] The weekly mortality statistics for influenza and pneumonia combined cast doubts on the wisdom of the commissioner's decision:[107] week ending December 7, 375; week ending December 14, 469; week ending December 21, 293; week ending December 28, 129.

The epidemic in St. Louis continued through March 15, 1919, and was responsible for a total of 3,691 lives.[108] For the state of Missouri, there were 12,250 deaths from influenza and pneumonia during the last four months of 1918 and 5,694 deaths in the first six months of 1919, making a total of 17,944.[109] This figure represented an excess of 389.5 deaths per 100,000 population over the estimated normal death rate from influenza and pneumonia.[110]

4. Better Care of the Mentally Ill

The administration of Dr. Edward C. Runge at the St. Louis Insane Asylum from 1895 to 1904 constituted an enlightened era in St. Louis's stewardship of its mentally ill. Dr. Runge transformed the methods of treatment at the institution. He educated the public regarding the hospital's problems and needs. By enlisting public interest in the asylum, he conditioned the voters in 1906 to approve funds for a major enlargement and improvement of the sanatarium's accommodations.

Prior to Dr. Runge, the care provided in the overcrowded asylum was mainly custodial. There was little individual counseling. All categories of patients were housed in the same building. The result was that the atmosphere was noisy and disorderly, making rest and recovery almost impossible.

By segregating the unruly patients, Dr. Runge was able to assure a quiet hospital at night. Sleepless inmates were given warm baths, perhaps some extra food and in a few cases a hypnotic. Physical restraints were kept to a minimum.[111]

Dr. Runge relied on art, music, outdoor exercise, light work and the counsel and encouragement of doctors and nurses for effecting improvement of patients. He had a deep personal interest in his patients. He treated them as human beings, trusted them and gave them increasing degrees of responsibility.[112]

This program would work most effectively if the serious overcrowding at the asylum could be eliminated. This would involve educating the citizens of St. Louis regarding the asylum's needs. For this task, Dr. Runge was admirably equipped. He was an excellent writer. Instead of limiting his annual reports to dull details of administrative housekeeping, he told human interest stories of individual cases and how they were successfully treated.[113] This campaign of education of the city council and the voters of St. Louis paid off. In 1906, the proposition to issue $1,000,000 in bonds to enlarge the insane asylum was approved.[114]

Two new wings were constructed at the east and west ends of the hospital making it one of the largest and best equipped in the country.

Beginning in 1877, the state legislature each biennial period made an appropriation for the partial support of the St. Louis institution. In addition to treating its own insane, the St. Louis hospital cared for scores of out-state patients, many of which were brought to the city for the sole purpose of receiving treatment. The amounts appropriated ranged from $30,000 to $85,000. St. Louis felt that the help given was too little. The state legislature was offended by the city's inability to specify the number of state patients it was caring for and also to explain how the money was expended.

In 1901, Governor Alexander M. Dockery vetoed the appropriation for the St. Louis institution. Since St. Louis was no longer receiving funds from the state, the municipal assembly passed a law that no patient should be admitted to its asylum who had not established six months of residence in St. Louis.[115]

Dr. Runge was followed at the asylum in 1904 by Dr. H. S. Atkins. He employed motion pictures not only for entertainment but also as a therapeutic agency.[116] Although psychiatrists in private practice were acquainted with, and beginning to apply, the teachings of Jean Martin Charcot and Sigmund Freud, there is no evidence that psychoanalysis was being used at the St. Louis Insane Asylum or in the state institutions.[117]

In 1911, the additions to the St. Louis Insane Asylum were completed, and the first 250 patients moved in. The completed structure was 1,233 feet wide. The original building and the two new wings were four stories high. However, on the extreme end of the west wing, because of the slope of the ground, the new part was five stories high; on the east end the new part rose six stories. The addition provided 536 more small rooms and eighty-eight large rooms to accommodate 1,500 patients.[118]

5. Toward Improving the Quality of Life

In addition to providing better care for its physically and mentally ill, St. Louis strove to improve the quality of life for all its citizens. This effort was concentrated on providing three major necessities — pure drink, food and air. The campaign enlisted the support of the local government, civic organizations and the press.

The battle for a wholesome milk supply for the city had been carried on since 1871 when a pioneer ordinance gave the board of health power to inspect milk sold for consumption and to condemn any found impure or adulterated.[119] This law was rendered inoperative by an alliance of hundreds of dairymen carrying on business in backyard sheds and barns. Eventually, a dairy inspection bill was passed which was designed to improve the healthfulness of conditions under which the city's milk was produced. However, it did not provide for inspection of milk sold to consumers, with provisions for the condemnation of supplies failing to meet high standards of healthfulness and butter fat content.[120] For this task, the board of health had to rely on a weak ordinance enacted in 1887.[121]

This ordinance established the office of milk inspector, with a salary of $1,500 a year. The inspector was required to be skilled in analytical and synthetical chemistry. He was expected to visit all dairies in the city twice a year and report to the municipal assembly annually a summary of his findings. The inspector was given authority to enter upon the premises of all milk dealers and to take samples of their products. The ordinance prescribed quality standards for milk and cream. The sale of impure or adulterated milk was punishable by a fine.[122]

The inadequacy of this ordinance was apparent to Mayor Wells. The city's population, by 1901, had grown to nearly 600,000 persons. Its milk supply was provided by a wide variety of dairy farms and plants. Two hundred and fifty dairy farms operated within the city limits.[123] They occupied cramped and often filthy quarters,[124] and lacked facilities for refrigeration and pasteurization of their product. Their milk was sold from carts, mostly in their immediate neighborhood.[125]

More than 4,000 dairy farms in Eastern Missouri and Western Illinois shipped milk to St. Louis by railways. The best of these were models of scientific dairying and sanitary operation. An example was the Maple Hill Dairy of Roodhouse, Illinois, which was conducted under the supervision of the St. Louis Pure Milk Commission and produced a premium quality of "certified milk" for the metropolitan market. This milk was not pasteurized or sterilized. It was guaranteed to contain no more than 30,000 bacteria per cubic centimeter[126] and at least 3.25 percent of butter fat.[127]

The majority of the dairies supplying the St. Louis market were small operations carried on as part of a balanced farming program. These dairies operated without electricity, refrigeration or running water. They were not subject to regulation by St. Louis's ordinances. Milk fresh from the cows was hauled to the nearest railway station for shipment. Much of it spent hours on the railway platform and in an unrefrigerated railway car.[128]

The demand for more rigid inspection was reinforced by the discovery, in July 1902, that milk supplied under contract with the city hospital was impure and causing sickness among the patients.[129] The city's milk inspector was blamed for neglecting his duties, and a move developed in the board of health to fire him.[130]

On August 27, 1902, the municipal assembly passed a strong inspection bill in which responsibility was transferred from the milk inspector to the city chemist's office. The law enlarged the inspection staff. In place of a single inspector, the law provided for a chief chemist, two assistant chemists, two milk inspectors and a clerk. Before beginning business, milk vendors were required to register in the office of the health commissioner and purchase a license. The cost for registering was one dollar a year. The semi-annual license fee was $2.50 for every wagon or vehicle used in the business. The sale of adulterated or impure milk, or milk not kept under proper refrigeration, was declared a misdemeanor. The city chemist was required at least once a month to visit the dairies where city milk was produced and to make recommendations for improvement. Dairies, which failed to implement these recommendations, would have their milk barred from sale. The ordinance set quality standards. Milk was required to contain at least three percent butter fat, eight and five-tenths percent non-fat solids and seven-tenths of one percent ash.[131]

Under Governor Joseph Folk the state became involved in assuring the wholesomeness of its milk supply. Missouri was an important dairy state. On April 8, 1905, the legislature passed an act creating the office of state dairy commissioner. The commissioner

had to have a "practical knowledge and experience in the manufacture of dairy products." He was authorized to appoint one deputy. The necessary analytical work of his office was to be done by the chemist of the state agricultural college in Columbia. The commissioner was empowered to enter all dairies and creameries for inspecting and taking samples. The sale of milk and milk products containing any foreign substance injurious to health was punishable by a fine of from $10 to $100.[132]

Following the passage by the United States Congress of the Pure Food and Drug Act of 1906, the general assembly abolished the position of dairy commissioner and created the state dairy and food office. The office chief could appoint a deputy and six inspectors. He was responsible for enforcing all laws relating to the production and sale of dairy products and the adulteration of food or drugs. He could seize and destroy any food, drug or dairy product that was adulterated or misbranded.[133]

The state standards for milk, based on a bulletin from the United States Department of Agriculture, were slightly higher than those established by ordinance in St. Louis. State law prescribed that milk contain not less than eight and three-fourths percent non-fat solids and not less than three and one-quarter percent of milk fat.[134]

The efforts of state and local inspectors wrought little improvement in St. Louis's milk supply. The Russell Sage Foundation, in a careful study conducted in 1910, found samples of bottled milk that contained 7,000,000 bacteria per cubic centimeter. The allowable maximum was 1,000,000. Much of the "loose" or unbottled milk showed bacterial counts of 35,000,000 bacteria. The investigation also revealed widespread watering of milk and cheating on butter fat content.

Much of the loose milk was sold at temperatures above 50 degrees.[135]

The failure of St. Louis to secure pure milk was blamable not on inadequate legislation or incompetent inspectors, though there were certainly too few of the latter. The fault lay with the disorganization of the dairy industry with four or five thousand dairies contributing to the city's milk supply. It was impossible for the average small dairy in the city or surrounding countryside to comply with the standard of sanitation set by city and state laws. Such a dairy lacked means for assuring that its product would be kept cooled to legal requirements during the long journey from cow to customer.

Two ordinances passed by the municipal assembly, on March 30, 1916, strengthened the system of milk inspection and effected a marked improvement of the city's milk. They authorized the appointment of an expanded inspection staff including the city chemist, an assistant city chemist, two assistant chemists, two milk inspectors and two clerks.[136]

Every person who sold milk in St. Louis had to have a permit issued by the board of public service. Permits were not automatically granted; they could be refused or revoked for cause. The sale of adulterated or misbranded milk was prohibited, and specific examples of adulteration were spelled out to guide the inspectors in their work. Milk was considered adulterated if it contained pathogenic bacteria or if subsequent to pasteurization it had more than fifty thousand living bacteria per cubic centimeter. Milk was termed adulterated too if it had been taken from any cow which had been fed on garbage, sour distillers' or brewery waste or other improper food.[137]

All milk offered for sale in the city had to be pasteurized, then immediately cooled to 45 degrees Fahrenheit or less. The only exception was for "certified milk," produced under stringent sanitary conditions.[138]

Sanitary officers of the health department were made responsible for the inspection of stables and barns where cows were kept. Detailed requirements were prescribed for cow stables in regard to space, ventilation and disposal of wastes. Existing stables not meeting these standards would be declared nuisances, and their owners would be subject to loss of their permits to operate dairies.[139]

The health commissioner was instructed to appoint two practical veterinary surgeons as inspectors. They and the city's sanitary officers were accorded access to all places where dairying was carried on. They were ordered to examine all cows for disease or exposure to contamination. The veterinary surgeons were authorized to go outside the corporate limits of St. Louis to any locality within a radius of 150 miles to examine cows whose milk was brought into St. Louis for sale.[140]

The stringent new rules had the desired effect of weeding out the insanitary and inefficient dairies. In 1912, there were 217 dairies operating in St. Louis. However in 1917, the year after the rules went into effect, the number had dropped to 156; the next year the count was 146.[141]

St. Louis, in early 1901, was still drinking muddy water from its plant at the Chain of Rocks on the Mississippi River. The water was pumped into settling basins and allowed to stand for about thirty-six hours before being sent into the mains for distribution throughout the city.[142] A filtration system, which had been an essential part of the original plan for the Chain of Rocks waterworks, had never been built.[143] Not only was the water unsightly but it was contaminated by the sewage of upriver cities and by the discharges of some of St. Louis's own sewers and creeks. The result was a high rate of typhoid fever and other diseases.[144]

Mayor Wells, shortly after his election, met with a representative group of businessmen and civic leaders to get their ideas and support for a campaign to secure pure water for St. Louis.[145] It was generally agreed that to avoid embarrassment and possibly the failure of the fair, the city would have to improve its water supply.[146]

Public discussion of the water problem centered around two possible solutions. One option was to go to the Meramec River for water. The Meramec was a small, clear stream, flowing through a predominantly rural country some ninety miles southwest of St. Louis. To smooth out seasonal variations in its water level, the river would have to be impounded.[147]

The second option was to construct a filtration system to purify and clarify the water from the Mississippi River at the Chain of Rocks. There were two types of filters. The "slow sand filter" consisted of a bed of fine sand, five feet deep, underlaid by drain tiles leading to the distribution mains. This type of filter was recommended where the water supply was reasonably clear though polluted by human and industrial wastes. In the operation of the filter, a gelatinous film of bacteria and other impurities formed on its surface. This film was the major agency in straining out the impurities.[148]

The "mechanical filter" was more complicated. It required a preliminary settling of the water to remove the major portion of suspended matter. The water was then treated with a coagulant. Percolation through a coarse sand filter followed. When the filter became clogged with silt, the course of water could be reversed. Its upward pressure cleansed the sand bed.[149]

Mayor Wells, supported by the board of public improvements, strongly opposed going to the Meramec River for water. The cost of the impoundment and of a ninety-mile conduit, parts of which would require tunneling, was estimated at $30,000,000.[150] The move would require the abandonment of the plant at Chain of Rocks, in which the city had invested about $10,000,000.[151] Although the water of the Meramec was reasonably pure, the growth of population in its watershed would in time make filtration necessary. Finally, the volume of water available in the Meramec was inadequate for St. Louis's prospective needs.[152]

Pending a decision on the type of filtration to be employed at the Chain of Rocks, the water commissioner received approval and funding for a rearrangement of the city's six settling basins. Under the existing plan, the water from the river passed through only one settling basin before going into the distribution system. By the new plan the sedimentation process was changed so that the water passed through all six basins. Each succeeding basin was slightly lower than its predecessor, so that the water tumbled over a series of waterfalls. To increase the fall and the consequent aeration of the water, a line of bricks on end was placed on the forward edge of each basin. The time spent in the settling process was increased to approximately seventy-two hours. To avoid the sediment that naturally collected in the bottom of the basins, the water for distribution was siphoned from near the surface. The new plan was successful in clarifying the city's water. [153] But the improvement was merely cosmetic; the removal of the bacteria and other impurities had not been achieved.

Mayor Wells, in 1903, assigned the problem of purifying the city's water to a new water commissioner, Ben C. Adkins. Adkins had served previously in the water department as the engineer in charge of distribution. In his instructions to the new commissioner, the mayor informed him that the solution to the problem must be inexpensive and, in view of the approaching World's Fair, had to be operational within a year's time.[154]

Fortunately, John F. Wixford, a scientist in the water department, had been experimenting with coagulation as a means of purifying water. Because of a popular prejudice, alum could not be used for this purpose. Wixford discovered that ferrous sulphate (iron) and calcium hydrate (lime), in proportions of one grain of ferrous sulphate and seven grains of calcium hydrate to a gallon of river water, would produce the desired result. The chemical reaction precipitated the iron in the form of ferrous hydrate, which slowly sinking to the bottom carried with it bacteria and other sediment. The process was found to eliminate over ninety percent of the bacteria and other impurities, and thus to equal or exceed the results of the most effective filters.[155]

The new process was credited with giving St. Louis one of the finest water supplies in the country. The improvement showed up in the city's health statistics. Cases of typhoid fever during the five years following the installation of the coagulation process were only half of the number of those for the five year period preceding the new purification system.[156]

A temporary blockage, in January 1912, of one of the inlet gates at the intake tower in the Mississippi River during an ice jam forced the water department for several days to pump unpurified water into the mains. To avoid an epidemic of disease, the public was warned to boil all its drinking water.[157]

This crisis alerted the citizens of St. Louis to the fact that its waterworks had no emergency or back-up capability. They were also surprised to learn that at times they were using 120,000,000 gallons of water daily, while their plant could pump only 80,000,000; the excess consumption was being made up out of reserves.[158]

To take care of St. Louis's immediate water needs, the municipal assembly appropriated funds for the construction at the Chain of Rocks of a sand-box or mechanical filter plant. The filtration plant went into operation in 1915 and constituted the third step in the purification process. The incoming water from the river was first subjected to the coagulation treatment, then passed through the descending system of settling basins and finally underwent the sand-box filtration before being pumped into the mains. The filtration step permitted the time spent in the settling basins to be cut in half and increased the daily capacity of the waterworks from 80,000,000 to 160,000,000 gallons daily. Besides, filtration enhanced the purity of the water so far as bacteria and chemical residues were concerned.[159]

Looking to the future, the water commissioner recommended the construction of a second intake tower at the Chain of Rocks and eventually a new plant on the Missouri River at a point nine miles above St. Charles. The new works would have a capacity of 200,000,000 gallons a day. With the removal of the main source of St. Louis's supply from the Mississippi to the Missouri River, the city would be assured of purer water, free from contamination by the wastes from Chicago and other upriver cities.[160]

St. Louis continued to be a dumping place for tainted meat and meat products from surrounding states, particularly Illinois. Animals, which were rejected because of injury or disease by packing house buyers at the East St. Louis Stockyards, were purchased at reduced prices by small uninspected concerns. Meat from these animals, known in the trade as "downers," was sent across the river at night and sold in shops in the poorer sections of the city of St. Louis.[161]

Government inspection of meat was at a minimum. St. Louis operated under a law which provided for the inspection of meat, fish, game and poultry sold to consumers in local stores and markets. The former inspection by St. Louis veterinarians at the slaughterhouses had been abandoned.[162] There was no state legislation on the subject. Federal inspection was limited to those cattle and hogs whose meat and meat products were destined for foreign markets. However, there was no inspection of meat products as they were being processed following slaughter. [163] The number of inspectors provided by the city of St. Louis and the federal government was inadequate for the tasks assigned.

The publication, in 1906, of Upton Sinclair's *The Jungle*, describing conditions in Chicago packing houses, created interest and concern regarding the wholesomeness of the nation's food. President Roosevelt sent two investigators to Chicago who confirmed Sinclair's account. The result was the passage, in 1906, of the Federal Meat Inspection Act. The law mandated the inspection of cattle after as well as before slaughter. This legislation applied to meat destined for interstate as well as foreign commerce.[164]

St. Louis had a number of independent packers which bought their animals in the St. Louis Independent Stockyards. These animals were subject to federal inspection before and after slaughter.[165] The independent packing houses, the largest of which was the St. Louis Union Packing Company, were conducted under thoroughly sanitary conditions. The local companies did not engage in the canning of meat products.[166]

6. Garbage Collection and Disposal

St. Louisans demanded clean air as well as pure food and drink. Smoke from industrial plants was a cause for complaint. The major contaminant, however, was the stench arising from the city's system of garbage disposal. In June 1903, Mayor Wells proposed that, in a coming election, bonds should be issued to establish a municipal garbage collection and a disposal plant.[167] For years this service had been provided by a private contractor, Ed Butler, through his two companies, the Excelsior Hauling and Transfer Company and the St. Louis Sanitary Company. These two profitable contracts were perquisites of the city boss and provided a regular income to supplement his occasional boodling fees. The St. Louis Sanitary Company established a large reduction plant at 3958 Missouri Avenue, on the bank of the Mississippi River in Southeast St. Louis, in the vicinity of the city workhouse. On Forest Park Boulevard near Vandeventer Avenue, upon a group of adjoining lots, Butler located the headquarters of the Excelsior Hauling and Transfer Company. Here were the stables, wagons, draft animals and other equipment used in making the weekly rounds of garbage collection.[168]

Complaints against Butler's system were numerous. The mayor and many members of the municipal assembly considered that Butler's charge of $257,196 a year for collecting and incinerating the garbage was excessive.[169] In cities with more efficient systems, the valuable by-products from reduction lowered the compensation demanded by the operating company. The loudest complainants were the homeowners, churches and schools that had to endure the malodorous fumes from Butler's "Stink Factory."[170]

In August 1903, a commission, including the Committee of Sanitary Affairs of each house of the municipal assembly, the board of public improvements and the health commissioner was appointed to investigate the garbage issue and to make recommendations. The commission, in its report, advocated[171]

a municipal collecting and hauling system; a private reduction plant; two municipal incinerating plants, and the separation of garbage and waste by householders.

Private operation of the reduction works was preferred in order to avoid having the city compete with business enterprise in the selling of the valuable by-products of the reduction process. The commission also considered that the task of reduction required specialized knowledge and skills not possessed by city workers.[172]

In line with the recommendations of the special commission, an ordinance was introduced in the city council, on March 1, 1904, providing for the payment of $145,000 for the purchase of Butler's garbage collection company. The price was attractive, so Butler readily accepted the offer. He calculated that after the city purchased his collecting agency, it would have to haul the garbage to his reduction plant. But to his surprise, the city rebuffed all his efforts to secure a renewal of his garbage disposal contract when it expired November 14, 1904.[173] Mayor Wells and Hiram Phillips, president of the board of public improvements, had other plans.

Twenty-two miles south of St. Louis, just off the western shore of the Mississippi River, lay Chesley Island, an uninhabited, 400-acre tract of sandy soil. A survey of the island by Hiram Phillips convinced him that it would be an ideal garbage disposal site.[174] Mayor Wells, fearful that any ordinance to acquire the island would be blocked in the house of delegates where Butler's combine still had a strong vote, purchased it with his personal funds.[175]

Three loading docks were established on the St. Louis levee. The garbage was hauled to these sites and loaded on barges which were towed to Chesley Island. The garbage was strewn over a selected area and then turned under by plows. Later a herd of hogs was settled on the island to perform at least the preliminary work of disposal. [176] The Chesley Island plan was intended as a temporary expedient.

During August 1907, the municipal assembly enacted an ordinance authorizing the board of public improvements to negotiate a ten-year contract for the reduction of the city's garbage. The contract specifications called for two loading stations in the city, which must be kept clean and free of odors. The reduction plant had to be outside the city limits, on a river or a railroad, and not less than one mile or more than twenty miles from the city.[177] The contract was awarded to the Standard Reduction Company.

In searching for a site, the company took options on three tracts of land south of Jefferson Barracks. But Captain Soulard Turner, quartermaster at the camp, warned the city of St. Louis that the location of the disposal plant in the vicinity of Jefferson Barracks might force the army to close the installation.[178]

Blocked from locating on the Mississippi, the company chose an area on the Missouri River opposite St. Charles. Access to the site was available by the Wabash Railway as well as by the river.[179] From the standpoint of St. Louisans, the arrangement was just perfect. However, the well-being of citizens of St. Charles had not been considered.

Two stations within the city were established to receive the garbage collected by the new company. At these stations, the wagons would drive up a long incline to a platform, from which they would dump their loads into a waiting rail car below. The cars were of boiler iron, in the shape of half a cylinder, and mounted on a flat bed carriage. When filled, trapdoors on top of the cars could be closed to retain the odors. Upon the arrival of the loaded cars at the reduction works opposite St. Charles, the cars could be tilted on their rockers to discharge their contents.[180] The reduction company expected to utilize all the possible by-products, including grease from the meat scraps in the garbage and also the residual sludge containing potash, ammonia and alcohol.[181]

Whatever good will might have existed originally toward a local industry which created new jobs was lost when the citizens of St. Charles had to endure the nauseating odors emanating from the plant during the spring and summer months. Civic groups protested but to no avail. Then the women of St. Charles took up the fight. The reporter for the St. Louis *Republic*, in a flight of classical fancy, compared their efforts to those of the women of ancient Carthage who, when the Roman legions were besieging their city, cut off their long tresses to make bowstrings for their husbands and sons who were manning the walls. The heroic women of St. Charles, in defense of their city, took up their pens and drafted a petition to Governor Herbert S. Hadley demanding that he do something to abate the nuisance in their neighborhood. To see that the letter reached the governor, it was hand carried and delivered.[182]

The issue of whether the St. Charles plant was a nuisance was submitted to the State Board of Health. The board's decision went against the plant. In implementation of the board's finding, Attorney General Elliott W. Major began a suit to enjoin the Standard Reduction and Chemical Company from receiving any more garbage at its St. Charles works.[183] On January 16, 1911, Judge B. A. Wurdemann at Clayton issued a temporary injunction restraining the reduction company and the Wabash Railway from further garbage disposal operations. Since only three weeks were allowed before the order went into effect, the St. Louis Board of Public Improvements was in a quandary as to how to dispose of the city's garbage after the ban began. The low stage of the Mississippi River made it impossible to resume transportation to Chesley Island.[184] In the emergency, the city proceeded to dump its garbage into the river.

A group of former mayors interviewed by the St. Louis *Republic*, recommended that the city assume the responsibility of collecting and disposing of its garbage.[185] This advice was disregarded and a contract was awarded to a private company to reduce the garbage at a plant in South St. Louis, probably Ed Butler's old works. The contract contained a provision that the process must emit no objectionable odors. The company violated this pledge, and once more the citizens of South St. Louis were up in arms. The city of St. Louis ordered the closing of the reduction plant and resumed dumping its garbage into the river.[186]

The St. Louis Board of Public Service, in 1916, awarded a contract to the Indiana Reduction Company, which had its plant in Illinois, just south of East St. Louis. The company charged St. Louis eighty-seven cents a ton to dispose of the garbage. Citizens of South St. Louis still got the stench when the breeze was from the east. The company, in August 1918, rejected a request from St. Louis to reduce its garbage rate.[187]

7. *The St. Louis* Republic's *Health Campaign*

On September 15, 1913, the St. Louis *Republic* launched a campaign to improve the city's health. At that time, St. Louis ranked fourth in healthfulness as the following statistics compiled by the New York Department of Health showing deaths per 1,000 inhabitants indicated:[188]

Cleveland	13.50
New York	14.11
San Francisco	14.24
St. Louis	14.50

The paper's public relations effort had two phases. First, there was a series of articles analyzing the factors responsible for St. Louis's standing as fourth among great American cities. This was accompanied by a drive to enlist all major groups in making St. Louis the healthiest city in the United States.[189]

Good, abundant and cheap food supplies contributed to the health of St. Louisans. A circle centered on St. Louis, with a 400-mile radius, included the major meat and cereal production areas of the United States. Vegetables from the Mississippi River bottoms, fruit from Southeast Missouri and the Ozarks, milk from Illinois, supplemented the locally ground flour and home-packed meats.[190]

St. Louis enjoyed the distinction of having more detached houses than any other great city in the world. Its building code required at least three feet of open space between two adjoining houses, thus guaranteeing a minimum of sunlight and fresh air. Most houses had backyards for gardening and other recreational uses. A modern four-room cottage in a decent neighborhood sold for $2,600 to $3,200, a capital investment within the capability of working-class families.[191]

In 1904, in preparation for the World's Fair, St. Louis transformed its water system to one of the finest in the nation. A system of weirs was installed to accelerate the sedimentation process in the settling basins. To this was added a coagulation step using iron sulphate and lime. In a final purification, the water was passed through sand filters. A flat rate encouraged St. Louisans to use water freely for bathing and cooking purposes as well as for sprinkling outdoors.[192]

St. Louis schools were models of scientific sanitation and ventilation. A system of air conditioning provided each classroom with air which had been washed, warmed and delivered through registers eight feet above floor level. School children were inspected daily for incipient diseases. If they stayed home sick, the school nurse visited them.[193]

Personal and group hygiene was taught in the schools from kindergarten through high school. Playgrounds were an essential part of each school's physical plant. The high schools had cafeterias where the children could secure warm, balanced meals at cost. The effectiveness of these sanitary arrangements was indicated by a dramatic drop in annual deaths among children as soon as they reached the age of six and entered school.[194]

St. Louis's health was protected by a well-organized system of private and public hospitals. In 1914, the city had approximately sixty private institutions, including the recently opened Barnes Hospital.

Its municipal organization comprised the city hospital and the female hospital with a combined patient load of approximately 700; the isolation hospital for highly contagious cases; the infirmary (or former poorhouse) where homeless and indigent persons were housed; the Robert Koch Hospital at quarantine for advanced cases of tuberculosis; the sanitarium, which accommodated 2,000 insane patients; and finally five dispensaries, each with a staff of physicians, to provide emergency medical care. Treatment in municipal hospitals was efficient and free to patients unable to pay.[195]

St. Louis had an excellent corps of doctors, many of them educated in the new scientific medicine in the laboratories and classrooms of Washington University and St. Louis University. In these schools, departments of social service had recently been established to train workers to supplement the efforts of professional medical personnel. The social workers went into the homes of needy families to assist them in solving problems of employment, nutrition, child care, health and money management. The social service workers also acted as referral agents in placing families in touch with other organizations that could help them.[196]

Dr. Max C. Starkloff, health commissioner, Dr. G. A Jordan, assistant health commissioner, and Dr. Louis H. Behrens, president of the St. Louis Medical Society, on September 15, 1913, heartily indorsed *The Republic*'s campaign as a means of increasing awareness of St. Louis's health needs and promoting cooperation in solving them.[197]

Samuel B. McPheeters, president of the St. Louis Board of Police Commissioners, pledged the support of his department's 1,600 patrolmen in bettering health conditions. The patrolmen were intimately acquainted with their beats and would be valuable reinforcements of the health department's limited force of sanitary inspectors. To guide their efforts, the health commissioner collected in a handbook the various laws dealing with nuisances and violations of the pure food and milk ordinances. A copy of this handbook was furnished to each policeman, who was required to familiarize himself with the contents.[198]

The police and Health Department inspectors began a campaign to force compliance with the city's code regarding tenement houses. They found widespread violation of the requirements to provide a hydrant on each floor and to make sewer connections with the city's sanitary system. Owners of tenements were informed of violations and were given an opportunity to make improvements before being fined.[199]

The Federation of Women's Clubs of America and the Consumers' League sent representatives to a meeting, on October 20, 1913, to arrange for participation in *The Republic*'s campaign.[200] During the last week of October, a committee, consisting of Frederick H. Fricke, state pure food and drug commissioner, John H. Ritter, head of the meat inspection organization of the city Health Department, Mrs. E. T. Senseney of the Consumers' League, and a reporter from *The Republic*, made a two-day inspection of meat markets in St. Louis. Their conclusion was that the city's meat supply was wholesome and was handled in a generally sanitary manner.[201] Earlier inspections had been made of restaurants, confectioneries and bakeries.

It was not possible to judge statistically the success of *The Republic*'s health campaign. But the general effects were certainly beneficial. The public became interested and involved in the promotion of good health. Women through their recently organized clubs assumed an activist role. Butcher shops, restaurants, confectioners and other food-handling establishments were put on notice that they must conduct their operations in a sanitary manner. Prosecutions for violations of health ordinances became the rule rather than the exception.

8. A Crisis in Medical Education

Major changes occurred in medical education during the first two decades of the twentieth century. The proprietary medical college was passing out of existence. The costs of teaching the new scientific medicine rendered the proprietary schools unprofitable.[202] Besides the State Board of Health was raising the standard of "a reputable medical college" by demanding longer academic programs, more laboratory equipment and greater opportunities for clinical instruction.[203] To meet the pressure exerted by the state board, proprietary schools were merging. The Homeopathic College in 1910 dropped completely out of the competition. While the proprietary institutions were declining, the medical schools of St. Louis University and Washington University were making spectacular progress.

In the spring of 1903, St. Louis's six medical schools graduated 355 doctors, distributed as follows: Washington University, 55; Marion-Sims-Beaumont, 96; Barnes, 115; Physicians and Surgeons, 61; American Medical College, 18; and Homeopathic College, 10. St. Louis was the recognized medical capital of the South and Southwest.[204]

The Medical Department of Washington University had been formed in 1899 by the union of St. Louis's two oldest medical institutions, the Missouri Medical College and the St. Louis Medical College.[205] The following year, Washington University received a $3,000,000 gift from Samuel Cupples and Robert S. Brookings that made it one of the most richly endowed universities in the country.[206]

William K. Bixby, Adolphus Busch, Edward Mallinckrodt and Robert S. Brookings, in April 1910, contributed $2,000,000 to a fund to finance the establishment of a $5,000,000 medical school affiliated with Washington University. The plan was to make it the equal of Johns Hopkins Medical School. The new school would include the Barnes Hospital, the Children's Hospital, as well as administrative, teaching and research facilities.[207] The Abraham Flexner report on medical education in the United States and Canada picked Washington University Medical School as destined to be the leading institution in the Southwest for the training of physicians.[208]

St. Louisans were stunned to read in the newspapers of July 28, 1910 that radical changes would be made in the university medical staff. Among those slated to go was Dr. Herman Tuholske, one of the city's most distinguished doctors.[209] In September 1910, the new medical school dean Dr. George Dock, formerly a professor at Tulane University, arrived. The reorganization of the faculty was one of his first responsibilities.

The plan was to make an almost clean sweep of the existing faculty. This was the group of doctors which had been acquired by the merger of two rival schools to form the university's medical department.[210] Unfortunately, these doctors had brought to the university the rivalry and animosity which had characterized their prior relationship. While employed by their former proprietary schools, they had built up large private practices from which they drew their major income. They considered their medical lecturing as a sideline, performed mainly for the professional experience and prestige involved. The older ones had not been educated in the research methods of the new scientific medicine.

The university wanted bright young men, trained in research, willing to spend their time in teaching and investigation, and satisfied to depend upon their salaries rather than private practice for their livelihood. To secure this type of doctor, the dean went to the campuses of the leading Eastern medical schools and to the staff of neighboring St. Louis University Medical School.[211]

Students entering the Washington University Medical School in the fall of 1910 had to present a diploma from an accredited high school and also certification of completion of one year of college work, embracing English, physics, chemistry, biology and one elective. Students matriculating in 1912 must have two years of college work.[212]

The St. Louis University School of Medicine was also the outgrowth of two previously existing medical institutions. The Beaumont Hospital Medical College had commenced operations in 1886 at Sixteenth and Walnut streets. The college moved into a modern and well-equipped building at the southwest corner of Jefferson and Pine streets in 1890. In that year, a group of doctors established the Marion-Sims Medical School. These two colleges merged in 1901. St. Louis University in 1902 bought for $115,000 the Marion-Sims-Beaumont establishment. [213] The contract provided that the staff of local clinical specialists would remain unchanged until June 1911.[214] As of the fall of 1903, the name St. Louis University School of Medicine supplanted the title of Marion-Sims-Beaumont Medical School.

On May 8, 1905, the medical school graduated 108 doctors. The commencement speaker was Dr. John M. Dodson, dean of the Medical Department of the University of Chicago. He spoke on the subject "The Research Idea and Method in Medical Education and Practice." St. Louis University claimed the honor of being the local pioneer in introducing research methods in its medical program.[215]

Dr. Young H. Bond, dean of the St. Louis University School of Medicine and founder of the Marion-Sims Medical College, resigned in 1907. He was succeeded as dean by Dr. Elias Potter Lyon.[216] For the improvement of medical education in St. Louis, he proposed that St. Louis University, Washington University and the University of Missouri at Columbia pool their resources and establish a single institution in St. Louis for the clinical instruction of the third and fourth years of the medical program. The three institutions would limit their classes to the first and second years of medical education, principally the scientific background.[217]

A major reorganization of administration of the university was effected in April 1909 with the appointment of an advisory board of laymen to supervise its affairs. The board was composed of twenty-four members, leading citizens of St. Louis both Protestant and Catholic. The president of the university was ex officio chairman. He and Archbishop John J. Glennon were the only clergymen.[218]

One of the first major projects planned by the new board was the establishment of a modern hospital, with the finest staff and equipment. The hospital would be operated under the auspices of the medical college of the university. The Sisters of the Incarnate Word, who maintained a hospital in San Antonio, Texas, were to furnish the building and provide the nursing services. The university would be obligated to secure a suitable building site. The medical school was to provide the staff, which would consist only of physicians of established reputation.[219]

Tightened education requirements were announced for the entering class of medical students for the year beginning in the fall of 1910. Each matriculant must have one year of college work in physics, chemistry and biology in addition to a four-year high school course. The medical course itself was of four years duration.[220]

The high quality of the training at St. Louis University Medical School was evidenced by the fact that only three percent of its 1909 graduates failed their examinations before state boards. This was the lowest percentage of any of the nation's medical schools, including Johns Hopkins and Harvard.[221]

The approaching end of the contract, which had preserved the status quo of the faculty, enabled St. Louis University to begin a major reorganization of the medical school. The first step in this process was the appointment of Dr. Charles Hugh Neilson to the chair of medicine, a post next to the dean in importance. Dr. Neilson had acquired a Ph.D. in chemistry and physiology before earning his M.D. from Rush Medical College in Chicago. He had been on the faculty of St. Louis Medical School for six years. Dr. Neilson was put upon a salary so that he could devote full time to his university work. This was a departure from the practice in medical schools where the clinical chairs were usually filled by physicians who gave their services to the school. Unlike the situation at Washington University, no wholesale changes in the teaching faculty were planned although their duties would be modified.[222]

The improvements carried out at both St. Louis University and Washington University were so thorough-going and promising as to justify the phrase the "renaissance of medicine in St. Louis."[223]

The will of James Campbell, public utility magnate, filed in probate court, June 16, 1914, left his entire fortune worth an estimated $35,000,000 to $40,000,000 to the St. Louis Medical School. The money would become available at the end of a short trust period.[224]

Barnes University, a proprietary school, sought without much success to find a suitable marriage partner. In 1905, it offered its medical school and the adjoining Centenary Hospital to the Missouri State University free of charge. Barnes's offer was prompted by a rival tender to the state school made by the University Medical College of Kansas City. The state university, which operated a two-year course at Columbia, was handicapped by its inability to provide clinical instruction for third- and fourth-year students. The Barnes gift, if accepted, would endow the state institution with a college building, a hospital, a staff of clinical specialists and a supply of patients.[225] The total value of the property offered was $300,000.

On June 29, 1907, the board of curators of the Missouri State University, in a conference with the Barnes University board of trustees, initialed the acceptance of the proffered gift. September 1, 1908 was set as the date of transfer of the property. The donation was made without conditions. The University of Missouri had the privilege of retaining the Barnes faculty members or putting in its own selected staff. The plan of the university was to teach the first two years of medicine at Columbia and the junior and senior years in St. Louis.[226]

Dr. Pinckney French, president of the Barnes University board of trustees, in explaining the generous donation, said that:[227]

the Barnes University found itself unable longer properly to finance the institution it had built up, and, rather than close the school, the board had decided to transfer it to the State, which had funds for its continued operation.

The University of Missouri failed to carry through with the transfer agreement. No official reason was given. There are several plausible explanations. Just before the planned transfer, the Barnes Medical School was discredited by the State Board of Health, and its 1908 graduates were refused permission to take the board's qualifying examinations.[228] A further consideration was the prospect of having to compete with the Washington University Medical School and the St. Louis University School of Medicine. Finally, there is the likelihood that the university curators had signed the agreement without making sure that the state could generate and would provide the necessary funding.[229]

On July 25, 1909, it was announced that Barnes University had passed into the hands of the Baptist Church of America and was to be made the central university of a national network. Several smaller educational institutions of the Middle West were expected to consolidate with the university. New officers and directors were elected resulting in a complete change of management. In addition to operating schools of medicine, dentistry and pharmacy, it was planned to establish schools of law, business and fine arts.[230]

Several weeks later Barnes University absorbed the staff of a new institution, which had planned to operate under the name of the Humboldt Medical College. These doctors were formerly members of the faculty of the College of Physicians and Surgeons who had become dissatisfied and resigned. Barnes University also was carrying on negotiations looking to the absorption of the faculty of the College of Physicians and Surgeons who had remained after the exodus. The list of trustees of the reorganized Barnes University was embellished with the names of various judges, clergymen, military officers as well as doctors.[231]

Before the first term of the reorganized university had ended, dissension had broken out.

The election to the faculty of Dr. W. H. Mayfield, who had been expelled from the St. Louis Medical Society for violation of provisions of the code of ethics against advertising, was resented by a number of the university faculty who turned in their letters of resignation.[232] Dr. Mayfield, who was president of the board of trustees, severed his connection in August 1911.[233]

On October 1, 1911, the announcement was made that Barnes University Medical School and the College of Physicians and Surgeons had merged. This good news was offset by the notification by the State Board of Health that their work was substandard and that their students would get no credit for their 1911-1912 classes.[234] Later in the month, Barnes Medical College was taken over by the American Medical College. Since the American Medical College was in good standing with the state board, the merger restored credit to the work being done by Barnes University students for 1911-1912.[235] By 1912, American Medical College was the sole remaining proprietary school in St. Louis.[236] American Medical College, in 1914, was supplanted by the St. Louis College of Physicians and Surgeons.[237]

9. The Medical Legacy of the Nineteenth Century

The nineteenth century witnessed giant advances in the field of medicine. This was the era in which modern scientific medicine was born, as Dr. William W. Keen in his article on "The Progress of the Century," published in the February 3, 1901 issue of the St. Louis *Republic*, indicated:[238]

The old student of medicine went from case to case, heard many a good maxim and learned many a useful trick but, after

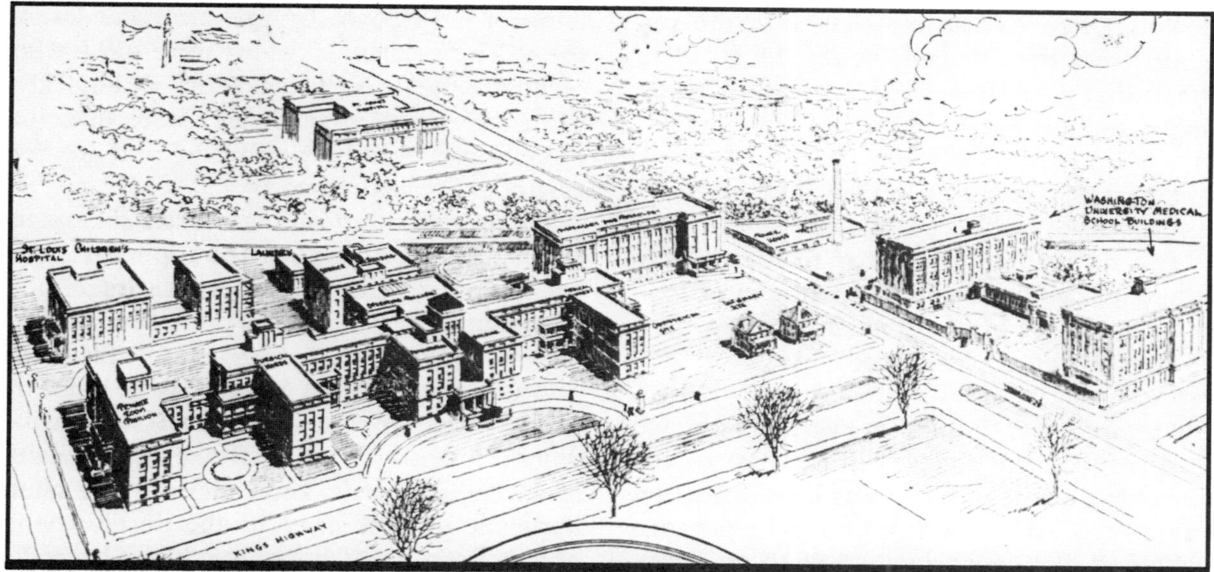

Barnes Hospital. Courtesy of the State Historical Society of Missouri.

all, it was only an empirical knowledge which he obtained. It did not go to the foundation of things; it was not scientific, as is the collegiate instruction of today.

The foundation of modern medical science was laid with the discovery by Louis Pasteur and Robert Koch that diseases are caused by germs or bacteria — infinitely small plant agents. Previously, certain fanciful speculations regarding disease causation had been advanced; but these did not lead to successful methods of treatment. With the discovery that each disease was caused by a specific germ, the search was initiated to find these specific causes and to take steps for their neutralization or eradication.[239]

Through careful laboratory work, it was established that bacteria form two principal classes, the cocci and the bacilli. The cocci, with their name derived from the Greek word coccus meaning "berry," are of two kinds. These are the staphylococci, which come in bunches, and the streptococci, which occur in long chains. The second class of bacteria, the bacilli, are rod-shaped.[240]

In 1883, Theodor Albrecht Klebs and Friedrich Loeffler identified the *bacillus diphtheriae* and successfully cultivated it on an artificial medium. Robert Koch found the tuberculosis bacillus and the cholera spirillum. Other important identifications of disease germs followed.

The nature and role of hospitals changed during the century. At the start they were charitable institutions, catering to indigent persons who were ill and homeless. The care was basically custodial. Hospital diseases induced by the crowded conditions abounded. The new style hospitals provided healthful and comfortable accommodations and served all classes of people. They were equipped with modern diagnostic and therapeutic equipment. Often they were closely associated with medical colleges.[241]

Laboratories for research and instruction in each branch of the new medicine were established. Of particular importance to the surgeon were the laboratories for the study of pathology or diseased tissue. Dr. Keen explained this relationship:[242]

So surgical pathology is the study of the processes of disease, the alterations in the minute structure of tissues and organs, without which no surgeon can be fitted for his task, much less can he be called an accomplished surgeon.

One problem of medical instruction which had plagued the colleges in the past — the obtaining of cadavers — was solved through state legislation making bodies of persons who had died in prisons, hospitals and mental institutions available to the medical schools. This eliminated the practice of grave robbing by professors and students.[243]

Dr. Keen pointed out how Darwin's theory greatly had enriched medical research:[244]

Largely owing to the doctrine of evolution, we now recognize the fact that, so far as his body is concerned, man is kindred to the brutes; that his diseases, within certain limitations, are identical with similar diseases of the lower animals; that his anatomy and physiology are, in essence, the same as the anatomy and physiology of the lower animals, even the very lowest; and that many of his diseases can be best studied in the lower animals, because upon them we can make exact experiments which would be impossible in man.

The practice of surgery was revolutionized by the development of anaesthesia. Previously, only the bravest patients were willing to undergo the excruciating pain of major surgery. They had to be strapped to the table or held down by the surgeon's attendants. The greatest surgeons were those who could use the knife most skillfully and quickly. With the use of anaesthesia, more difficult operations could be performed and greater care could be exercised.[245]

The introduction of anaesthesia increased the number of operations performed. Unfortunately, the post-operative infections from blood poisoning, erysipelas, tetanus and gangrene also rose. The remedy for this situation was found by Dr. Joseph Lister, who, in 1865, introduced a method of sterilizing wounds, bandages and instruments by means of antiseptic sprays and dressings. He later improved his technique by the development of aseptic surgery, which excluded bacteria in wounds by a scrupulous cleanliness of the operating theater and the surgical instruments. Dr. Lister's methods, which quickly spread, resulted in a dramatic increase in the safety of surgical operations.[246]

The transfer of the site of surgical operations from the home to well-equipped hospitals was another significant step in improving medical care. The delivery of babies was the last major operation to follow the trend from home to hospital care.

In the field of cures for diseases, the big break-through was the development of serum therapy. It was discovered that the liquid part of the blood of an animal, that has survived a certain disease, contains an antidote (or antibodies) against further infection. This serum from a laboratory animal can be used to confer immunity on human patients or to assist in curing patients who have acquired the disease. In 1890, Emil Adolph von Behring and Shibasaburo Kitazato pioneered in developing the serum employed in combatting diphtheria. Serums also were produced for treating tetanus, typhoid fever and spinal meningitis. The treatment of diseases by drugs lagged.

Only citrus juice, opium, quinine, and digitalis did what was expected of them. [247] Dr. William Travis Howard, Jr., in his work *Public Health Administration and the Natural History of Disease in Baltimore, Maryland 1797-1920,* declared:[248]

> There is no evidence that any drugs or other medicaments now or ever used are capable of exerting specific curative effects upon any of the exanthematous diseases, nor upon typhus and typhoid fevers, whooping-cough, pneumonia, bacillary dysentery, cholera, diarrhoeas and tuberculosis, nor, until the specific antisera came into use, upon diphtheria, epidemic meningitis, and tetanus.

Sanitary science wrought miracles in preventing diseases. The provision of wholesome supplies of water and of milk, the enforcement of pure food and drug laws, the installation of flush toilets and the treatment of human wastes in disposal plants, these and other similar measures helped to confer upon city populations a collective immunity.

Aided by the techniques of anaesthesia and asepsis, surgery made rapid progress. Operations on the head, the chest and abdomen, previously barred because of the danger of post-operative infections, became routine.[249]

New instruments and tools enhanced the efficiency of the surgeon. These included the ophthalmoscope, to examine the interior of the eye; the rhinoscope, to look into the nose; the hemostatic forceps for clamping arteries; the clinical thermometer and many others. Of the new instruments, none was more important than the X-ray machine, which produced pictures of the body's bones, muscles and organs.[250]

This rich legacy provided the curriculum for the progressive medical schools of the twentieth century and became the basis for spectacular new discoveries and inventions.

10. The Medical Profession's Progress From Powerlessness to Authority

The medical profession entered the twentieth century in a disorganized state. It was badly overcrowded, with many of its practitioners the products of diploma mills. The monetary return of its members was low in comparison with other professions. Its public image was unflattering. Despite recent scientific advances in surgery and in serum therapy, its efficiency in curing disease was not impressive. Two major sectarian systems, the Eclectics and the homeopaths, created dissension in the ranks of the profession. The American Medical Association, the national organization of the regulars, was supported by only a fraction of the eligible doctors.[251]

During the first two decades of the twentieth century, this situation was dramatically changed. The Eclectics and the homeopaths, in culmination of a process that had been gradually taking place, merged with the regulars.[252] In St. Louis, the Good Samaritan Hospital, the citadel of the homeopaths, became allopathic in 1902.[253] The Homeopathic Medical College of St. Louis, following an unfavorable evaluation by the State Board of Health, closed its doors in 1910.[254] The American Medical College (Eclectic), in 1910, joined the regulars.[255]

The Medical Practice Act, approved by the Missouri legislature March 12, 1901, tightened the licensing requirements for physicians. No longer was the possession of a diploma from a medical college sufficient to enable a person to practice. The new law required a candidate for a license to pass, with a grade of at least seventy-five percent, an examination given by the State Board of

Health.[256] By an amendment to the law, enacted in 1907, an applicant must also possess a certificate of graduation from an accredited high school or college and a diploma from a reputable four-year medical college.[257] These laws, with the resultant closing of several of the state's marginal medical schools, reduced the influx of poorly trained doctors into the profession.

The American Medical Association, in a major reorganization carried out in 1901, changed the basis for representation in its house of delegates. Previously, county and regional chapters as well as state organizations could send representatives to the national governing body. Under the new constitution, only state associations could elect delegates to the national assembly, which was reduced in size to 150 members. To belong to the American Medical Association, a doctor had to hold membership in his county and state organizations. The new plan made the county medical societies "the foundation of the whole superstructure."[258] The failure of a doctor to join his local medical society brought serious consequences, such as "denial of hospital privileges, loss of referrals, loss of malpractice insurance, and, in extreme cases, loss of a license to practice."[259] The new constitution vitalized the national as well as the state medical organizations. Membership in the American association jumped from 8,000 in 1900 to 70,000 in 1910. The Missouri society, reorganized in 1903, witnessed its membership grow in one year from 258 to 1,600 and its revenues expand from $774 to $3,200.[260]

The growing authority of the medical profession coincided with a radical change in the role of hospitals, as described by Paul Starr in *The Social Transformation of American Medicine:*[261]

But in a matter of decades, roughly between 1870 and 1910, hospitals moved from the periphery to the center of medical education and medical practice. From refuges mainly for the homeless poor and insane, they evolved into doctors' workshops for all types and classes of patients. From charities, dependent on voluntary gifts, they developed into market institutions, financed increasingly out of payments from patients. What drove this transformation was not simply the advance of science, important though that was, but the demands and example of an industrializing capitalist society, which brought larger numbers of people into urban centers, detached them from traditions of self-sufficiency, and projected ideals of specialization and technical competence. The same forces that promoted the rise of hospitals also brought about changes in their internal organization. Authority over the conduct of the institution passed from the trustees to the physicians and administrators. Nursing became a trained profession, and the division of medical labor was refined and intensified, as conceptions of efficient and rational organization prevailing elsewhere in the economy were applied to care of the sick. The sick began to enter hospitals, not for an entire siege of illness, but only during its acute phase to have some work performed upon them. The hospital took on a more activist posture; it was no longer a well of sorrow and charity but a workplace for the production of health . . . .

The access that private practitioners gained to hospitals, without becoming their employees, became one of the distinctive features of medical care in America, with consequences not fully appreciated even today. In Europe and most other areas of the world, when patients enter a hospital, their doctors typically relinquish responsibility to the hospital staff, who form a separate and distinct group within the profession. But in the United States, private doctors follow their patients into the hospital, where they continue to attend them.

11. Increase of State Responsibility in Medical Matters

The Missouri legislature, in the early twentieth century, abandoned the passive role it had maintained in regard to public health issues. The licensing of physicians had been left to the medical colleges, with the possession of a diploma the only prerequisite for practice. The function of the State Board of Health had been limited to deciding which colleges were reputable. The state board had authority to quarantine districts in which contagious diseases existed in order to prevent contacts by residents from outside. But it had no power to send its agents into infected areas to combat and control disease outbreaks. The State Board of Health, operating on a pitifully small annual budget, was an advisory rather than an administrative body.[262]

With the passage of the Medical Practice Act of March 12, 1901, the state assumed control of medical licensing through the establishment of an examining board, which passed on the qualifications of applicants. A decision of the Missouri Supreme Court, in 1897, had denied the right of the Missouri State Board of Health to decide what out-of-state medical schools were reputable. The diplomas of out-of-state medical schools, approved by their own state boards, had to be accepted without question.[263] The prejudicial effects of this decision were overcome by requiring that all candidates for a license must pass successfully an examination before the Missouri Board of Health.

Since the 1901 law did not specify the preliminary education required of medical students, many candidates for the M.D. degree were coming before the board with inadequate educational prerequisites. For some groups of applicants, the failure rate was as high as fifty percent.[264] Legislation, enacted by the Missouri Assembly on June 14, 1907, spelled out the preliminary requirements which a candidate must satisfy. He must have a certificate of graduation from an accredited high school or its equivalent. Further, he must have earned a diploma from a four-year medical college that was accredited by the Missouri State Board of Health. The St. Louis *Republic*, in its issue of September 15, 1907, summarized the state of Missouri's tightening of its requirements for the licensing of physicians:[265]

Up to and including the year 1894, a good moral character and a diploma from some reputable medical college of two years' requirements. From the close of 1894 to 1901, the applicant for a license to practice must have presented a diploma from a reputable medical college of three years' requirements. From March 12, 1901 to June 14, 1907, the applicant was required to take an examination before the State Board of Health, and secure an average of 75 per cent of such questions as were asked. Since June 14, 1907, the applicant must have the preliminary qualifications, be a graduate of a reputable medical college of four years' requirements before he is allowed to take the examination.

The dates of Missouri's two major laws dealing with medical licensing, i.e., 1901 and 1907, indicate that the state had begun to eliminate its inefficient proprietary medical schools considerably before the publication in 1910 of the Carnegie Foundation report on medical education by Alexander Flexner. Those proprietary schools that survived into the first decade of the twentieth century had already ceased to be profitable and were closing voluntarily.[266] In St. Louis, a major factor hastening their demise was the formidable competition of their richly endowed competitors, the Washington University Medical School and the St. Louis University School of Medicine.

In 1905, the Missouri assembly established a sanatorium for the treatment of incipient cases of tuberculosis at Mt. Vernon, the county seat of Lawrence County in southwest Missouri. This was one of the first instances of the state of Missouri crossing the imaginary line between public health and private practice. The medical profession of St. Louis, in 1901, had fought the efforts of the local board of health to persuade the municipal assembly to declare tuberculosis a contagious disease and thus subject to quarantine and other public health measures.

The bill to establish the Mt. Vernon sanatorium was introduced by Dr. James Stewart of Warren County and apparently encountered no organized opposition from the medical societies. Tuberculosis was one of the state's most lethal diseases. The medical profession had no drugs that could cure or even halt it. The only proven remedy was to treat it in the incipient stage in a sanatorium, which provided open-air living, rest and plenty of nourishing food. The treatment might extend over months or even several years. A mountain location was preferable. The sanatorium at Mt. Vernon was at an elevation of 1,200 feet above sea level and consisted of a hospital-administrative building and a group of villas spaced in an irregular pattern. Each villa had a long covered portico, on which the patient slept except in the coldest weather. The sanatorium served paying as well as charity patients.[269]

Missouri's plan for the care of its insane was to provide in each of the four corners of the state a mental hospital; in addition there was the Fulton hospital in the center of the state. The population of the four state institutions at the dates indicated was as follows: State Hospital No. 1 (Fulton), as of December 31, 1912, 1,003 patients; State Hospital No. 2 (St. Joseph), as of August 1, 1913, 1,505 patients; State Hospital No. 3 (Nevada), as of June 1, 1913, 1,249; State Hospital No. 4 (Farmington), as of August 1, 1913, 594 patients. Each hospital with its extensive acreage was a cooperative farm, producing much of its food and dairy products.[270]

The methods of treatment employed in the state hospitals thus were described by the superintendent of State Hospital No. 4 in his second biennial report for the years 1903-1904:[271]

Drugs are not specially indicated in the treatment of insanity. Outdoors exercise, baths and good wholesome food, instead of drugs, are relied upon almost entirely to promote sleep.

There are other measures of inestimable value. I refer particularly to amusements of various kinds. There is no doubt of the therapeutic value of amusements and employment. The beneficial results obtained by diversion is recognized by all who are conversant with the advanced methods of treatment of insanity. It serves the purpose of destroying the monotony of hospital life, stimulates the mind to greater activity and greatly improves the general health.

The twelfth biennial report of Hospital No. 3 for 1910-1911 indicated no major changes in treatment procedures:[272]

The long line of mechanical restraints and heroic drug treatments have been displaced by hydrotherapy, massage, proper food, outdoor life, occupation and rest, with indicated medical treatment.

Missouri, in 1901, moved toward the establishment of a public health system. The major cities and some counties had boards of health and health officials. But many small towns and rural counties lacked these agencies.[273] In outbreaks of smallpox, diphtheria and other contagious diseases, they had to rely on the uncoordinated efforts of their local doctors. Many of these practitioners were unprepared to identify, much less to treat, these epidemic diseases.[274]

The legislature, by a law passed on January 25, 1901, ordered the establishment in each county of a board of health consisting of the judges of the county court and a reputable physician appointed by them. The county board was endowed with the same powers and authority given to the State Board of Health in relation to the prevention of spreading of contagious diseases. The county board was to act as a subsidiary to the state board and enforce the regulations of the parent body.[275] An important omission in the law was that it did not specifically require the county boards to register and report the names of those sick of contagious diseases.[276]

The State Board of Health commented on this damaging deficiency in its twenty-ninth annual report covering the years 1911-1912:[277]

There will be little progress made in this State in the matter of conserving the health and lives of its citizens until legislation is had placing the local health officers under the jurisdiction of the State Board of Health and, until by statute, with a penalty clause attached, contagious and infectious diseases shall be reported to local and State health authorities.

The recommendations of the State Board of Health were implemented in a law approved by the legislature, May 21, 1919. The experience of the state during the influenza epidemic of 1918-1919, when many communities were without leadership in the fight against the disease, may have prompted the general assembly to act. The law provided for the appointment of a commissioner of health to enforce the rules of the state board, a task formerly carried out by the secretary of the board. The commissioner must have had experience in public health administration. The State Board of Health was given the responsibility "to safeguard the health of the people in the state, counties, cities, villages and towns." Each county court every third year was to appoint a reputable physician as a deputy state commissioner. If the county court failed to act, the State Board of Health was empowered to make the appointment. The deputy commissioners were charged to enforce the rules and regulations of the state board. Dereliction of duty was punishable as a misdemeanor. All rules and regulations made under the new law by the State Board of Health were to supersede local ordinances and were to be enforced by local and state authorities. Cities of more than 75,000 population that maintained organized health departments would not be affected by the law provided they furnished the State Board of Health with regular reports of the incidence of contagious diseases.[278]

Hospitals, like health agencies, were concentrated in the large cities. Most were affiliated with religious denominations and private universities. The general assembly, on March 19, 1907, passed a law authorizing the county court of each county to levy a tax or issue bonds to build and operate a county hospital. It was the intent of the legislature that the counties should place in their hospitals the poor for whom they were responsible.[279] Gradually, this restricted mission of the hospitals was abandoned.

An effective public health program requires accurate and comprehensive statistical information. To provide such data, the State Board of Health, in conformity with an act of the general assembly approved May 9, 1909, established the Central Bureau of Vital Statistics. This law required the prompt registration of all births and deaths. The central bureau was to be located in Jefferson City. The secretary of the State Board of Health was to serve as the state registrar of vital statistics.[280]

For the collection of data, the state was divided into registration districts. Each city and each incorporated town comprised a separate district. For the portion of each county outside of incorporated communities, the state board was authorized to designate the boundaries of rural registration districts. For each registration district, the State Board of Health was to appoint a registrar. The local registrars were entitled to be paid twenty-five cents for each birth certificate and each death certificate turned in by the attending physicians for registration.[281]

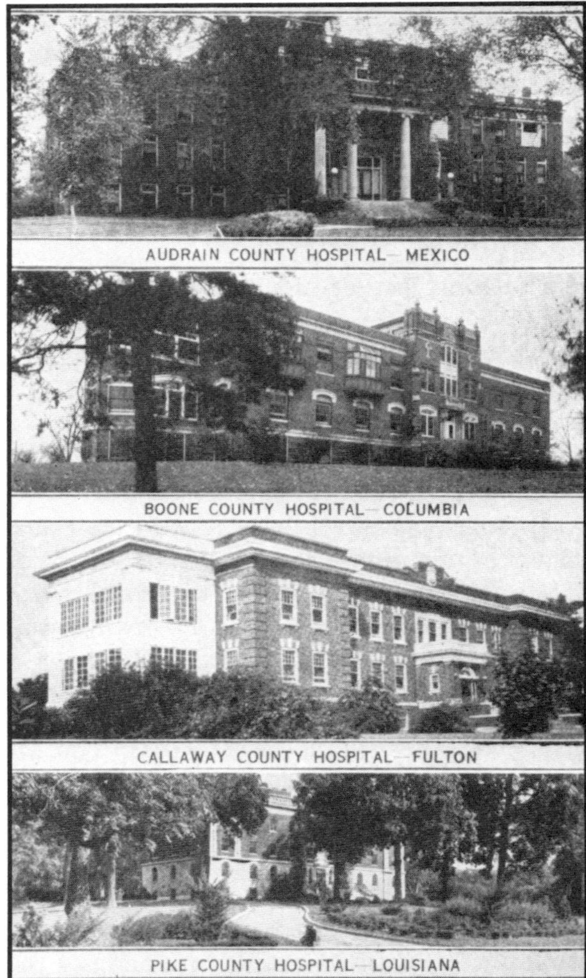

Early couty hospitals. Courtesy of the State Historical Society of Missouri.

The administration of the law was so satisfactory that, after a thorough survey of the state office and a checking of its returns by a representative of the National Bureau of the Census, Missouri was admitted to the United States registration area as of January 1, 1911.[282]

The budget of the State Board of Health increased steadily as new responsibilities were assigned to the board:[283]

1901-1902 ....$15,000
1903-1904 ....$10,000
1905-1906 ....$13,000
1907-1908 ....$15,000
1909-1910 ....$15,000
1911-1912 ....$62,300
1913-1914 ....$62,000
1915-1916 ....$67,250
1917-1918 ....$52,550
1919-1920 ....$55,000

The biennial appropriation of $15,000 for 1901-1902 provided $5,000 for the secretary's salary, office expenses and collecting statistics. Ten thousand dollars of the appropriation were allocated for eradicating smallpox.[284] The $13,000 appropriation for 1905-1906 contained funds for a bacteriologist and for controlling infectious diseases.[285] These were items in addition to the former expenses of the board.

The 1909-1910 law included funds for the payment of a $10 per diem to members of the State Board of Health while engaged in official business.[286] The 1911-1912 appropriation provided financial support for the Central Bureau of Vital Statistics.[287] This was the major item of the board's expenditures for the remainder of the decade.

The state board was in part self-supporting. Fees charged for administering the medical licensing examinations and also for furnishing information from the Bureau of Vital Statistics regarding births and deaths contributed toward meeting the expenses of the board.

By 1920, the State Board of Health was a firmly established part of the bureaucracy, with a biennial budget of $55,000 and a staff of a dozen officials, clerks and stenographers.[288] A 1919 directive had commissioned it to bring the benefits of scientific medicine into every city, county and town of the state. In preparation for this task, it added to its two administrative divisions of vital statistics and laboratories new ones for preventable diseases, child hygiene and venereal disease.[289]

12. Miscellaneous Examining Boards

By an act of March 27, 1903, the general assembly accorded professional status to a new school of medical practice — the osteopaths. It created a board of osteopathic registration and examination, consisting of five osteopathic physicians. This was the first instance of the legislature setting up a separate examining board for a specialized medical group; the homeopaths and the Eclectics took their examinations before the State Board of Health. The osteopathic board was authorized to elect a secretary, who could receive a salary of not more than $1,500 a year. Members of the board would receive compensation not exceeding $10 a day for time spent in discharge of their duties.[290]

A person desiring to practice osteopathy was required to apply to the secretary of the board for a certificate. His application must show that he had completed a course of not less than four terms of five months each in a reputable osteopathic college. He must then successfully pass an examination prepared by the board covering general medical courses and also specific osteopathic offerings. A successful candidate received a certificate, which he had to present for recording in the office of the county clerk of the county in which he expected to practice.[291]

The advances made in medicine and surgery in the nineteenth and early twentieth centuries created a need for highly trained nurses. Those nurses, who by education and experience had enhanced their professional skills, were entitled to some mark of distinction, corresponding to the doctor's "M.D."

By an act of May 6, 1909, the general assembly established the board of examination and registration of nurses, consisting of five members. The majority of the appointees had to be chosen "from those actually engaged in nursing and who have graduated from reputable training schools, giving not less than a two years' course of training, who have had at least five years' experience in nursing and caring for the sick and afflicted, including one year's teaching in a training school for nurses."[292]

Every applicant for registration must be at least twenty-one years old, of good moral character, with a general education equivalent to that obtained by the completion of a grammar school course of study.[293]

Any applicant could be registered to practice nursing, without taking an examination, who possessed a diploma issued before December 1, 1912, by a training school connected with a general hospital giving a two or more years' training course, with systematic instruction in the hospital wards.[294]

For older nurses, an alternative method of obtaining registration was provided. Any applicant would be registered, without an examination, who prior to 1895 had received one year's training in a general hospital and who was actually engaged in professional nursing at the date of passage of the act.[295]

After 1912, the applicant would be registered if he or she had a diploma from a training school connected with a general hospital requiring a course of two or more years training, with systematic experience in a general hospital, and upon passing such an examination before the board as might be considered necessary to determine the fitness and ability of the applicant to give efficient care of the sick.[296]

Every applicant for registration must pay a fee of five dollars. Upon receipt of a certificate to practice, each nurse must file a copy with the county clerk of the county in which he or she resided. Any person who had complied with the provision of the law and received a certificate would be known as a "registered nurse" and qualified to use the designation "R.N."[297]

Chapter VII
An Era of Progress and Reform, 1900-1920

1   Rolla Wells was born in St. Louis, June 1, 1856. He was educated at Washington University and at Princeton. Upon the death of his father, he assumed the management of the former's large business and property interests. Rolla Wells was recognized as one of the leaders of the Democratic party of St. Louis and the nation. His two terms as mayor of St. Louis were among the most constructive in the city's history. He served as treasurer of the Democratic National Committee from 1912 to 1916 and as chairman of the board of the Federal Reserve Bank of St. Louis for the term beginning in September 1929. Walter Williams and Floyd C. Shoemaker, eds. *Missouri Mother of the West.* Revised edition. (The American Historical Society, Chicago, 1930), Vol. IV, pp. 33-34.

2   The report of the grand jury which investigated the boodling activities of Ed Butler's combine gave the following description of St. Louis' law makers: "We have had before us many of those who have been, and most of those who are now, members of the House of Delegates. We regret to report that we have found a number of these utterly illiterate and lacking in ordinary intelligence, unable to give a better reason for favoring or opposing a measure than desire to act with the majority. In some no trace of mentality or morality could be found. In others, a low order of training appeared, united with base cunning, groveling instincts and sordid desires. Unqualified to respond to the ordinary requirments of life, they are utterly incapable of comprehending the significance of an ordinance, and are incapacitated both by nature and by training to be the makers of laws." St. Louis *Republic,* Apr. 6, 1902, part I, p. 1:6.

3   James N. Primm, *Lion of the Valley: St. Louis,* Missouri (Boulder, Colorado, Pruett Publishing Co., 1981), pp. 385, 390.

4   St. Louis *Republic,* Apr. 25, 1901, p. 4:3.

5   *Idem.*

6   *Ibid,* Aug. 15, 1900, p. 14:1.

7   *Idem.*

8   *Ibid,* Dec. 25, 1904, part III, p. 3:1-4.

9   *Ibid,* Jan. 24, 1903, p. 7:3.

10   *Ibid,* Aug. 9, 1905, p. 14:1; *ibid,* Aug. 11, 1905, p. 3.

11   *Ibid,* Aug. 13, 1905, part II, p. 8:3-4.

12   *Idem.*

13   *Idem; ibid,* May 7, 1911, part I, p. 10:2-4.

14   *Ibid,* May 28, 1906, p. 10:2.

15   *Ibid,* May 7, 1911, part I, p. 10:2-4.

16   *Ibid,* June 9, 1909, p. 9:2; *ibid,* Apr. 1, 1910, p. 8:1.

17   *Ibid,* June 9, 1909, p. 9:2.

18   *Ibid,* Apr. 1, 1910, p. 8:1.

19   *Idem.*

20   *The Revised Code of St. Louis, 1912,* ed., by Edgar R. Rombauer, p. 741.

21   St. Louis *Republic,* June 11, 1910, p. 1:5.

22   *Ibid,* June 15, 1910, p. 1:7.

23   *Ibid,* June 11, 1910, p. 1:5. In the text of the article, the number of visiting doctors was given as thirty-six. However, in a box in which the doctors were named the number was thirty-seven.

24   *Ibid,* June 15, 1910, p. 1:7.

25   *The Revised Code of St. Louis, 1912,* p. 743.

26   *Ibid,* p. 745.

27   St. Louis *Republic,* Dec. 22, 1906, p. 14:3.

28   *Ibid,* Jan. 6, 1908, p. 12:4.

29   *Ibid,* May 26, 1910, p. 12:4.

30   *Ibid,* May 21, 1907, p. 14:2.

31   *Ibid,* Oct. 9, 1910, part V, p. 6.

32   *Ibid,* May 19, 1902, p. 7:2.

33   *Ibid,* Aug. 18, 1901, part I, p. 7:2-3.

34   *Ibid,* Apr. 5, 1907, p. 5:2.

35   *Idem.*

36   *Ibid,* June 2, 1908, p. 1:1.

37   *Ibid,* Dec. 10, 1910, p. 2:4.

38   *Ibid,* May 12, 1912, part II, p. 9:2-5.

39   *Ibid,* Dec. 20, 1914, part II, p. 1:1-5.

40   *Ibid,* Dec. 20, 1914, part II, p. 1:5.

41   Additional buildings have been erected since 1914.

42   St. Louis Children's Hospital was a separate corporation with its own governing board. The north and south laboratories and the administration building east of Euclid Avenue were the property of Washington University. The title to the buildings west of Euclid Avenue, excluding the St. Louis Children's Hospital, was vested in the Methodist Episcopal Church, South. St. Louis *Republic,* Dec. 20, 1914, part II, p. 1:2-3.

43   St. Louis *Republic,* Dec. 20, 1914, part II, p. 1.

44   *Ibid,* July 13, 1913, part IV, p. 1:6.

45   St. Louis *Republic,* Dec. 20, 1914, part II, p. 1:4.

46   *Ibid,* Dec. 20, 1914, part II, p. 1:6.

47   *Ibid,* Oct. 30, 1902, p. 5:2-4.

48   *Ibid,* June 20, 1905, p. 4:2.

49   *Ibid,* Dec. 10, 1905, part I, p. 10:4.

50   *Ibid,* May 8, 1911, p. 10:4-6.

51   *Ibid,* Aug. 2, 1902, p. 8:2.

52   *Ibid,* June 11, 1906, p. 6:4.

53   *Ibid,* Feb. 3, 1910, part I, p. 1:4.

54   *Ibid,* May 12, 1912, part II, p. 9:5.

55   The names of the major hospitals and their patient capacities were as follows: city hospital, 300; female hospital, 300; quarantine hospital, 150; emergency hospital, 100; Alexian Brothers Hospital, 250; St. Mary's Infirmary, 150; Missouri Baptist Sanitarium, 150; St. Luke's Hospital, 135; Lutheran Hospital, 125; St. Louis Mullanphy Hospital, 150; Jewish Hospital, 100; Washington University Hospital, 125; Mayfield Sanitarium, 106; St. Anthony's Hospital, 200; Bethesda Incurables' Hospital, 30; St. Louis Skin and Cancer Hospital, 25; Evangelical Deaconesses' Hospital, 90; St. Louis Children's Hospital, 90; Mount St. Rose Sanitarium, 65; St. Ann's Maternity Hospital, 60; St. Louis Baptist Hospital, 60; Jefferson Hospital, 55; St. John's Hospital, 50; association hospital, 50; Martha Parsons Free Hospital for Children, 50; Protestant Hospital, 40; Christian Hospital, 30; Josephine Hospital, 30; Rebekah Hospital, 35; Provident Hospital (for Negroes), 15; Missouri Pacific Railway Hospital, 80; Frisco Railway Hospital, 70. St. Louis *Republic,* Dec. 2, 1906, part II, p. 2:2. Besides its numerous hospitals, St. Louis had twenty-five institutions for the relief and care of neglected children, thirteen institutions for aid of the aged poor, four organizations for the relief of

defectives, six institutions for the rehabilitation of delinquents. There were also some sixty miscellaneous institutions for "preventive, social, supervisory and educational work in charity." St. Louis *Republic,* May 20, 1906, p. 34:1-4. Probably at no time in St. Louis's history has the "safety net" for its unfortunates, provided by private organizations, been more comprehensive and adequate than in the first decade of the twentieth century.

56 St. Louis *Republic,* Dec. 2, 1906, part II, p. 2:2.

57 Morris J. Vogel, *The Invention of the Modern Hospital, Boston 1870-1930* (Chicago, the University of Chicago Press, 1980), pp. 52, 100-101.

58 St. Louis *Republic,* Feb. 13, 1902, p. 1:6-7.

59 *Ibid.,* Nov. 2, 1901, p. 1:5-7; *ibid.,* Dec. 27, 1901, p. 2:3-4.

60 *Ibid.,* Nov. 20, 1901, p. 7:5; *ibid.,* Dec. 27, 1901, p. 2:3-4; *ibid.,* Feb. 13, 1902, p. 1:6-7.

61 *Ibid.,* Feb. 13, 1902, p. 1:6-7.

62 *Ibid.,* Feb. 4, 1906, p. 6:2-3.

63 *Ibid.,* Feb. 19, 1907, p. 1:4.

64 *Ibid.,* Apr. 1, 1910, p. 8:1.

65 *Ibid.,* Jan. 15, 1905, part II, p. 8:4.

66 *Ibid.,* Oct. 30, 1910, part V, p. 6:7; Primm, *opus cit.,* pp. 345-418.

67 St. Louis *Republic,* Nov. 10, 1901, part III, p. 1:3.

68 *Idem.*

69 *Idem.* The doctors feared that under the proposed law their patients suffering from tuberculosis would be removed from their homes to county almshouses or to state sanitaria. Many tuberculosis patients shared this fear. St. Louis *Republic,* May 19, 1911, part V, p. 2:1.

70 *Ibid.,* Nov. 10, 1901, part III, p. 1:3.

71 *Idem.*

72 *Ibid.,* July 4, 1909, part V, p. 5.

73 *Ibid.,* Jan. 15, 1905, part II, p. 8:1.

74 *Ibid.,* May 11, 1905, p. 2:1-2; *ibid.,* Jan. 15, 1905, part II, p. 8:3.

75 *Ibid.,* Jan. 15, 1905, part II, p. 8:1-2.

76 *Ibid.,* May 24, 1907, p. 3:2.

77 *Revised Code of St. Louis, 1914,* ed. by Hugh K. Wagner (St. Louis, Von Hoffman Press, 1918), pp. 1236-1237.

78 St. Louis *Republic,* Oct. 30, 1910, part V, p. 6:7.

79 *Ibid.,* Dec. 18, 1910, part V, p. 2:1.

80 *Ibid.,* Oct. 30, 1910, part V, p. 6:7. Deaths in St. Louis during the first decade from other diseases were as follows: smallpox, 144; measles, 518; scarlatina, 625; diphtheria, 1,582; croup, 327; whooping cough, 591; cerebro-spinal fever, 166; typhomalarial and other fevers, 729; puerperal fever, 241; diarrhoeal diseases, 2791; erysipelas, 573; septicaemia, 814; syphilis, 283; other zymotic diseases, 400; phthisis and tuberculosis, 11, 521; marasmus and scrofula, 2,365; hydrocephalus and tubercular meningitis, 1198; rheumatism and gout, 397; bronchitis, 3,546; pneumonia, 9,971; heat stroke, 377; cirrhosis of liver, 1,980; alcoholism, 348; diseases of generative organs, 402; la grippe, 230; other diseases of respiratory organs, 2,529; typhus fever, 1; suicide, 1,845; homicide, 848; accident, 4,346. Total 53,093. The 1,615 deaths from typhoid are included in this figure. Several of the individual disease totals were badly blurred on the source consulted so may have been misread. St. Louis *Republic,* Oct. 30, 1910, part V, p. 6:7.

81 *Ibid.,* Feb. 20, 1906, p. 3:1.

82 On this point, the court declared: "Where, as here, the plaintiff has sovereign powers and deliberately permits discharges similar to those of which it complains, it not only offers a standard to which the defendant has the right to appeal, but as some of these discharges are above the intake of St. Louis, it warrants the defendants in demanding the strictest proof that the plaintiff's own conduct does not produce the result, or at least so conduce to it that courts should not be curious to apportion the blame." St. Louis *Republic,* Feb. 20, 1910, p. 3:3.

83 St. Louis *Republic,* Feb. 20, 1906, p. 3:3; *ibid.,* Feb. 20, 1906, p. 3:4.

84 Primm, *opus cit.,* p. 401.

85 The 1918 influenza attack was a pandemic, with an estimated 30 to 40 million deaths. Alfred W. Crosby, Jr., *Epidemic and Peace 1918* (Westport, Connecticut, Greenwood Press, 1976), p. 207.

86 St. Louis *Republic,* Oct. 3, 1918, p. 5:1-2.

87 *Ibid.,* Oct. 4, 1918, part II, p. 1-2. The bill was passed Oct. 14.

88 *Idem.*

89 *Idem.*

90 *Idem.*

91 *Ibid.,* Oct. 8, 1918, part I, p. 1:2-3.

92 *Ibid.,* Oct. 9, 1918, p. 1:2-3.

93 *Idem.*

94 *Ibid.,* Oct. 20, 1918, part II, p. 5:2.

95 *Ibid.,* Nov. 9, 1918, p. 1:1.

96 *Ibid.,* Oct. 10, 1918, p. 1:4.

97 *Idem.*

98 *Ibid.,* Oct. 15, 1918, part II, p. 1-7.

99 *Ibid.,* Oct. 28, 1918, part II, p. 1:2.

100 Crosby, *opus cit.,* These figures are for influenza and pneumonia combined.

101 *Ibid.,* p. 8.

102 *Ibid.,* p. 7.

103 In Philadelphia, the local branch of the Council of National Defense coordinated the defense against influenza. Crosby, *opus cit.,* p. 79.

104 *Ibid.,* p. 60; St. Louis *Republic,* Nov. 13, 1918, p. 1:2.

105 St. Louis *Republic,* Nov. 28, 1918, p. 2:4-5.

106 *Ibid.,* Dec. 7, 1918, part II, p. 1:4.

107 Crosby, *opus cit.,* p. 61. The students permitted to return to classes were probably as safe in school as they would have been at home. Their teachers in the early weeks of the epidemic had acquired valuable experience as nurses' aides. They could be expected to enforce proper ventilation and the banning of crowds in the schools. Regular medical checks could identify pupils in the early stages of colds and influenza. These could be sent home.

108 Crosby, *opus cit.,* p. 61.

109 *Ibid.,* p. 212 (unnumbered)

110 *Idem.* This was one of the lowest rates for which statistics were available.

111 St. Louis *Republic,* Sept. 6, 1903, part II, p. 1:1-4.

112 *Idem; ibid.,* June 8, 1902, magazine section, p. 7.

113 *Ibid.,* June 8, 1902, magazine section, p. 7.

114 *Ibid.,* Oct. 26, 1906, p. 6:2-6.

115 *Ibid.,* Apr. 24, 1901, p. 8:1.
116 *Ibid.,* Jan. 23, 1904, p. 1:1; *ibid.,* June 12, 1910, part V, p. 4.
117 *Ibid.,* Nov. 6, 1910, part V, p. 6.
118 *Ibid.,* Oct. 26, 1906, p. 6:2-6.
119 St. Louis *Missouri Republican,* Mar. 21, 1871, p. 2:6.
120 St. Louis *Republic,* Mar. 28, 1896, p. 11:6.
121 *Municipal Code of St. Louis,* ed., by Eugene McQuillin 1901 (St. Louis, Mo., Woodward and Tiernan Printing Co., 1901) p. 533.
122 *Idem.*
123 St. Louis *Republic,* Feb. 25, 1906, part IV, p. 1:5-6.
124 *Ibid.,* Oct. 23, 1906, p. 10:1.
125 The city chemist, in December 1902, stated that 4,500 dealers supplied St. Louis with milk. Approximately 250 of these operated within the city limits. St. Louis *Republic,* Dec. 4, 1902, p. 16:6.
126 *Ibid.,* July 29, 1906, part I, p. 2:1. Much of the milk sold in St. Louis contained 8,000,000 to 10,000,000 bacteria per cubic centimeter. *Ibid.,* part I, p. 2:4.
127 *Ibid.,* part I, p. 2:1.
128 *Ibid.,* May 13, 1911, p. 5:1.
129 *Ibid.,* July 10, 1902, p. 14:4.
130 *Ibid.,* Aug. 1, 1902, p. 14:4.
131 *Revised Code of St. Louis* 1907, ed. by William F. Woerner (St. Louis, Mo., Samuel F. Myerson Printing Co., 1907) pp. 671-680.
132 *Laws of Missouri, Passed at the Regular Session of the Forty-Third General Assembly, Begun and Held at the City of Jefferson, January 4, 1905* (Jefferson City, Mo., The Hugh Stephens Printing Co., 1905) pp. 133-135.
133 *Laws of Missouri, Passed at the Regular and Extra Sessions of the Forty-Fourth General Assembly, Regular Session Begun and Held January 2, 1907. Extra Session Begun and Held April 9, 1907 at the City of Jefferson* (Jefferson City, Mo., The Hugh Stephens Printing Co., 1907) pp. 246-251.
134 *The Revised Statutes of the State of Missouri, Revised and Promulgated by the Forty-Fifth General Assembly* (Jefferson City, Mo., The Hugh Stephens Printing Co., 1909) Vol. I, p. 324. In the case of *St. Louis v. Dairy Co.* (213 Mo. 148), the Missouri Supreme Court decided that "a city may fix standards of purity and strength equal with or less than those by state law, but not greater." *Revised Code of St. Louis 1914,* ed. by Hugh K. Wagner (St. Louis, Mo., 1918) p. 1196 footnote.
135 St. Louis *Republic,* Oct. 11, 1911, p. 5:2.
136 *Revised Code of St. Louis 1914,* ed. by Hugh K. Wagner (St. Louis, Mo., 1918) p. 1196.
137 *Ibid.,* pp. 1199-1201, 1203.
138 *Ibid.,* pp. 1204-1205.
139 *Ibid.,* pp. 1207-1209.
140 Ibid., pp. 1211-1212.
141 Statistics from St. Louis city directories.
142 St. Louis *Republic,* Nov. 17, 1903, p. 1:6. Under the new weir system in which the water flowed through all six basins, the flowing time was increased to approximately seventy-two hours. *Idem.*
143 St. Louis *Republican,* Mar. 20, 1878, p. 2:4-5. This was the plan developed by James P. Kirkwood after visiting a number of waterworks in Europe during 1865 and

1866.
144 St. Louis *Republic,* Apr. 4, 1909, part V, p. 4:2.
145 *Ibid.,* Mar. 26, 1909.
146 *Idem.*
147 *Ibid.,* Apr. 4, 1909, part V, p. 4:1.
148 *Ibid.,* Sept. 9, 1900, part II, p. 1:1.
149 *Ibid.,* Sept. 9, 1900, part II, p. 1:2.
150 *Ibid.,* Apr. 4, 1909, part V, p. 4:1.
151 *Idem; ibid.,* June 1, 1902, part III, p. 6:1.
152 *Ibid.,* Jan. 16, 1902, p. 4:1-2.
153 *Ibid.,* May 17, 1903, part V, p. 2:2-6; *ibid.,* Nov. 17, 1903, p. 1:4-6.
154 *Ibid.,* Apr. 4, 1909, part V, p. 4:1.
155 *Ibid.,* Feb. 12, 1905, part II, p. 1:4-7; *ibid.,* Mar. 5, 1905, part I, p. 17:2-4; *ibid.,* May 26, 1909, p. 6:2.
156 *Ibid.,* Apr. 4, 1909, part V, p. 4:2.
157 *Ibid.,* Jan. 10, 1912, p. 1:1.
158 *Ibid.,* Apr. 6, 1913, part I, p. 1:3.
159 *Idem; ibid;* Jan. 1, 1916, p. 1:6-7.
160 *Ibid.,* Jan. 19, 1913, part II, p. 2:5.
161 *Ibid.,* June 3, 1905, part III, p. 6:1-2.
162 *Ibid.,* June 2, 1906, p 2:2.
163 *Ibid.,* June 5, 1906, p. 2:1.
164 *Idem.*
165 *Ibid.,* June 24, 1906, part I, p. 13:6.
166 *Idem.*
167 *Ibid.,* June 27, 1903, part I, p. 4:2.
168 *Ibid.,* Mar. 2, 1904, p. 1:4.
169 *Idem.*
170 *Ibid.,* Apr. 2, 1905, part V, p. 1:2-3.
171 *Ibid.,* Aug. 28, 1903, p. 6:1-2; *ibid.,* Nov. 16, 1903, p. 6:2.
172 *Ibid.,* Nov. 16, 1903, p. 6:2.
173 *Ibid.,* Nov. 15, 1904, p. 14:4.
174 Ibid., Dec. 11, 1904, part IV, p. 1.
175 Primm, *opus cit.,* p. 385.
176 St. Louis *Republic,* Dec. 11, 1904, part IV, p. 1:1-7; *ibid.,* Feb. 5, 1905, part I, p. 10:1-7.
177 *Ibid.,* Aug. 7, 1907, p. 1:2.
178 *Ibid.,* Apr. 12, 1908, part I, p. 1:7.
179 *Ibid.,* Nov. 15, 1908, part I, p. 9:4-6.
180 *Idem.*
181 *Ibid.,* Mar, 7, 1909, part V, p. 4.
182 *Ibid.,* June 19, 1910, part V, p. 4.
183 *Ibid.,* Apr. 27, 1910, p. 6:2.
184 *Ibid.,* Jan. 17., 1911, p. 13:2.
185 *Ibid.,* Nov. 21, 1913, p. 2:3.
186 *Ibid.,* Jan. 7, 1916, p. 4:4.
187 *Ibid.,* Aug. 7, 1918, part II, p. 1:3.
188 *Ibid.,* Sept, 15, 1913, p. 1:2-4.
189 *Idem.*
190 *Ibid.,* Sept. 17, 1913, p. 5:1-2.
191 *Ibid.,* Sept, 19, 1913, p. 4:3-4.
192 *Ibid.,* Sept. 18, 1913, p. 2:3-4.
193 *Ibid.,* Sept. 20, 1913, p. 5:2-3.
194 *Idem.*
195 *Ibid.,* Sept. 23, 1913, p. 5:3-4.
196 *Ibid.,* Sept. 25, 1913, p. 5:1-2.
197 *Ibid.,* Sept. 16, 1913, p. 1:1.
198 *Ibid.,* Sept. 17, 1913, p. 1:1; *ibid.,* Sept. 20, 1913, p. 1:1.
199 *Ibid.,* Oct. 1, 1913, p. 3:3.
200 *Ibid.,* Oct. 21, 1913, p. 1:1.
201 *Ibid.,* Nov. 2, 1913, part I, p, 1:1-7.

202 *Ibid.*, Feb. 20, 1908, p. 9:7.

203 *Ibid.*, Sept. 15, 1907, part I, p. 2:4-5.

204 *Ibid.*, Apr. 1, 1903, p. 6:6.

205 *Ibid.*, May 24, 1903, mag. sect. p. 2:1.

206 *Ibid.*, May 30, 1900, p. 1:3-4.

207 *Ibid.*, Apr. 27, 1910, p. 1:7.

208 *Ibid.*, Aug. 7, 1910, part IV, p. 22:7.

209 *Ibid.*, July 28, 1910, p. 1:7.

210 *Ibid.*, July 28, 1910, p. 1:7; *ibid.*, July 30, 1910, p. 3:3.

211 *Ibid.*, July 30, 1910, p. 3:3.

212 Ibid., Aug. 7, 1910, part IV, p. 227.

213 William B. Faherty, *Better the Dream: St. Louis, University and Community 1818-1968* (St. Louis University, 1968), pp. 212-214.

214 St. Louis *Republic*, Feb. 6, 1911, p. 9:4.

215 *Ibid.*, May 8, 1905, p. 12:2-3.

216 *Ibid.*, May 4, 1907, p. 1:2.

217 *Ibid.*, July 7, 1909, p. 6:2.

218 *Ibid.*, July 7, 1909, p. 12:4.

219 *Idem.*

220 *Idem.*

221 *Ibid.*, June 8, 1910, p. 8:1-2.

222 *Ibid.*, Feb. 6, 1911, p. 9:4.

223 *Ibid.*, June 8, 1910, p. 8:1-2.

224 *Ibid.*, June 17, 1914, extra edition, p. 1:6-7.

225 *Ibid.*, July 1, 1905, p. 4:3; *ibid.*, June 30, 1907, part III, p. 2:1; *ibid.*, Sept. 7, 1907, p. 5:6.

226 *Ibid.*, June 30, 1907, part III, p. 2:1.

227 *Ibid.*, Feb. 20, 1908, p. 9:7.

228 *Ibid.*, Oct. 28, 1908, p. 12:3.

229 In its biennial report to the 48th General Assembly for the two years ending Dec. 31, 1910, the University of Missouri Board of Curators declared: "Men in the medical profession are now calling upon the university and even demanding that the Board of Curators re-establish medical instruction in the laws two years of the medical course. This cannot be done until the State is willing to provide additional hospital facilities for clinical instruction." University of Missouri, "Biennial Report of the Board of Curators to the 46th General Assembly for the Two Years Ending December 31, 1910," (Jefferson City, Mo., The Hugh Stephens Printing Co., 1911), p. 26. Included as Serial No. 37 in *Appendix to the House and Senate Journals of the 46th General Assembly of the State of Missouri, 1911* (Jefferson City, Mo., The Hugh Stephens Printing Co., 1911)

230 St. Louis *Republic*, July 25, 1909, part I, p. 1:3.

231 *Ibid.*, Aug. 8, 1909, part I, p. 1:2.

232 *Ibid.*, Feb. 20, 1910, part I, p. 1:5.

233 *Ibid.*, Aug. 18, 1911, p. 7:5.

234 *Ibid.*, Oct. 1, 1911, part I, p. 1:2.

235 *Ibid.*, Oct. 22, 1911, part I, p. 5:6.

236 Gould's *St. Louis Directory, 1912*, p. 2571.

237 *Ibid.*, 1914, p. 2657.

238 St. Louis *Republic*, Feb. 3, 1901, magazine section, p. 4:3.

239 *Ibid.*, Feb. 3, 1901, magazine section, p. 4:4-5.

240 *Ibid.*, Feb. 3, 1901, magazine section, p. 4:5.

241 *Ibid.*, Feb. 3, 1901, magazine section, p. 4:1.

242 *Ibid.*, Feb. 3, 1901, magazine section, p. 4:3.

243 *Ibid.*, Feb. 3, 1901, magazine section, p. 4:2. The cadavers, which were made available for medical research, were of persons who died in state institutions and lacked friends or relatives willing to claim their bodies for burial.

244 *Ibid.*, Feb. 3, 1901, magazine section, p. 4:2.

245 *Ibid.*, Feb. 3, 1901, magazine section, p. 4:3.

246 *Encyclopedia Americana*, 1953 edition, Vol. XVII, pp. 467-468.

247 *Columbia Missourian*, Mar. 9, 1986, p. 5C:2.

248 William Travis Howard, Jr., *Public Health Administration and the Natural History of Disease in Baltimore, Maryland 1797-1920* (Washington, D.C., Carnegie Institution of Washington, 1924, p. 538.

249 St. Louis *Republic*, Feb. 3, 1901, magazine section, p. 4:7.

250 *Idem.*

251 Paul Starr, *The Social Transformation of American Medicine* (New York, Basic Books, Inc., Publishers, 1982), pp. 79-110.

252 *Ibid.*, pp. 100-102.

253 St. Louis *Republic*, Aug. 2, 1902, p. 8:2.

254 *Twenty-Fifth Annual Report of the Board of Health of Missouri to the Governor and the 45th General Assembly 1907-1908* (Jefferson City, Mo., The Hugh Stephens Printing Co., 1909), p. 26. Included in the *Appendix to the House and Senate Journals of the 45th General Assembly of the State of Missouri 1909* (Jefferson City, Mo., The Hugh Stephens Printing Co., 1909).

255 St. Louis *Republic*, Aug. 7, 1910, part IV, p. 8:2. Dr. J. J. Link, who owned a majority of the stock, offered to sell his stock to any group of physicians interested in continuing the institution as an Eclectic medical college. When, after a six months period, his offer had not been taken up, he announced the change to a regular medical program. *Idem.*

256 *Laws of Missouri, Passed at the Session of the Forty-First General Assembly Begun and Held at the City of Jefferson, January 2, 1901.* Regular Session (Jefferson City, Mo., Tribune Printing Co., 1901), pp. 207-208.

257 *Laws of Missouri, Passed at the Regular and Extra Session of the Forty-fourth General Assembly. Regular Session Begun and Held January 2, 1907. Extra Session Begun and Held April 9, 1907 at the City of Jefferson* (Jefferson City, The Hugh Stephens Printing Co., 1907), pp. 359-360.

258 Starr, *opus cit.*, p. 109.

259 *Ibid.*, pp. 111-112.

260 *Ibid.*, p. 110.

261 *Ibid.*, pp. 146-147.

262 "Twenty-Ninth Annual Report of the State Board of Health of Missouri, 1911." (Jefferson City, Mo., The Hugh Stephens Printing Co., 1913), p. 7. Included in *Appendix to the House and Senate Journals of the 47th General Assembly of the State of Missouri, 1913* (Jefferson City, Mo., The Hugh Stephens Printing Co., 1913), Vol. II.

263 St. Louis *Republic*, January 4, 1897, p. 1:7. This case, that of Charles E. Johnston, a graduate of the Physio-Medical College of Cincinnati, Ohio, *vs. the State Board of Health of Missouri* was decided by the Missouri Supreme Court in favor of the plaintiff. Harold W. Eickhoff, "The Organization and Regulation of Medicine in Missouri, 1883-1901." (Ph.D. dissertation,

University of Missouri, 1964), p. 154. But the decision did not nullify the power of the board to determine what Missouri colleges were reputable. This authority had been established by the decision in the case of *E. G. Granville vs. the State Board of Health of Missouri* (1884). St. Louis *Republican*, Dec. 4, 1884, p. 10:3-5. Eickhoff, *opus cit.*, pp. 121-122. The Johnston decision, however, did diminish the control of the board over graduates of out-of-state medical colleges. For this reason, it contributed to the growing support among doctors and public officials for the establishment of a board of medical examiners. Another factor working toward the same end was the concern in the medical profession over the threat posed by osteopathy, Christian Science and Weltmerism, the latter a mind-cure system. Eickhoff, *opus cit.*, pp. 230-231.

264 "Twenty-Fifth Annual Report of the Board of Health of Missouri to the Governor and the 45th General Assembly 1907-1908" (Jefferson City, Mo., The Hugh Stephens Printing Co., 1909), p. 8. Included in *Appendix to the House and Senate Journals of the 45th General Assembly of the State of Missouri, 1909* (Jefferson City, Mo., The Hugh Stephens Printing Co., 1909)

265 St. Louis *Republic*, Sept. 15, 1907, part I, p. 2:4-5.

266 Starr, *opus cit.*, p. 118.

267 St. Louis *Republic*, Feb. 17, 1907, part I, p. 1:1-7.

268 *Ibid.*, Nov. 10, 1901, part III, p. 1:3.

269 *Ibid.*, Feb. 17, 1907, part I, p. 1:1-7.

270 *Official Manual of the State of Missouri, For the Years 1913-1914, ed. by Cornelius Roach, Secretary of State* (Jefferson City, Mo., The Hugh Stephens Printing Co., 1914), pp. 287-296.

271 "Second Biennial Report of State Hospital No. 4, Farmington, Mo., to the General Assembly of the State of Missouri 1903-1904." (Jefferson City, Mo., Tribune Printing Co., 1905), p. 15. Included in *Appendix to the House and Senate Journals of the 43rd General Assembly of the State of Missouri 1905* (The Hugh Stephens Printing Co., 1905).

272 "Twelfth Biennial Report of Hospital No. 3, Nevada, Missouri to the Forty-Sixth General Assembly, 1911" (Jefferson City, Mo., The Hugh Stephens Printing Co., 1911) p. 10. Included in *Appendix to the House and Senate Journals of the 46th General Assembly of the State of Missouri, 1911* (Jefferson City, Mo., The Hugh Stephens Printing Co., 1911) as Serial No. 16.

273 St. Louis *Republic*, Aug. 14, 1888, p. 12:5.

274 "Biennial Report of the State Board of Health of Missouri, 1905-1906" (Jefferson City, Mo., The Hugh Stephens Printing Co., 1907), p. 6. Included in *Appendix to the House and Senate Journals of the 44th General Assembly of the State of Missouri, 1907* (Jefferson City, Mo., The Hugh Stephens Printing Co., 1907).

275 *Laws of Missouri, Passed at the Session of the Forty-First General Assembly Begun and Held at the City of Jefferson January 2, 1901.* Regular Session. (Jefferson City, Mo., Tribune Printing Co. 1901), p. 180.

276 "Twenty-Ninth Annual Report of the State Board of Health of Missouri, 1911" (Jefferson City, Mo., The Hugh Stephens Printing Co., 1913), p. 9. Included in *Appendix to the House and Senate Journals of the 47th General Assembly, State of Missouri, 1913,* (Jefferson City, Mo., The Hugh Stephens Printing Co., 1913), Vol. II.

277 *Idem.*

278 *Laws of Missouri, Passed at the Session of the Fiftieth General Assembly Which Convened at the City of Jefferson, Wednesday, January 8, 1919,* ed. by John L. Sullivan, Secretary of State, 1919 (Jefferson City, Mo., The Hugh Stephens Printing Co., 1920), pp. 372-274.

279 *Laws of Missouri, 1907*, pp. 194-198.

280 *Laws of Missouri, Passed by the 45th General Assembly, 1909 Which Convened at the City of Jefferson January 6, 1909* (Jefferson City, Mo., The Hugh Stephens Printing Company, 1909) pp. 538-539.

281 *Ibid.*, pp. 539, 547.

282 "Twenty-Ninth Annual Report of the State Board of Health of Missouri," p. 11.

283 The biennial appropriations are from *Laws of Missouri* for the years indicated.

284 *Laws of Missouri*, 1901, pp. 6-7.

285 *Laws of Missouri*, 1905, pp. 6-7.

286 *Laws of Missouri*, 1909-1910. p. 17.

287 *Laws of Missouri Passed at the Session of the Forty-Sixth General Assembly Which Convened at the City of Jefferson January 4, 1911* (Jefferson City, Mo., The Hugh Stephens Printing Co., 1911) pp. 11-12.

288 *Offical Manual of the State of Missouri For the Years 1919-1920, ed. by John L. Sullivan, Secretary of State* (Jefferson City, Mo., The Hugh Stephens Company, Printers, 1920), p. 190.

289 *Laws of Missouri*, 1919-1920, p. 372.

290 *Laws of Missouri, Passed at the Session of the Forty-Second General Assembly, Begun and Held at the City of Jefferson*, January 7, 1903), p. 218.

291 *Ibid.*, p. 219.

292 *Laws of Missouri, 1909-1910*, p. 669.

293 *Ibid.*, p. 670.

294 *Idem.*

295 *Ibid.*, pp. 670-671.

296 *Ibid.*, p. 671.

297 *Ibid.*, pp. 671-672.

Chapter 8

Expansion of Activities by the State Board of Health

1. A Slow Start

THE STATE BOARD OF HEALTH, during its first thirty-five years, had made little impact on the life of the average Missourian. It is likely that few outside of the medical profession were aware of its existence.[1] The state board conducted examinations of applicants to practice medicine, surgery and midwifery, and granted state licenses to successful candidates. It also operated the Bureau of Vital Statistics for the registration of births and deaths. When an epidemic broke out in a local community, the board, in the absence of a physician on its staff, dispatched one of its medical members to advise and work with the doctors of the affected area.[2]

However, a start had been made toward the goal of bringing the benefits of scientific medicine into every city, town and county of the state. In 1901, the Missouri legislature had enacted a law requiring each county to establish a board of health consisting of the judges of the county court and a reputable physician appointed by them.[3] This law remained as something of a dead letter until 1919, when spurred by the experience of the state during the influenza epidemic, the general assembly appointed the secretary of the board of health as the state health commis-

sioner; the physicians on the county boards of health were instructed to function as deputy state commissioners. The state health commissioner and his deputies were responsible for enforcing health laws.[4] At about the same time, state authorization was given for the establishment of county hospitals. A number of counties, including Audrain, Boone, Callaway and Pike counties, took advantage of the opportunity.

Two areas of particular need in Missouri were child hygiene and rural sanitation. The high rates of infant mortality prompted the creation, in 1919, of a Division of Child Hygiene in the Department of Health. Since the Missouri Department of Health lacked trained public health officials, it requested assistance from the United States Public Health Service. This organization dispatched to Missouri a field team consisting of a surgeon (or doctor), three public health nurses, a field organizer, a schedule supervisor, a secretary and a clerk. The group, with the cooperation of the American Red Cross, the Missouri Tuberculosis Association and the Missouri Division of Child Hygiene examined 125,000 school children in thirty-nine towns and in the rural districts of nineteen counties.

A survey of 5,610 homes in twenty-three towns was made to determine the percentage of births that had been properly reported and also to secure data regarding the sanitary condition of homes, the amount of milk used, relative income, and prenatal examinations conducted with their bearing on the physical condition of the children and the rates of infant mortality.[5]

For work in the area of rural sanitation, the fifty-first general assembly appropriated $20,000. The United States Public Health Service and the International Health Board, a branch of the Rockefeller Foundation, supplied matching funds. Dr. Thomas Parran, Jr., of the United States Public Health Service, was assigned to serve temporarily as director of the Missouri health board's Division of Rural Sanitation. He was assisted by Dr. M. V. Ziegler of the United States Public Health Service as consultant. The International Health Board also provided consulting personnel. An extensive survey was made of seven southeast Missouri counties, with particular reference to the prevalence of malaria and the best methods of combatting it. Besides this localized study, every county in the state was offered financial and technical assistance in the establishment of model health departments, one half of the cost to be provided by the county governments and the other half to be shared equally by the state of Missouri, the international board, and the United States Public Health Service. Under this program, model county health departments were established in Greene, Jasper, Polk and Monroe counties.[6]

The Division of Sanitary Engineering was organized in 1922. The areas of its responsibility were: improved rural school sanitation; purity of water supplies, municipal and private; safety of milk supplies; and improved sewerage.[7]

A department for the control of contagious diseases was established in 1925. For working in this field, the board hired a physician trained in epidemiology to spend his time consulting and working with local physicians in the suppression of contagion. To facilitate this undertaking, a central diagnostic laboratory was founded with adequate personnel to provide prompt and efficient analysis of specimens sent in by physicians and public health nurses.[2]

The work undertaken by the board of health in the control of venereal disease was both clinical and educational. A total of 214,387 persons were treated at twenty-two permanent clinics set up by the board. Free salvarsan, the most effective remedy then available, was provided in indigent cases.[9]

Missouri, for a number of years, had been in the federal death registration group of states. It gained in 1927 admission to the federal birth registration area. This recognition was accorded to states that reported as high as ninety percent of their births. Thenceforth, Missouri's reports of both births and deaths would be reported in federal census statistics.[10]

The expanded volume of the board's service in the field was reflected in its personnel roster for 1927. Of the twenty-three employees, eight were in the professional and technical category, including an epidemiologist, a bacteriologist, two sanitary engineers, one sanitary inspector and three laboratory technicians. The other employees were clerical and stenographic workers.[11]

As the board of health increased its staff and operations, it found it necessary to draw up a workable organizational plan. Up to this time its organizational chart had shown the State Board of Health with a number of divisions loosely grouped below it. Some of these had been created by the board as need arose, others by law. In the latter case, they represented merely the intent of the legislature, since no funding was immediately provided. The new organizational plan, developed during the 1929-1930 biennium, placed the following seven divisions subordinate to the board: (1) Administration; (2) Vital Statistics and Licensure; (3) Contagious Disease Control; (4) Public Health Laboratories;(5) Sanitation; (6) Child Hygiene and Public Health Nursing; (7) Cooperative County Health Service.[12]

Even though the state's annual appropriation for the work of the board of health increased gradually in the 1920s, this amounted in 1929 to only $168,750. A report of the State Survey Commission on public health needs and costs recommended that the state spend $586,100 yearly for this purpose. Although Missouri was tenth in the United States in population, it ranked forty-first in its per capita appropriation for health conservation. Its expenditure was only $.0763 per biennium per person.[13]

A flooding of the Ohio and Mississippi rivers just below their confluence, in January 1937, provoked a disaster of a magnitude that the State Board of Health had not previously experienced. Approximately 25,000 persons were driven from their homes in the southeast Missouri counties of Scott, Mississippi, Butler, Dunklin, Stoddard, Pemiscot and Cape Girardeau. The inundation occurred in the depth of winter when the roads and fields were covered by ice and snow.

The American Red Cross, United States Public Health Service, the Missouri National Guard, the State Highway Patrol, and the State Board of Health rushed relief teams to the crisis area. These were augmented by the services of local doctors, nurses and sanitarians. For purposes of administration, four districts were established in the affected group of counties, with a sanitarian at the headquarters of each district. Temporary quarters for refugees were set up in churches, schools, armories and post offices. Emergency feeding arrangements were put into operation, and badly needed supplies, such as cots, blankets and warm clothing distributed.

Various hospitals in St. Louis sent some of their internes for duty; also three physicians of the United States Public Health Service were made available. These officers immunized refugees against smallpox, typhoid fever and diphtheria. Respiratory diseases, particularly pneumonia, and frozen limbs were major problems. Emergency water and sewerage facilities in the refugee camps were set up.[14]

Following the recession of the flood waters, sanitary activities centered on disinfecting private water supplies that had been flooded. This was accomplished by pumping out the contaminated water and disinfecting the wells with chlorine.[15]

As a result of the state's experience in the handling of an emergency involving a number of different agencies, the state health commissioner made the following proposal:[16]

It is recommended that the State Board of Health as the official health agency of the State should in times of emergency have complete control and supervision over disease prevention, sanitation and hospitalization. Necessarily considerable cooperation from other agencies such as the Red Cross and local doctors and nurses will always be necessary to handle the health and medical hazards incident to an emergency. However, effective organization of such services indicates strongly, as a result of past experiences, that the administration of this work should be under one official head and logically this should be the State Board of Health.

On December 22, 1937, the State Board of Health passed a regulation governing the sale of graded and labeled milk requiring that:

the production, transportation, processing, handling, sampling, examination, grading, labeling, regrading, and the sale of milk and milk products sold for ultimate consumption within the State of Missouri as labeled or graded milk shall be regulated in accordance with the terms of the 1936 edition of the United States Public Health Milk Ordinance.

The Department of Health recognized that the attainment of the stated goal would require the cooperation of local county and city health departments. In the case of St. Louis and Kansas City, interstate cooperation would be needed, since their milk supply territories cross state boundaries.[17]

During 1937, a substantial increase in budgets due to matching grants from the federal government and also the organization of new health districts provided an opportunity to put into effect revised administrative policies, as described in the following statement:[18]

Under the present program the actual field activities of the Health Department will be delegated to District Health Units which will function in their respective localities essentially as a small state health department. The administration of these district units, each constituting a health officer, a public health engineer and two or more nurses, and the full-time county health departments is the function of the Division of Local Health Work.

Through the institution of the new organizational plan, the central office divisions of the board of health gave up their operational functions and became advisory and supervisory in nature, transmitting their advice and requests to the district health units and the county health boards through the channel of the Division of Local Health Work.[19]

2. The State Board and the Problem of Licensing

While the state board was busy with its new task of bringing scientific medicine to the people, it was also engaged in controversy regarding one of its oldest roles — the licensing of physicians. New systems of healing — chiropractic, osteopathic and Christian Science — were demanding recognition and accreditation. The expansion of medical science was forcing the extension of training and the downgrading of lectures as the main source of instruction. The hospital had emerged as the major center for the treatment of acute medical problems.

By the 1920s, Missouri had six colleges engaged in the training of doctors. The Washington University Medical School, the St. Louis University Medical School and the Medical School of the University of Missouri at Columbia were modern institutions with excellent buildings, staffs and laboratories. They were rated as Class A medical centers by national agencies. The St. Louis College of Physicians and Surgeons, the Kansas City University of Physicians and Surgeons and the Kansas City College of Medicine and Surgery were proprietary institutions of Class C rating.[21] The more stringent entrance requirements, the longer courses and higher standards of the first three schools had the unintended effect of creating a market for the cheaper, shorter and inferior type of medical

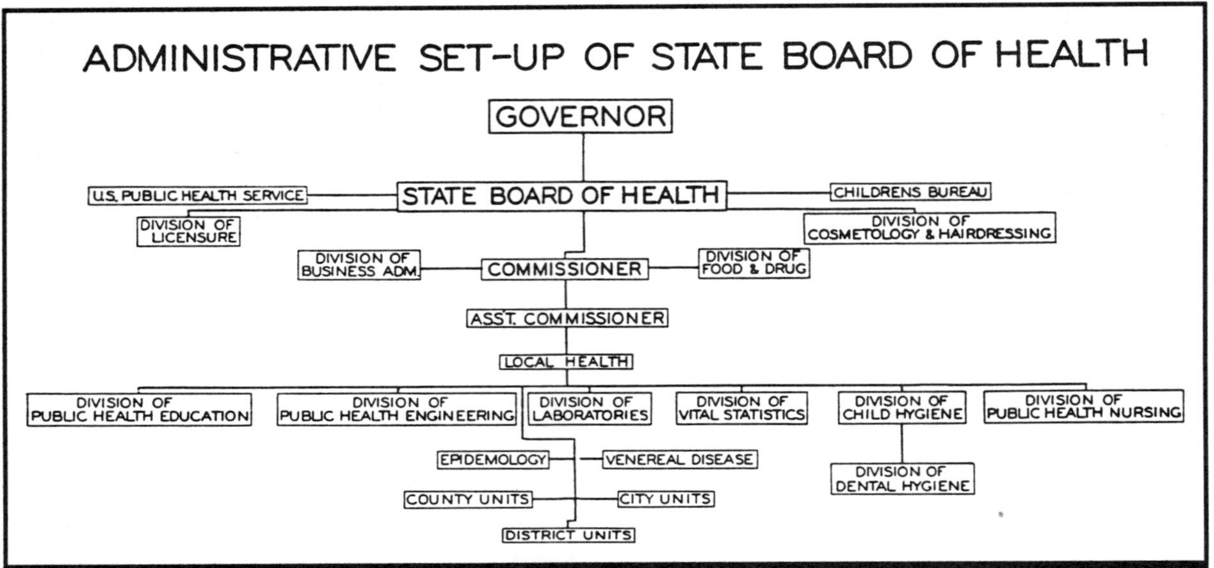

(For the source of the organizational chart, see footnote No. 20)

education provided by the three proprietary colleges.

These colleges could occasionally generate a lot of support in Jefferson City. By their friends, they were viewed as the necessary means for providing replacements for the traditional country doctor and also for keeping the road to professional status open to the sons of poor families.[22]

The issue came to public attention in 1921 when the Missouri legislature enacted Senate Bill 433, which made significant changes in medical practice requirements. It eliminated the adjective "reputable" from the existing legal provision that a candidate for licensing had to be a graduate of a reputable four-year medical college. It also made the action of the State Board of Health, in permitting or denying access to medical examinations, subject to review in the local circuit courts.[23]

The state and local medical organizations were roused to action by the bill and urged Governor Arthur M. Hyde to veto it. Instead, the governor, listening to the advice of the representatives of the Class C medical schools, signed the act. This law effectively robbed the State Board of Health of its authority to determine which institutions were diploma mills, whose graduates could legally be denied the privilege of licensing. [24]

Dr. Nathaniel Allison, dean of the Washington University School of Medicine, and Dr. Hanau W. Loeb, dean of the St. Louis University Medical School, wrote to Governor Hyde, requesting that he have a team of scientists from the University of Missouri conduct a survey of the three proprietary schools.[25]

On March 27, 1923, the state legislature reversed its action of two years previously, which had opened the floodgates to poorly trained practitioners. It returned the word "reputable" to the section of the medical practice act, which required that persons applying to take licensing examinations must furnish proof of having received "a diploma from some reputable medical college of four years' requirements, including two years' experience in operative and hospital work."[26]

With its authority to scrutinize the operations of medical schools restored, the state board asked Dr. F. C. Waite of Western Reserve University, Cleveland, Ohio, an authority in the field of medical education, to conduct a survey of all six of Missouri's teaching institutions, beginning November 1, 1923. The matters to be looked into were "the buildings, equipment, curriculum, arrangement of courses, personnel of faculty and the entrance credentials of students."[27] Dr. Waite, in his final report, called attention particularly to the careless record keeping of the class C colleges and their negligence in checking the high school credentials of the matriculants.[28]

Meanwhile, the state board was conducting a comprehensive investigation of the allegedly unlawful activities of the proprietary schools, including bribery, falsification of high school credentials and the granting of fraudulent diplomas.[29]

At the same time the medical schools were being surveyed, the state board was conducting an investigation of doctors' licenses, to determine which physicians were practicing without licenses or on the basis of false certificates, or were guilty of unprofessional or dishonorable conduct.[30] Police officers, with questionnaires for compiling data from all persons throughout the state who were treating the sick, were assigned to conduct door to door canvasses. Those found guilty were threatened with loss of their licenses.[31] As a result of this investigation, sixty physicians were cited by the state board. Those cited had the right of appeal to local circuit courts if they challenged the findings of the board.[32]

Attorney General Robert William Otto, on June 16, 1925, filed quo warranto proceedings in the Missouri Supreme Court, seeking to revoke the charters of the St. Louis College of Physicians and Surgeons and the Kansas City College of Medicine and Surgery. The St. Louis College of Physicians and Surgeons was incorporated on August 8, 1879; the Kansas City College of Medicine and Surgery secured its charter as a medical institution on January 26, 1916.

Charges in the twin suits were practically identical and included the following:[33]

That the colleges are violating their charter privileges, and selling diplomas to prospective applicants to practice medicine.

That the required records of the proceedings of the colleges are not being kept.

That the colleges are being maintained for private profit and gain, contrary to their stated purposes of incorporation to educate and fit students for the practice of medicine and surgery.

That instruction is largely by students themselves, who are alleged to be incompetent to give such instruction.

That they have failed to maintain a properly organized curriculum of four years instruction and have not provided a dispensary or hospital for instruction of students.

The quo warranto proceedings in the Missouri Supreme Court were successful in forcing the closing of the Kansas City College of Medicine and Surgery.[34] However, the seals and records of the college were not turned in but were used by a former official and his colleagues to prepare and sell bogus diplomas. For this offense, they were tried and convicted in federal court of mail fraud.

On October 18, 1943, the state board requested the attorney general to institute ouster proceedings against the Kansas City University of Physicians and Surgeons. The charges were not criminal in nature, but rather that the college lacked the staff and apparatus to qualify as a first-class medical school. The college had received its charter in 1922 but had not operated continuously since that time. The institution was not recognized as a reputable college by the State Board of Health, and its graduates were not permitted to take state licensing examinations.[35] The St. Louis College of Physicians and Surgeons had discontinued operations earlier.

With the powerful aid of the United States postal inspectors, Missouri was gradually overcoming its reputation as a haven for the operation of diploma mills.

The closing of the three Class C medical colleges created a need for additional training opportunities for physicians in the state. In 1909, the paucity of funds provided by the general assembly had forced the University of Missouri to eliminate the last two years of the four-year medical program and discontinue granting the M.D. degree. Students, having completed work at the University of Missouri, transferred to some other medical school for their final years of training.

The development at the outbreak of World War II of a serious shortage of doctors, both for the armed forces and civilian society, prompted a revival of consideration by the board of curators of the reestablishment of a full four-year program. But by this time, Kansas City, as well as Columbia, was bidding for the privilege of providing the site for the hospital and instructional facilities in which the third and fourth year of training would be conducted. After several years of heated argument in the state legislature, in the press and in medical circles, the board of curators, on July 27, 1945, adopted a resolution ordering that the four-year medical school be reestablished on the University of Missouri campus as soon as funds were made available by the general assembly. However, no immediate action was taken by the legislature to carry out the board's wishes.

In April 1951, the board of curators asked the assembly for $13,500,000 to construct a medical center in Columbia. The figure was trimmed to $6,000,000 in the legislature and approved by the governor, with the understanding that additional funds would be requested later. A site in Columbia south of Rollins field was selected.

The arguments which determined the contest between Columbia and Kansas City for the medical complex were, first, the central position of Columbia in the state; second, the advantage of having the medical school in close relationship with the various science departments of the university; and finally, the constitutional argument that the board of curators, not the legislature, was responsible for the government of the university.[36]

3. A New Constitution for Missouri

The 1945 Missouri constitution, in Article IV, Section 37, provided for the establishment of a new department to coordinate all health and welfare services of the state as follows:

The health and general welfare of the people are of primary public concern; and to secure them, the General Assembly shall establish a department of public health and welfare, and may grant power with respect thereto to counties, cities or other political subdivisions of the state.

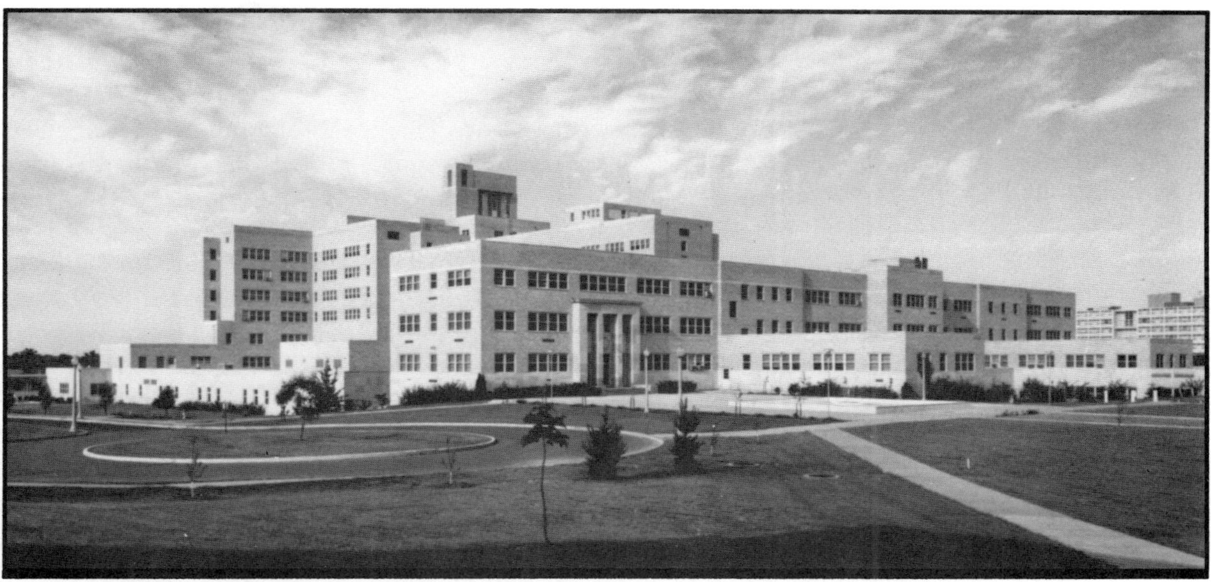

University of Missouri Medical School. Courtesy of the State Historical Society of Missouri.

In compliance with this constitutional provision, the sixty-third general assembly passed Senate Bill 349, which created the new department, the scope and purpose of which was:

to improve and protect the health of the people of the State of Missouri; to care for the mentally ill and those who are ill from other causes, so far as the laws of Missouri can provide; to provide care and maintenance for certain other purposes, as provided by law; to administer laws concerning social welfare, including certain social security laws.

The law further specified that the department should have three major divisions: the Division of Health, the Division of Mental Diseases and the Division of Welfare. The State Board of Health, the board of managers of the State Eleemosynary Institutions, and the State Social-Security Commission were abolished. The powers and duties over activi-

ties and institutions, formerly controlled by and administered through them, were transferred to the Department of Public Health and Welfare together with any additional powers which might be assigned to the department.

The new constitution provided that all employees in the state eleemosynary institutions, and other state employees as specified by law, should be selected on the basis of merit, ascertained by competitive examinations. A state merit system was established, which became effective July 1, 1946.

The Division of Health was the central health authority of the state. It exercised administrative supervision over the following programs and institutions:

Local Health and Hospital Administration; bureau of public health nursing; bureau of health education; hospital survey and planning service; epidemiology service; Waynesville General Hospital; Missouri Trachoma Hospital; section of laboratories; section of statistics; section of preventive medicine; bureau of maternal and child health; bureau of tuberculosis control; bureau of public health dentistry; bureau of venereal disease control; nutrition service; section of environmental sanitation; and bureau of food and drug inspection.

The 1945 constitution abolished the State Board of Health and transferred its licensing powers to the following professional boards: the State Board of Medical Examiners; the State Board of Nurse Examiners; the State Board of Osteopathic Examiners: and the State Board of Pharmacy.[36] The State Board of Medical Examiners is a bipartisan body of six members, three Republicans and three Democrats. All are practicing physicians.

On April 19, 1946, the state legislature enacted a comprehensive medical practice act designed to adjust Missouri's procedures to the 1945 state constitution and to make the prerequisites for licensing as strict as those of the most progressive jurisdictions. Under this law, a candidate for a license must have earned a diploma from an accredited high school. He also must have completed two years of premedical subjects in an approved college. Finally, he must have received a diploma from a reputable four-year medical college; this part of his training had to include two years experience in operative and hospital work. The licensing examination before the State Board of Medical Examiners was practical as well as written and involved testing in the major branches of medical science. The applicant had to achieve an average grade of seventy-five percent. The newly accredited doctor had to have his license recorded in the office of the clerk of the county where he resided. The practice of medicine without a license or with a fraudulent certification was prohibited and stiff

penalties prescribed. Licenses must be renewed every two years. The state board had authority to revoke licenses for unprofessional or dishonorable conduct. The accused physician could appeal the board's decision to the circuit court.[37]

4. *The State Government and the Responsibility for the Mentally Ill*

In the early period of the state's history, each county was responsible for its mentally ill citizens. After being adjudged incompetent in a trial in the county court, they became wards of the county, and their care was farmed out to some relative or interested party. In 1851, the first state mental hospital was opened at Fulton, Missouri, and the counties had the option of sending their patients there, or taking care of them in county poorhouses.[38]

St. Louis County in 1869, because of the transportation problems involved in getting its patients to Fulton, established its own asylum.[39] This was later transferred to the city of St. Louis and renamed the St. Louis Sanatarium. The state paid St. Louis varying amounts, the subject of continuing controversy, for taking care of thousands of patients who otherwise would have been a burden on the state treasury. In 1948, after a long period of negotiation, the city of St. Louis deeded the sanatarium to the State Department of Public Health and Welfare for a token payment of one dollar.[40] It was estimated the move would save the city annually at least one million dollars. The transfer of ownership had been opposed by relatives of the patients who feared the quality of care would decline.

A shift was made in the management of the state's mental institutions in 1921. A bipartisan board of managers, appointed by the governor, was substituted for the four separate institutional boards. The board was empowered to appoint a paid health supervisor who would direct the manner of treatment of the inmates of the state mental hospitals. It was anticipated that the change would promote better coordination of the policies of the four hospitals and also save money through competitive bidding and mass purchasing. The health supervisor would be an ex officio member of the board.

During the period 1920 through 1940, the population of Missouri's mental hospitals increased rapidly, as the following table shows:[41] 1920, 5,190; 1930, 7,113; 1940, 9,500. There was an increase between 1920 and 1930 of 37 percent of mental hospital inmates and only a 6 percent increase in the state's general population. Between 1930 and 1940, there was a gain of 33 percent in institutional patients and an increase of only 4 percent of the general citizenry. The statistics indicate that the inmate population was growing seven or eight times as rapidly as the group outside hospital walls.

Changes in society help to account for this development. The extended family, which provided home and support for relatives who could not make it on their own, was disappearing. Families were living in smaller quarters. Domestic help was affordable only by the rich. More wives were working and thus not available for home nursing care. Finally, there was the growing realization that mental disease, in many cases, was curable in appropriate treatment centers. By reducing the monthly charge for county patients in its institutions from $18 to $6, the state legislature encouraged the trend set by these sociological factors.[42]

New methods of treatment were becoming available in the 1920s and 1930s. Previously, the therapy had been limited to drugs designed to keep the patient reasonably quiet and controllable. Important among the new drugs were insulin and metrazol. Electric shock and heat therapy also were employed. The metrazol, insulin and electric shock treatments produce convulsions in the patient's brain which break up abnormal thought patterns. Heat therapy, involving a therapeutically induced spell of malaria or an electrically heated sweat box, was found effective in killing the germs of neurosyphilis. The rate of improvement of the new shock therapies, employed on selected groups, appeared to average from 50 percent to 60 percent. But many patients showed no improvement. A sizable percentage suffered fractures from the convulsions. A small injection of curare, a South American plant poison, eases the muscle strain which causes the fractures.[43]

There were other types of therapy. These include psychotherapy, group psychotherapy, hydrotherapy, recreational therapy, occupational therapy and industrial therapy. Because of staff and equipment constraints, the full potential of these treatment means has not been achieved in Missouri's institutions.

The voters of Missouri, in 1934, approved a bond issue of ten million dollars for the improvement of the state's eleemosynary and penal institutions. The federal government, as part of its national work relief program, added $3,778,000. This new funding provided means for the establishment at each of the four mental institutions of a psychiatric clinic, which served as a reception and diagnostic center. The atmosphere was that of a hospital, not an asylum. New patients were examined and, if the prognosis was favorable, were given intensive treatment and released to return home. Elderly patients and others, who failed to respond to treatment, were assigned to one of the wards.[44]

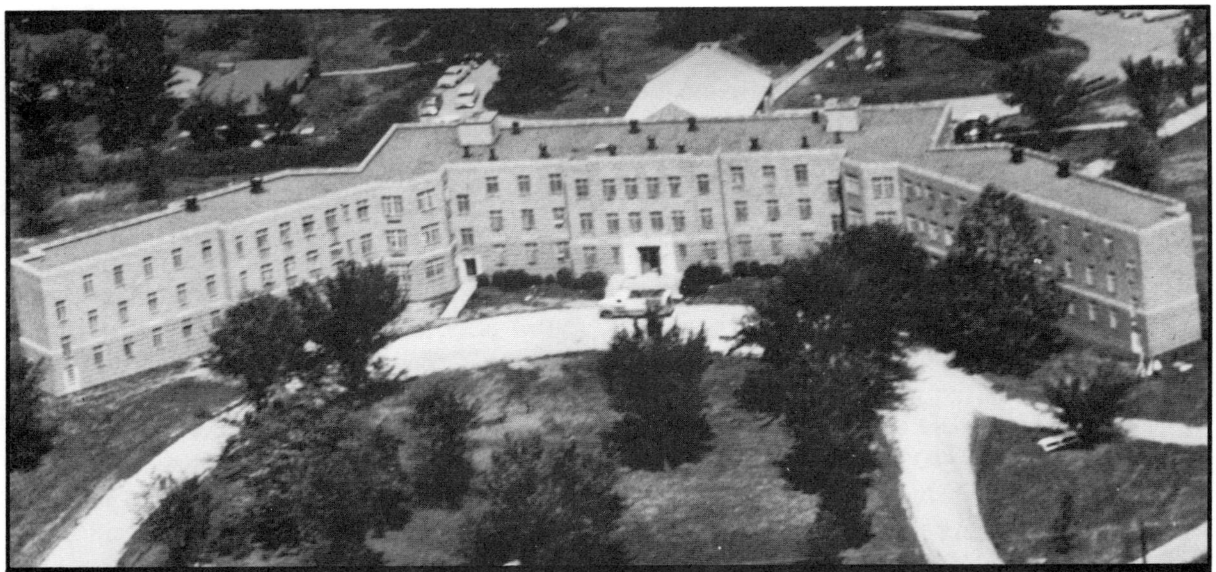

Admission and acute treatment center at the Fulton state hospital (operational in the middle 1930's). Courtesy of the hospital staff.

In May 1947, the Missouri House of Representatives commissioned a comprehensive survey of conditions in the state's mental institutions. The report revealed that only 5.4 percent of the residents were receiving active medical treatment. The large majority were senile patients, receiving minimal custodial care, including monotonous food, little recreation and endless hours of sitting and rocking under the watchful eyes of attendants, who quickly stifled any attempts at conversation or merriment. The report also disclosed the drastic shortage of doctors, nurses and other therapists necessary for an effective treatment program.[45]

More than a decade previously, Dr. Ralph Hanks, superintendent of Hospital No. 1 at Fulton, had called attention to the waste and futility of constantly enlarging mental hospitals, which were hardly more than warehouses for senile populations:[46]

The State cannot continue to build more and more buildings to house the more chronically insane patients, and the only way in which we are going to obviate this is by increasing our facilities in order that we will have adequate equipment and personnel, adequate number of properly trained physicians, psychiatric nurses, social workers and whatever personnel is necessary that the patients may receive the most intensive treatment, in order to shorten their hospitalization and turn a larger number back into society and industry.

A mental hygiene program for the State of Missouri is badly needed. This will necessitate a considerable amount of extramural activities in the form of mental hygiene clinics, child's guidance clinics and other additional programs which should be held from time to time in numerous communities and perhaps permanent clinics in the larger centers. The greatest amount of good to be derived in a program for the reduction of mental disease will come from a prevention program. The greatest amount of success in combating disease in general has come from programs of prevention rather than a cure, and while we will get the greatest amount of cures in the earlier care, eventually the greatest amount of success will be in the preventive field.

5. Important Advances in Medical Science

Medical science made noteworthy improvements during the 1930s and 1940s. These advances, coming at the time of World War II, revolutionized the treatment of battle injuries. Dr. Stuart Mudd, professor of bacteriology at the University of Pennsylvania School of Medicine and a former St. Louisan, in an interview with a *Post-Dispatch* reporter, thus described the changes:[47]

Two of the greatest causes of death in the last war were secondary shock and wound infection. Tens of thousands and hundreds of thousands of those fatally wounded could have been saved had plasma and sulfonamide drugs been in use from 1914 to 1918. Plasma is the most effective means ever devised for treating shock, while sulfonamide drugs are medicine's best answer to date for infection.

A third medicine, penicillin, was discovered to be effective in many cases where sulfa drugs failed. Penicillin, which quickly acquired the title, the "wonder drug," is obtained from a mold grown in an artificial liquid medium.[48]

The bacteria-retarding agent first had been noticed on a culture plate in 1929 by Dr. Alexander Fleming, an English bacteriologist. Dr. H. W. Florey, who had continued

Dr. Fleming's research, was able to make arrangements, in 1941, for the mass production of the drug, which became available for use in English and American military hospitals.[49]

The first public notice of the drug in the United States was in the testimony of Dr. A. Newton Richards of the Office of Scientific Research and Development before the House Appropriations Committee in the summer of 1943. Dr. W. Barry Wood, Jr., of Barnes Hospital, St. Louis, was one of a dozen physicians chosen to explore the clinical possibilities of the little known substance. Dr. Wood gave the following report regarding his findings:[50]

In addition to materially checking the growth of the staphylococcus bacteria, a common source of infection in battle wounds, penicillin has been found successful in treating infections caused by the pneumococcus and streptococcus bacteria . . . . At Barnes Hospital penicillin has been employed with good results in treating certain types of boils, abscesses, osteomyelitis (a bone disease), certain forms of meningitis, and putrid lung infections.

Other investigators at the hospital had employed penicillin to cure drug-resistant gonorrhea.

Dr. Wood warned that penicillin was not a cure-all. His research indicated that it had no effect on "such infectious diseases as typhoid fever, influenza, typhus fever, Rocky Mountain Spotted fever, brain abscesses or bacterial endocarditis (an infection of the heart valve).[51]

Penicillin, unlike the sulfa drugs to which some patients were allergic, appeared to have no unfavorable side effects.

In the period following World War II, when penicillin became available for widespread civilian use, it was found that various strains of bacteria were developing immunity to the drug.

Four options were available for overcoming this resistance. The first was to increase the dosage of penicillin. This was possible since it is not toxic. The second way was to combine penicillin with several other drugs. The third, and most successful method, was to discover new antibiotics. An example is streptomycin. The fourth approach was to prescribe supplementary chemical compounds that make the germs more sensitive to the penicillin.[52]

Surgery benefitted from the use of the new drugs. A major danger of surgery was post-operative infections. This risk was greatly diminished by the application of sulfanilamide or penicillin to the wound area.[53] The germicidal action of the drugs strongly reinforces the prophylactic procedures (scrubbing, sterilization of instruments, masks and surgical gowns) of the operating team. With the risk of infection practically eliminated, a number of the most frequent modern operations, including Caesarean sections, hernia repairs, prostatectomies and hysterectomies, have become fairly routine with a high rate of success.

The administration of anesthetics became a recognized medical specialty, as the following statement indicates:[54]

Just before World War II professional anesthesiologists came to replace the nurse-anesthetists. Nurses trained in anesthesia, and directly responsible to surgeons, occupied an important role in many teaching hospitals throughout the United States and were not readily displaced. Today trained nurses are again on the scene but directly responsible to the department of anesthesiology. The opposition of surgeons to professional anesthetists involved prestigious professors of surgery at The Hopkins and other institutions, but the battle for the professional anesthetist was gradually won . . . . The professional anesthetist is now essentially a clinical pharmacologist knowing considerably more about drugs than the nurse-anesthetist did at an earlier period, however skilled and experienced she might have been in the administration of an inhalation anesthetic.

During the early years of the twentieth century, St. Louis University Medical School and Washington University Medical School maintained close relationships with the Rockefeller Institute, the headquarters in the United States of medical research. In January 1921, Dr. John Auer, pharmacologist of the Rockefeller Institute, was chosen to head the newly organized department of pharmacology of the Medical School of St. Louis University.[55] Dr. Herbert S. Gasser, professor of pharmacology and physiology from 1921 to 1931 at the Medical School of Washington University, was selected as director of the Rockefeller Institute following the resignation of Dr. Simon Flexner.[56]

A number of St. Louis medical scientists have won international recognition. Dr. Edward A. Doisy of the St. Louis University medical faculty in 1943 received a Nobel prize for his work in synthetizing vitamin K.[57] The next year, Dr. Joseph Erlanger of the Washington University Medical School won a Nobel award for his research regarding the functions of nerve fibers.[58] Dr. Carl Ferdinand Cori and his wife Dr. Gerty Theresa Cori of the Washington University medical faculty in 1947 won Nobel honors for their discoveries regarding the manner in which starch is converted into sugar in the body.[59]

6. Distribution of the Benefits of Medical Science

Americans generally were in agreement regarding the excellence of scientific medical care. Serious questions, however, were being raised regarding its availability to large segments of the population. The expense of extended hospital stays was devastating to the resources of ordinary families. The gradual depletion of their physicians threatened to deprive rural areas of the South and Middle West of professional care. The consolidation of the power of the medical profession gave it the ability to delay or defeat experimental programs for the wider delivery of medical services.[60]

These and other issues prompted the establishment in Washington, D.C., in April 1926, of a group called the Committee on the Costs of Medical Care, consisting initially of prominent economists, physicians and public health specialists. It was later expanded to include representatives of various interest groups such as the medical profession, labor and private business. Dr. Ray Lyman Wilbur, a physician who was the head of Stanford University, was chosen chairman.[61]

The committee's extensive research revealed the following conditions:[62]

(1) Uneven distribution in the costs of medical care among families.

(2) General shortage of convalescent facilities.

(3) General shortage of dental care to meet the real needs of the people.

(4) Inadequacy of personal and financial support of our health department.

(5) Inability of many of our patients to obtain nursing services because of cost; actual shortage of nurses trained in obstetrics and public health; a surplus of private duty nurses, considering present inability of people to employ them.

(6) Extensive use of inferior types of treatment and widespread self-medication.

(7) Low, insecure, net incomes of many physicians, dentists and nurses.

(8) Insufficient utilization of preventive procedures.

(9) Inability of many people to differentiate accurately between good and poor medical service.

The committee was not able to agree on a unified report, so submitted majority and minority statements. The majority report endorsed group medical practice and group payment but opposed compulsory health insurance. It proposed that local governments, assisted where necessary by the federal and state governments, should contribute a share of the costs of group payment plans for low income persons.

The minority report, prepared by eight private physicians and a representative of Catholic hospitals, rejected compulsory health insurance. It also denounced voluntary insurance as a first step toward a compulsory system. The report demanded that government competition in the practice of medicine be discontinued; that government care of the indigent be increased with the aim of relieving the medical profession of that burden; and that the general practitioner be restored to the central place in medical practice.[63]

The American Medical Association, the Missouri State Medical Association and the St. Louis Medical Society endorsed the minority report.[64] The action of the St. Louis society is easily understandable since the Rev. Alphonse M. Schwitalla, dean of the St. Louis University School of Medicine, was a member of the Committee on the Costs of Medical Care as a spokesman for Catholic medical institutions and probably drafted the minority statement.[65]

The St. Louis Medical Society, at its meeting of October 10, 1933, established a Code and Contract Board consisting of three members appointed by the president. Its mission was to monitor agreements and contracts made by its members to render medical service for stipulated payments. The society was not opposed to all service contracts. Many of its members were beneficiaries of such arrangements. It opposed only agreements that involved:[66]

(1) Solicitation of patients, directly or indirectly.
(2) Underbidding to assure contracts.
(3) Compensation inadequate to assure good medical service.
(4) Interference with reasonable competition.
(5) Prevention of free choice of physician.
(6) Conditions inadequate for proper service to patients.
(7) Any provisions or practical results contrary to sound public policy.

It is obvious that any disciplinary action of the society would depend heavily upon the subjective judgment of its three-man investigative board. A contract to provide a certain occupational group, e.g., the employees of the Missouri Pacific Railroad, with medical services would eliminate this group from the pool of possible patrons of other St. Louis doctors. Would that be fair and "reasonable competition" with one's peers?

The failure of Congress to develop a national health system encouraged various occupational groups to establish their own plans. In Washington, D.C., in 1937, a number of government employees set up their Group Health Association, paying a small monthly fee in return for which they became entitled to medical and hospital benefits provided by salaried physicians. This violated the American Medical Association's veto of group medicine, which sets up a third party between doctor and patients. The doctors participating in the plan were threatened with dismissal from their county medical societies and with refusal of consultations and referrals by their medical associates. Washington hospitals refused to accept as patients members of the insurance cooperative. The Assistant Attorney General Thurman Arnold brought suit under the Sherman Anti-Trust Act against the American Medical Association and its subordinate medical societies, which had carried out the boycott. The suit went up on appeal to the United States Supreme Court which found the American Medical Association guilty of anti-trust violations.[67]

An earlier cooperative plan had more lasting consequences than the Washington experiment. In 1929, the Baylor University Hospital provided 1,500 school teachers a maximum of twenty-one days of hospital care for a yearly fee of $6 per person. This scheme is credited with being the original of the Blue Cross system. Several other Dallas hospitals adopted competitive plans. These early arrangements were direct service rather than indemnity systems.[68]

In February 1938, the St. Louis Medical Society, upon the recommendation of its Medical Economics Committee, launched a group hospital service plan. Participation at first was limited to its own members, their families and their office employees. Benefits included twenty-one days of hospital care in a semi-private room, medicines, nursing and routine laboratory work. The cost was $.75 per month for each individual, $1.50 for a family. This, like the Baylor plan, was a service arrangement.[69] Later the plan was made available to business and professional groups outside its own membership.

In a report issued on September 29, 1939, Dr. Carl F. Vohs, chairman of the society's Medical Economics Committee, told of the rapid expansion of the service. All approved hospitals of the St. Louis area were participating. The plan was governed by a board of trustees representing the public, the medical profession and the hospitals. It was operated by a staff of more than thirty employees, under the supervision of the executive director, Ray F. McCarthy. During its initial operations, the organization had paid the hospitals $425,000, representing 87 percent of the total bills of approximately ten thousand admissions. Total assets were in excess of a quarter of a million dollars, and unencumbered reserves were more than $165,000. One of every ten persons in St. Louis was a member. The St. Louis plan provided its benefits to all parts of the state except Jackson County; it also served Southern Illinois. The St. Louis organization provided assistance in the development of statewide plans for Arkansas and Oklahoma and Jackson County in Missouri.[70]

In January 1945, the Missouri Medical Service (Blue Shield) began operations. For a fee of $1.60 a month for individuals and $3.75 for families, a substantial portion of medical, surgical and hospital costs could be prepaid. Existing Blue Cross members could pay an additional $.85 a month for individual and $2.25 a month for family coverage under the combined plan. Unlike the original Blue Cross plan, Blue Shield, from the start, operated on an indemnity principle. The doctor could set his own fee. If in a particular case, it exceeded Blue Shield indemnification, the patient had to pay the difference.[71]

Though they operated under separate names, Blue Cross and Blue Shield were closely tied administratively:[72]

The Missouri Medical Service will share collection facilities and office staff with Blue Cross. Executive boards of the two organizations, both nonprofit, are separate, though there is some duplication.

In early May 1947, Senator Robert F. Wagner of New York and five other Democratic senators introduced a comprehensive health insurance bill. Already a number of European countries had installed such a benefit system.[83] The American Medical Association raised a war chest of $3,500,000 to defeat the plan. Instead of waging an entirely negative campaign, the association stressed the success of group insurance organizations, such as Blue Cross and Blue Shield, which it claimed made a national system unnecessary.

The *St. Louis Post-Dispatch*, which was strongly in favor of the proposed legislation, called attention to its beneficial features. It also pointed out the shortcomings of the Blue Cross-Blue Shield approach:[74]

It is actually impossible, in fact, for medical insurance groups to cover the whole population. Most of them must, for actuarial reasons, limit their membership to persons of certain age groups or certain income limits or to those in organized employment groups. Their services must be restricted to a certain number or type of calls, or extra premiums must be charged.

The Missouri Medical Society's plan, for instance, covers only physicians' and surgeons' fees in hospital cases, to the exclusion of office calls, home visits and preventive medicine. These latter are the services which cover the greater part of an average family's needs; hospital care is required in only a small percentage of cases.

The Wagner bill would include the entire working population. This would spread the cost of medical care to the point that would cause no excessive burden on anyone . . . .

In addition, the bill provides for expansion of public health facilities and for aid to medical education and research. It specifies that doctors may enter or remain out of the system, as they please, and that patients may continue to consult doctors on the present fee basis, if they wish. It provides for local and state councils to administer the system, thus establishing a sound decentralization.

Although Congress rejected the Wagner bill, it did pass a number of entitlement programs, which at least indirectly involved the nation's health and welfare. The most important of these was the Social Security Act of 1935. By making payments of 1 percent of his wages up to $3,000 a year, matched by equal payments by his employer, a worker could be assured of an old-age pension when he retired at age sixty-five. The plan gradually was improved by admitting new groups of employees and by increasing the amounts paid in by workers and employers.[75] The Social Security system was used as the basis of Medicare and Medicaid when these health care plans were set up in 1965.

7. St. Louis's Campaign For Pure Milk

Shortly after World War I, during which the inspection of the local milk supply was badly neglected, representatives of twenty St. Louis clubs and organizations formed the Citizens' Milk Committee to do something about the matter. Mrs. M. G. Seelig, wife of a prominent Washington University Medical School professor, was the leader of the group.

About eighty percent of St. Louis milk came from Southern Illinois. It was produced as a side line by farmers, most of which lacked the equipment or knowledge to provide clean milk. The farmers hauled their milk to depots or to railroad stations for transportation to St. Louis. The milk cans were carried in baggage cars to the city where often they remained for hours at Union Station before they were picked up by the milk distributors. A St. Louis ordinance required that all milk sold in the city be pasteurized and that it must not contain more than 50,000 bacteria per cubic centimeter after treatment. In only one of St. Louis's plants was the pasteurization process completely efficient. In a bacteriological test conducted at Children's Hospital, milk taken from doorsteps showed as high as 1,200,000 bacteria per cubic centimeter. St. Louis pediatricians warned parents against feeding local milk to their children, recommending that they substitute condensed or powdered milk.[76]

On December 9, 1920, Ernest Kelly, investigator of market milk for the Bureau of Animal Industry, United States Department of Agriculture, appeared before the Citizens' Milk Committee as an expert witness. He suggested that St. Louis set up a permit system by which the Health Department would have authority to ban milk produced on Illinois farms under unsanitary conditions. He also recommended that the temperature requirement for pasteurization be raised from 140 degrees Fahrenheit to 145 degrees, to be maintained for a period of thirty minutes.[77]

In April 1920, the tuberculin testing of approximately 2,000 cows producing 2,500 gallons of milk daily within the city limits had been abandoned by the City Health Department when this responsibility was officially taken over by the state.[78] Unfortunately, the State Board of Health was not adequately staffed for the task.

The Missouri Supreme Court, in April 1926, held that the St. Louis ordinance, requiring that all milk except Grade A certified must be pasteurized, was in violation of state law, which permitted the sale of raw milk. But the decision stated that the city might set up proper standards and safeguards guaranteeing that milk must be safe and wholesome. This ruling effectively eliminated St. Louis's control of its milk supply.[79]

A new ordinance, meeting the requirements of the supreme court's decision, was drawn up in the Committee of Public Welfare of the board of aldermen. The substance of the proposed act was thus described:[80]

The present bill proposes that the city embargo all milk except that taken from cows whose owners could show for them a certificate that they had been tested for and found free of tuberculosis. It sets up such stringent rules for the handling of raw milk that it likely would result in most plants installing pasteurizing plants rather than endeavor to meet these stringent rules.

The ordinance, which was passed on March 21, 1928, required that milk labeled pasteurized must be heated at 142 degrees Fahrenheit for thirty minutes. It also specified that certified raw milk must not contain more than approximately 50,000 bacteria per cubic centimeter. Enforcement was placed in the hands of the chief chemist, the assistant chemist and milk inspectors of the Department of Health. But the number of such inspectors was not specified.[81]

A 1933 ordinance restructuring the health department placed milk inspection under a new food control section. This section assisted pasteurization plants in modernizing their equipment and improving their pasteurization procedures.[82]

On November 16, 1934, the board of aldermen passed a compromise milk ordinance, which L. C. Frank, chief of the United States Milk Investigations Office, called a "progressive step" but inadequate. The bill contained no provision for a tax to pay for inspection; however, the city dairies and the milk producers of the district guaranteed a fund of at least $60,000 a year, based on a contribution of one cent for each 100 pounds of milk distributed in St. Louis. Payments would be made to a board consisting of representatives of the city, producers, distributors and consumers. The board was authorized to employ inspectors under the jurisdiction of the city health division. The plan would make possible a slight increase in the number of inspectors, many of them working at the milk producing farms.[83]

A report by the Federal Trade Commission, in mid-June 1936, that milk and cream from uninspected dairy farms had been sold in St. Louis energized a movement for the adoption of the United States Public Health Service's standard milk ordinance. The St. Louis Medical Society took the lead in this campaign. The ordinance provided for the grading of milk and would tax the industry to employ forty-two inspectors, instead of the nineteen then working.[84]

A hearing by the Public Welfare Committee of the board of aldermen on the afternoon of November 12, 1936, drew a crowd of supporters that likely set a record in the city's history.[85]

The representatives of sponsoring groups, gathered at the City Hall for the public hearing on the ordinance, were an impressive assemblage. They were spokesmen for progressive organizations of great variety and large membership. The medical and dental professional societies. Parent teacher groups. Consumers' organizations. Religious groups of several denominations. American Legion posts. Women's study clubs. Civic organizations. And all are groups without axes to grind, who support the movement only because they unite in an affirmative answer to the question at issue: Shall St. Louis have safe milk?

Individual spokesmen for the bill, which is based on the model ordinance of the United States Public Health Service, likewise were a group of high standing in the community. Medical leaders, religious leaders, public officials, members of university faculties and many others. Almost 100 local organizations and countless individuals have gone on record as favoring the measure. Total membership of the various clubs and societies is more than 180,000.

Despite objections by the milk producers and the dairies that the bill would require that they purchase expensive equipment, that it would drive many of them out of business, and that it would increase the price of milk to the public, the measure was passed.[86]

The standard ordinance embodied three major improvements over the previous compromise law. The new act made it possible for the board of public service to lower the grade of any dairy's milk that failed to come up to the required standard. The experience of other cities had indicated that this was a fairer and more effective way than using the power to close a dairy or to prosecute in the police court.

Second, the proposed tax of four cents per hundred weight of milk, amounting to one-eleventh of a cent per quart, was more equitable than using city funds or relying on contributions by the dairy industry to pay for inspection. This eliminated the conflict of interest which was unavoidable when the inspectors had to look to those they inspected for their pay.[87]

Third, the new ordinance lowered the permissible bacterial count of Grade A pasteurized milk to 200,000 bacteria per cubic centimeter before pasteurization and 30,000 bacteria after treatment.[88] This change, dictated by urgent public health considerations, was expected to dispel the unsavory reputation of St. Louis milk as being "bacterial soup."

The United States Public Health Service reported on August 24, 1938, that with the exception of sixteen small towns and cities, St. Louis was the only community in the United States in which all the market milk was pasteurized. Other towns in St. Louis County with a high percentage of pasteurized milk were: Clayton, 99.9 percent; University City, 99.6 percent; Ferguson, 80 percent; Kirkwood, 94 percent; and Webster Groves, 93 percent.[89]

8. Increased Use and Demand For Hospitals

By the mid-1920s, the hospital had become the key factor in medical practice. Home visits had drastically declined as doctors conducted more of their consultations in their offices and sent their patients to the hospital for acute and chronic illnesses. Operations, including the delivery of babies, which had been performed at home, were transferred to a specialized ward of a hospital. The institution of effective systems of germ control and aseptic surgical procedures removed the danger of contagion which hospitals formerly had harbored. Middle- and upper-class families led the movement toward greater hospital dependency.

Hospitals became, not only safer, but more convenient and comfortable. In the newer hospitals single or double rooms, with lavatories attached, replaced the old open wards. Central air conditioning made hospital life endurable in the hot Missouri summers. X-ray services, radiation equipment and pathological laboratories for speedy identification of disease germs, supplemented the ministrations of the family doctor as he treated his hospitalized patients. In the larger cities, the general hospital was faced with competition by specialized institutions, dealing with a limited range of ailments.

St. Louis, as a major medical center which attracted a large volume of non-resident patients, experienced a chronic shortage of hospital beds. A large proportion of its hospitals continued to be affiliated with religious denominations, particularly the Catholic church. But various secular groups, e.g., national railway systems and social organizations, also participated in the establishment and operation of hospitals.

The Ancient Arabic Order, Nobles of the Mystic Shrine (popularly known as Shriners) in 1920 decided to add a charitable mission to their society. In addition to conducting their mystical ceremonies and colorful parades, they would sponsor a national system of free orthopedic hospitals for crippled children. The hospitals would be financed by an annual contribution of $2 made by each of its 600,000 members. The first of these hospitals was built in St. Louis and was opened for patients in June 1924. It was a $550,000 building with a capacity of eighty patients. The facility was designed as a unit of the Barnes Hospital system and would be staffed and operated by the Washington University Medical School faculty. It became the central unit of a Shrine hospital network with later branches in Shreveport, Louisiana; Minneapolis, Minnesota; San Francisco; and other American cities. In the St. Louis hospital, research work and instruction for the other Shrine hospitals would be conducted.[90]

Contracts for the new Missouri Pacific Railroad hospital, to be located at Grand and Shaw avenues, were let on September 14, 1921, with construction to begin within ten days. The structure, costing approximately $850,000, consisted of a main building of six stories for white employees and a two-story annex for black workers. The total capacity of the two buildings was between three and four hundred patients. The 40,000 employees on the Missouri Pacific lines contributed from forty to ninety cents a month to the hospital maintenance fund. In the event of sickness or accident, they were entitled to medical and hospital care without further cost. The hospital plan was managed by a board consisting of representatives of workers and the railroad.[91]

A survey, conducted in December 1923, indicated that St. Louis had a shortage of 2,500 to 4,000 beds in private hospitals. Except for urgent cases, it was impossible to get a room in a private hospital, with less than a month's waiting. At the time of the survey, the number of patients at the St. Louis

City Hospital was nearing its optimum capacity of 800.[92]

St. Mary's Hospital, in a six-story structure at Clayton Road and Bellevue Avenue, was dedicated June 10, 1924, in a ceremony conducted by Archbishop John J. Glennon. It was the third hospital opened locally by the Catholic nursing order, the Sisters of St. Mary, which had begun its existence in 1871 at Third and Gratiot streets, St. Louis. The $1,600,000 structure was located on an eighteen-acre wooded tract just beyond the city limits.[93]

The new hospital contained 300 rooms, single and double, but no wards. In case of emergency, the number of beds in a room could be doubled, giving it a maximum capacity of 600 patients. Beds in double rooms were $3.00 a day, in a private room $5 to $8 daily. Free treatment would be extended to deserving poor patients.

Although the nursing sisterhood was in charge of administration, St. Louis University provided medical and educational services. The medical school furnished ten full-time resident physicians for the hospital and infirmary, and a visiting staff of sixty-seven physicians for the hospital. This arrangement, similar to that between Barnes Hospital and the Washington University Medical School, transformed St. Mary's into a university-related teaching institution.[94]

The new Christian Hospital at Carter and Newstead avenues was opened in late October 1925. It had a capacity of 140 beds and was the only general hospital in North St. Louis, serving a population of more than 200,000. The new institution was not associated with a religious denomination. Its orientation was more philanthropic and feminist than religious. The $400,000 cost of its building had been raised by public subscription. Miss Elizabeth Gill was the superintendent;

Mrs. Evalyn Davis of Washington University served as president of the corporation.

The hospital was operated by eighteen regular nurses, fifteen alumni nurses on call, and twenty-two student nurses. Its accommodations were open to the entire medical profession. Its own staff did not include resident physicians. It was equipped especially to handle obstetrical cases.[95]

A campaign was conducted from September 24 to October 4, 1926 to raise $700,000 to build a new Evangelical Home and Hospital, with a capacity of 175 beds, on Oakland Avenue west of Clayton Avenue, just across from Forest Park. The St. Louis Medical Society, the Chamber of Commerce and other civic organizations endorsed and participated in the drive. The building was estimated to cost $1,000,000, of which $300,000 was already in hand. The new hospital would replace the outgrown Deaconess facility at West Belle Place and Sarah Street.[96]

In July 1928, funds were sought to make the Washington University Medical School a world center for research on diseases of the eye, ear, nose and throat. Under the will of Mrs. Eliza McMillan, approximately $1,000,000 had become available for this purpose. The General Education Fund, a Rockefeller foundation, provided $1,500,000. Further contributions were received from local donors to bring the amount available to $4,000,000. The new eight-story structure would be named "The McMillan Eye, Ear, Nose, and Throat Hospital" and would be located at Euclid and Scott avenues, directly opposite the medical school. To head the new hospital, Dean W. McKim Marriott of the School of Medicine selected Dr. Harvey J. Howard as professor of ophthalmology and Dr. Lee Wallace Dean as professor of otolaryngology. Dr. Howard was for ten years in charge of eye research for the Rockefeller

Institute at Union Medical College in Pekin, China, and a recognized leader in this field. Dr. Dean was formerly head of the medical school of Iowa University and served as editor of the *Annals of Otolaryngology*, the most respected journal concerned with diseases of the ear, nose and throat.[97]

The McMillan hospital would fill an important vacancy in the medical school's system of satellite research centers, as the following statement indicates:[98]

> In the Washington University medical unit there is now Barnes Hospital for adult medical and surgical patients; St. Louis Children's Hospital for children suffering from medical and surgical conditions; St.Louis Maternity Hospital has recently joined the group and the new Maternity Hospital will be erected during the present year. With McMillan Hospital the group will be complete except for the hospital of nervous and mental diseases and there will be few institutions in the country with equal facilities for teaching and research.

The 113th commencement of St. Louis University, on June 2, 1931, coincided with the laying of the cornerstone of the new $1,000,000 Firmin Desloge Hospital located at Grand Boulevard and Rutger Street. Commencement speakers appropriately pointed out that the new institution filled three long recognized needs of St. Louis:[99]

> a hospital particularly dedicated to the service of persons of moderate means; a teaching hospital adjacent to the School of Medicine; and, by relieving St. Mary's Infirmary of its present use for white persons, a hospital for Negroes, which is to include a nursing school for Negro college women.

The hospital was named in honor of Firmin Desloge, a deceased lead magnate, who with his widow and two sons were generous benefactors of Catholic charitable enterprises.

The Homer G. Phillips Hospital, located on a tract comprising most of two city blocks and bounded by Whittier Street and St. Ferdinand, Kennerly and Goode avenues, was dedicated February 22, 1937. Harold L. Ickes, secretary of the interior, was the featured program speaker. The hospital was named to honor a popular Negro lawyer and civic leader who had been assassinated in 1931.[100]

Funds for the hospital had been provided in the $87,000,000 local bond issue passed in 1923. A disagreement over the location of the structure delayed its construction. The hospital commissioner and the St. Louis Medical Society, for reasons of convenience and economy, wanted it located adjacent to the city hospital. Black leaders, however, insisted that it be built in the newer residential area surrounding Sumner High School, where many of their race had built homes. With the issue at an impasse, Negro patients were treated, under crowded and unsatisfactory conditions, in city hospital no. 2, conducted in the old Barnes Medical College building at Harrison Avenue and Lawton Boulevard.[101]

With the 1932 elections coming up, the board of aldermen yielded to the wishes of the black community and construction was started at the western residential site, using funds appropriated in the 1923 bond issue. The cornerstone was laid December 10, 1933, and the building was finally ready for occupancy in early March 1937.

The hospital consisted of an administrative building with two ward wings, a service building and a nurses' and a superintendent's

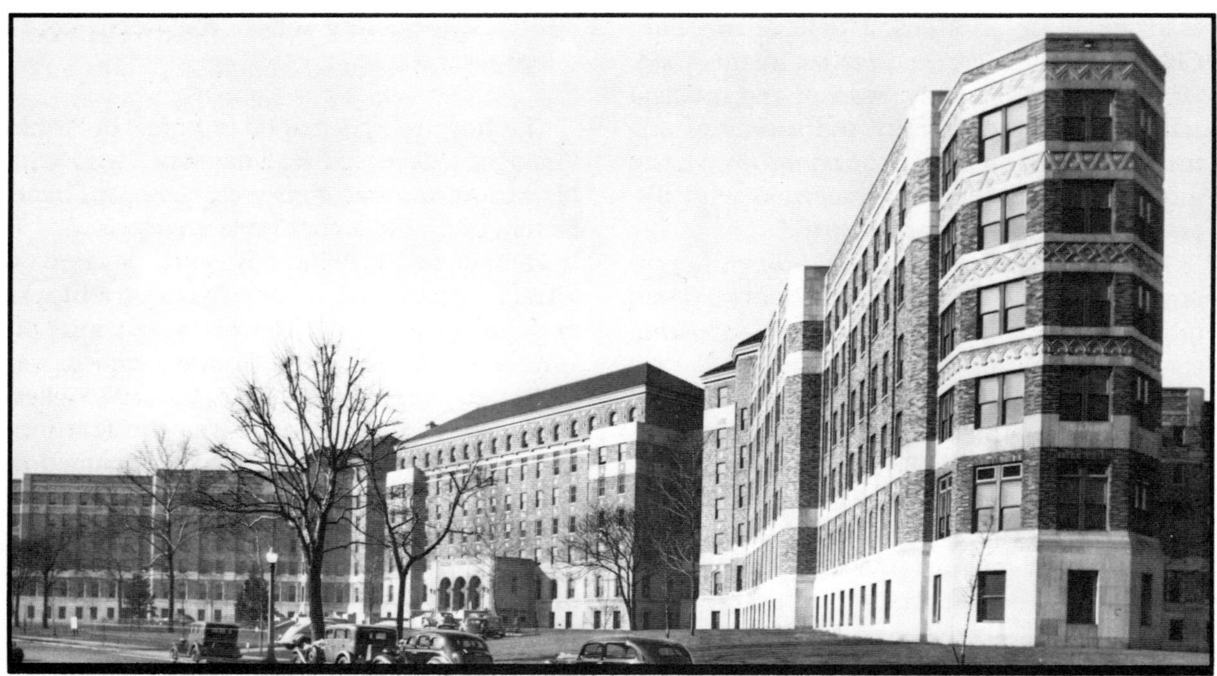

Missouri Historical Society. Homer G. Phillips Hospital, photo by W.C. Persons PB 582
Homer G. Phillips Hospital

residence in the rear. The central building and its wings were architecturally distinctive in that their fronts formed, not a straight line but a half circle, with the approach by a curving driveway off of Whittier Street. The capacity of each wing was 300 patients. The building was provided with the latest, state of the art facilities and equipment. The overall cost was slightly more than $2,000,000, of which thirty percent came from a PWA grant. The hospital would be operated by an all-Negro staff. The superintendent of hospital no. 2 proudly referred to the new facility as "the finest such institution for Negroes in the world."[102]

The Ellis Fischel State Cancer Hospital in Columbia was dedicated and opened for patients on April 26, 1940. This was the first such hospital in the United States designed exclusively for cancer treatment.[103] The same considerations that moved the state in 1905

to establish the state sanatorium for tuberculosis in Mt. Vernon were responsible for the inception of the cancer center. Cancer, like tuberculosis, requires extensive treatment. County hospitals lacked the required equipment and trained personnel. Many hospitals refused to accept cancer patients, fearing that the disease was highly contagious. Few families were able to afford the schedule of treatment. The Barnard Free Skin and Cancer Hospital in St. Louis, established in 1905, offered the best therapy available in the state.

The Columbia hospital was named for Dr. Ellis Fischel, a noted St. Louis oncologist, who was the prime mover in the establishment of the Columbia institution and the chairman of the original Cancer Commission, which exercised administrative oversight. He was the son of Dr. Washington E. Fischel, who had served as president of the staff at the Barnard hospital.

The Columbia institution occupied a 40-acre tract on old U.S. Highway 40, in the northern section of the city. It had seven stories of reinforced concrete, with a brown and cream-colored exterior. It was equipped to provide radiation, chemical and surgical treatment. Its mission was to serve indigent patients, free of charge. It began work with a staff of 115 members, headed by Dr. Harry Seekman, formerly of the Michael Reese Hospital of Chicago.

While the hospital was under construction, a cancer clinic and treatment center of thirty-six beds was operated at the Fulton state hospital. A similar unit was planned for the St. Joseph state hospital.[104]

The building to house the Malcolm A. Bliss Psychopathic Institute in St. Louis was ready for occupancy in June 1939. It was six stories high and formed part of the city hospital complex. It had facilities for 185 white and black patients. Funds from the 1934 state bond issue and a PWA grant paid the costs of construction. During the first eighteen months of its availability, the new structure would be put to general administrative and clinical use by city hospital personnel while several of the old hospital buildings were being replaced. At the end of that period, the psychopathic institute would assume the functions of the old observation ward of city hospital and provide modern facilities for research in the care and prevention of mental disorders. It would go into business with none of the associations of the old asylum or mental hospital.[105]

Thirty St. Louis hospitals received full approval by the American College of Surgeons in its 1945 hospital survey. Dr. Malcolm T. MacEachern, associate director of the college in charge of hospital matters, listed as follows the requirements upon which hospitals were approved:[106]

Modern physical plant; clearly defined organization, duties, responsibilities and relations; carefully selected governing board with supreme authority; competent, well-trained superintendent responsible to board; adequate and efficient personnel; organized medical staff of ethical physicians and surgeons; adequate diagnostic and therapeutic facilities; accurate complete medical records; regular group conferences of administrative and medical staffs and a humanitarian spirit.

St. Louis hospitals which received full approval were:[107]

Alexian Brothers, Barnard Free Skin and Cancer, Barnes, Bethesda, Christian, De Paul, Evangelical Deaconess Home and Hospital, Firmin Desloge, Frisco Employees, Homer G. Phillips, Jewish, Josephine Heitkamp Memorial, Lutheran, McMillan, Missouri Baptist, Missouri Pacific, Mount St. Rose Sanatorium, Peoples, St. Anthony's, St. John's, St. Louis Children's, City Hospital, City Sanitarium, St. Louis Maternity, St. Mary's, St. Luke's, St. Mary's Infirmary, St. Vincent's Sanitarium, Shriners' Hospital for Crippled Children.

Help in alleviating St. Louis's and Missouri's shortage of hospital beds was promised through the passage by Congress in 1946 of the Hospital Survey and Construction Act (known as the Hill-Burton program). Congress, having failed to enact a national health insurance plan because of conservative opposition, discovered in hospital construction a non-controversial way to do something to improve the nation's welfare. The program would create employment at a time when millions of World War II veterans were looking for work. Besides, the hospital industry and the professional medical organizations warmly supported it.[108]

Money for the construction program would be distributed to the states on the basis of population and per capita income. States with low per capita income would receive greater amounts to compensate for their poverty. The overall amount of the five-year program was initially estimated at $1.8 billion, for approximately 195,000 beds. The federal share eventually reached $3.7 billion. Matching funds provided by the states and localities were approximately $9.1 billion.[109]

To participate in the program, each state had to conduct a survey by its health department to determine its needs and then draw up a plan to meet these requirements. The federal government would pay the cost of the survey.

On December 10, 1946, Governor Phil M. Donnelly announced the names of the advisory council that would assist the health division in conducting the survey and in formulating a statewide plan for constructing new facilities. The members were: Ray F. McCarthy, former director of the group hospital service (Blue Cross) in St. Louis; Dr. Emmett F. Hoctor, superintendent of State Hospital No. 4, Farmington; Nell Morgan, president of the State Nurses' Association; L. O. Wallace, member of the executive board of the Missouri Farmers' Association; Mrs. Paul Palmer, member of the board of directors of the State Farm Bureau Federation; O. V. Jackson, Rolla; and Everett Johns, member of the State Board of Registration for architects and professional engineers.[110]

To get federal aid after the survey was concluded, an organization or community had to apply to its state board of health for approval before submitting its request to the federal government. If the request was in harmony with the survey, it had a good chance of being approved.

9. Expansion of St. Louis's Water Supply

The construction of the Chain of Rocks plant with its three-step process of sedimentation, coagulation and filtration assured St. Louis of a clear, wholesome supply of water. The problem of the future was to see that the city's pumping capacity kept pace with the demands of its growing population and industry.

In 1921, it was estimated that the Chain of Rocks works could supply 140,000,000 gallons of water each twenty-four hours. With the addition of one more high service engine, the total capacity could be raised to 160,000,000 gallons per day. If the projected growth of demand was realized, the city would be consuming the peak output of the Chain of Rocks source by 1928. In case a new plant was not started during 1922 or 1923, the city would face a serious water shortage from 1928 onwards.[111]

To avoid this calamity, it was planned to build a new waterworks at Howard Bend on the Missouri River, eight miles above St. Charles, where the stream curves to the eastward toward the St. Louis suburbs. There were several good reasons for building the new waterworks on the Missouri River rather than expanding the Chain of Rocks establishment. The Missouri River water was less polluted than that from the Mississippi and consequently more easily clarified and purified. Also, the cost of forcing the Missouri River water through the mains to city customers would be less.[112]

The first step involved in the transfer of pumping operations to the Missouri River was the purchase by the city of a fifty-three acre tract in St. Louis County between the Warson and Old Bonhomme roads, south of Olive Street road. The site, part of an area known as Strattman Hill, was the highest point in the county. On it the city planned to construct a giant reservoir for water piped from the Missouri River. Water from this reservoir would flow by natural gravity to all parts of St. Louis.[113]

On February 14, 1923, the voters of St. Louis approved a $77,300,000 civic bond issue, which included $12,000,000 earmarked for the new waterworks.[114]

By the fall of 1924, work on the new plant at Howard Bend was well underway. A row of dikes was constructed on the north side of the river opposite the plant site in order to force the main current of the river to flow past the waterworks on the south bank. Since the pumping engine pits and the water intake were to be built on the floor of the river, a cofferdam was constructed to temporarily drain the work site.[115]

The *Post-Dispatch* of November 24, 1928, had pictures of the new waterworks in near-completion state. Seated on the river bank were the pump house and the adjoining boiler house, with its huge smokestack. Coal from rail cars was brought to the boiler house on an inclined conveyor system.[116]

The intake consisted of a set of openings at various levels of the outer wall of the pump house, through which the river water poured into five interchangeable pools. From these the pumps would circulate the waters to the various steps of the purification process.[117] Following its sedimentation and clarification, the clear water would be forced by the high service pumps through the sixteen-mile main of five-foot pipe to the covered reservoir on Strattman Hill. The reservoir and the surrounding area were renamed Stacy Park. The new waterworks went into operation in February 1929.

The plant had two 60,000,000 gallon engines for pumping clear water. One pump would be held in reserve for emergencies. The 60,000,000 gallons from the new plant, with the 160,000,000 from the Chain of Rocks, would give the city a total of 220,000,000 gallons daily. This should take care of projected needs until 1940. [118]

10. Garbage Disposal

The disposal of its garbage was a problem that long plagued the city of St. Louis. The only period when this issue was handled with any continuity and a minimum of public outcry was when the contracts to collect and dispose of the unsavory stuff were regularly awarded to the city boss Colonel Ed Butler. Butler reduced the garbage in his plant on the Mississippi River in South St. Louis, charging the city a quarter of a million dollars annually for the service.[119] Citizens of the neighborhood objected to the odors from the plant. But they knew that they could do nothing about it, in view of Butler's tight control of city government. Like Chicagoans with the stockyard odors, St. Louisans learned to live with the stench from the garbage works. But with Butler's loss of power and also of the garbage contract, the citizens became more protective of the wholesomeness of their neighborhoods.

They were not concerned particularly where the city disposed of its wastes — provided it was in someone else's backyard. In this they were like folks everywhere. At various times St. Louis dumped its garbage into the Mississippi River; it shipped it down stream to a large island to be fed to hogs; it sent it over to the Illinois side for disposal; and it established a reduction plant on the

Missouri River opposite St. Charles until the State Board of Health halted the operation.

On April 14, 1922, a contract was let for the erection of a garbage incinerator plant on the Mississippi River at the foot of Choteau Avenue. The site was about three quarters of a mile south of Olive Street. The structure was to be one of four incinerators within the city. The other three were to be at Bissell's Point, at Kingshighway and McRee Avenue, and the third near the city workhouse. The Choteau Avenue plant was the first step of the city toward abolishing the prevailing method of disposing of garbage by hauling it down the river in barges, to be sold to hog farmers.[120] The city estimated that the cost of collecting the garbage and transporting it down the river was approximately $5.60 per ton. By incinerating it at plants located in north, south and central areas of the city, the cost could be reduced considerably. It was planned to use tractors and trains of trailers to collect the garbage and haul it to the nearest incinerator.[121]

On November 14, 1922, a committee of members of the board of public service and of the board of aldermen visited the new incinerating plant on Choteau Avenue and were favorably impressed by the claims of the contractor that the disposal operation would be odorless. In the process, powerful suction fans drew the air from the garbage bins and other interior areas and forced it through the furnaces.[122]

The apparent success of the first incinerating plant encouraged the board of aldermen to pass an ordinance providing for the establishment of the second plant on De Tonty Street and Kingshighway. The site was in an upper-class residential area and close to Shaw's Garden, Tower Grove Park and the Washington University Medical School. Real estate agents, businessmen, hospitals, citi-

zens' protective associations and other groups strongly protested, not only against the anticipated odors from the plant, but also against the traffic of garbage wagons that would be passing through their neighborhood. The opposition was so widespread and influential, as attested by petitions signed by 5,500 persons,[123] that the board of public service, on September 7, 1923, refused to act on the bids for the De Tonty plant.[124] The overall plan for four incinerators was abandoned. Only the Choteau Avenue plant, with a daily capacity of eighty tons, was operational.

With the collapse of the incinerator plan, the city returned to its previous practice of depending on hog farmers to dispose of its garbage. In a highly competitive round of bidding, the Jefferson Distributing Company got the contract, in February 1924, at a cost to the city of $1.03 a ton. The company explained that it had invested $60,000 for a barge and an island and had to have the contract even at an unprofitable rate of return.[125]

The following year, a five-year contract was awarded to Charles L. Rea of Kansas City, a hog farmer, for disposal of garbage at a rate of $.74 per ton. The operation of the contract, however, was delayed by an injunction brought by the Jefferson company and by Thomas Faudree. The two parties claimed that awarding of the contract to Rea had not been done in accordance with the city charter.[126] Before the case came to trial, however, the three contesting farmers had reached an out-of-court settlement.

According to the agreement, Rea would be the contractor in name only; the Jefferson company would haul the garbage and receive the money for their services. The garbage would be divided among the farmers — Rea, the Jefferson company and Faudree. By the terms of the five-year contract, the city would pay $.74 per ton for the hauling and disposal services.[127]

The granting of the contract to Rea did not remove the issue from public discussion and from political patronage. St. Louisans were surprised to learn that all garbage was not equal; that there was "good garbage" and "alley garbage." Good garbage was collected from hotels, restaurants and clubs and consisted exclusively of edible refuse. Alley garbage, in addition to food, contained paper, cans, dead animals, broken glass and ashes. Hog feeders, who threw alley garbage to their hogs, suffered regularly an eight to ten percent loss of animals from eating toxic substances. Rea, upon investigation of the operation of his contract, found that aldermen, city officials and other political personages, had been "getting a little garbage for a friend" who was feeding a few hogs. The result was that Rea was receiving no good garbage and little even of the alley sort.[128]

In July 1929, in anticipation of the expiration of Rea's contract in February 1930, a group of city officials spent a day in inspecting how Rea used his garbage. The tour started at the foot of Choteau Avenue, where city wagons backed on to the dock and dumped their contents into a 500-ton-capacity barge. A steamboat owned by Rea towed the loaded barge fifty-six miles down river to Establishment Island where Rea had his hog farm.

The *Post-Dispatch* thus described the next step:[129]

At the island, the garbage is distributed to different feeding pens by a steam- driven clamshell bucket and a narrow gauge railway. Bucket-loads of garbage are dropped through a hopper to cars, the cars are hauled to roofed feeding pens, and there the reeking grayish-brown mess is dumped.

Garbage which arrives on a barge at the island looks not at all like the refuse that was dumped into it 24 hours before. Heat and pressure on the trip down cook it into a sour mass that Rea says is more palatable for hogs than fresh garbage.

In 1930, Hog Haven Farms, Inc., received a five-year contract to dispose of the city's garbage. But residents of South St. Louis opposite the farm secured an injunction. The president of the company expressed his willingness to carry out the contract and dispose of the garbage at some other site.[130]

Although most of the sites, where St. Louis garbage had been dumped, were on large Mississippi River islands, the odors from thousands of hogs and their food supplies were carried by varying winds to communities on both river banks. Offended citizens of the communities affected were displaying an increasing determination to resort to the courts to halt these nuisances.

The growing resistance of communities to having hog farms in their vicinity prompted St. Louis's director of streets and sewers Frank J. McDevitt to devise a new plan. This was to grind the garbage and discharge it into the Mississippi River through the sewer system. The War Department, which had jurisdiction over navigable streams, gave its approval; its sole concern was the assurance of freedom of navigation.[131]

Seth Gordon in Washington, president of the American Game Association, using test results arrived at by the Bureau of Fisheries, foretold the environmental results that would follow from McDevitt's plan:[132]

U.S. Bureau of Fisheries experts, who have made a careful study, report that this added burden of filth will destroy all aquatic life for at least 190 miles below St. Louis. Instead of further destroying the public waters which flow by the front door of St. Louis, your city should install a modern sewage treatment plant to eliminate the rotten mess which is already being dumped into the Father of Waters. Other progressive cities with civic pride are doing just this.

If St. Louis stoops to this proposal it will seriously hinder and delay the movement for clean streams throughout the land.

Despite this adverse report, McDevitt proceeded with the establishment of a pilot garbage grinding plant. In defense, he cited the approval of the War Department. His own tests, he asserted, had revealed no serious effects on aquatic life.[133]

By 1936, St. Louis had a mixed system of garbage disposal. Approximately 100 tons a day were being ground up and flushed away in the sewers. The incinerator at Choteau Avenue was still available. There were also a number of licensed and unlicensed garbage collectors with their particular routes. Finally, the city, instead of granting an overall contract for disposal, was conducting a retail business of selling its garbage directly to hog farmers.[134] The city was doing its own collecting, mostly with a fleet of mule-drawn wagons. The move to tractor-trailer trains apparently had not been implemented.

Chapter VIII
The State Board of Health Expands Its Activities

1   State of Missouri, *Official Manual for Years Nineteen Twenty-seven and Nineteen Twenty-eight* (Jefferson City, Mo., The Hugh Stephens Press, 1927), p. 705.
2   *Idem.*
3   *Laws of Missouri, Passed at the Session of the Forty-first General Assembly Begun and Held at the City of Jefferson, January 2, 1901.* Regular Session (Jefferson City, Mo., Tribune Printing Co., 1901), p. 180.
4   *Laws of Missouri, Passed at the Session of the Fiftieth General Assembly Which Convened at the City of Jefferson, Wednesday, January 8, 1919.* Edited by John L. Sullivan, Secretary of State 1919, (Jefferson City, Mo., The Hugh Stephens Printing Co., 1920), pp. 372-374.
5   *Official Manual for the State of Missouri, for the Years 1921-1922* (Jefferson City, Mo., 1922), p. 841.
6   *Ibid.,* pp. 841-842
7   *Official Manual of the State of Missouri for the Years 1923-1924* (Jefferson City, Mo., The Hugh Stephens Press, 1923), p. 774.
8   *Official Manual of the State of Missouri for the Years 1925 and 1926* (Jefferson City, Mo., The Hugh Stephens Press, 1926), p. 867.
9   *Idem.*
10 *Official Manual of the State of Missouri for the Years Nineteen Twenty-seven and Nineteen Twenty-eight* (Jefferson City, Missouri, The Hugh Stephens Press, 1927), p. 705.
11 *Ibid.,* p. 703.
12 *Official Manual of the State of Missouri for the Years Nineteen Twenty-nine and Nineteen-thirty* (Jefferson City, Mo., Botz-Hugh Stephens Press, 1929), p. 847.
13 *Report of the State Survey Commission to the Honorable Henry S. Caulfield, Governor of Missouri, Nov. 30, 1929,* pp. 44-45. Contained as Serial No. 47 in *Appendix to the House and Senate Journals of the Fifty-sixth General Assembly, State of Missouri* (Jefferson City, Mo., 1931), Vol. I.
14 Missouri State Health Department, Henry F. Parker M.D., State Health Commissioner, *Annual Report* 1937 (Jefferson City, Mo., Midland Printing Co., 1939). Contained as Serial No. 22 in *Appendix to the House and Senate Journals of the Sixtieth General Assembly, State of Missouri* (Jefferson City, Mo., Midland Printing Co., 1939) Vol. 2, pp. 31-32.
15 *Ibid.,* pp. 36-37.
16 *Ibid.,* p. 39.
17 *Ibid.,* p. 69.
18 *Ibid.,* p. 59.
19 *Idem.*
20 *Annual Report of the State Board of Health of Missouri for the Year 1939,* by Dr. Harry F. Parker, State Health Commissioner, p. 6. Contained as Serial No. 22 in *Appendix to House and Senate Journals of the Sixty-first General Assembly, State of Missouri, 1941* (Jefferson City, Mo., 1941), Vol. I.
21 St. Louis *Post-Dispatch*, Oct. 20, 1923, p. 3:6.
22 *Ibid.,* Mar. 31, 1921, part II, p. 1:1-2.
23 *Ibid.,* May 1, 1921, part I, p. 3:4.
24 *Ibid.,* Apr. 16, 1921, p. 1:2-3; *ibid.,* May 1, 1921, part I, p. 3:4.

25   *Ibid.*, Mar. 31, 1921, part II, p. 1:1-2.
26   *Laws of Missouri, Passed at the Session of the Fifty-second General Assembly, Which Convened at the City of Jefferson, Wednesday January 3, 1923* (Jefferson City, Mo., The Hugh Stephens Press, 1924), p. 254.
27   St. Louis *Post-Dispatch*, Nov. 26, 1923, part I, p. 13:3.
28   *Ibid.*, Nov. 28, 1923, p. 3:5-6.
29   *Ibid.*, Dec. 12, 1923, p. 27:2.
30   *Ibid.*, Nov. 28, 1923, p. 3:5-6.
31   *Ibid.*, Dec. 4, 1923, p. 14:4.
32   *Ibid.*, Feb. 7, 1925, p. 3:4.
33   *Ibid.*, June 17, 1925, p. 2:4.
34   *Ibid.*, Mar. 5, 1935, part I, p. 3:3.
35   *Ibid.*, Oct. 19, 1943, p. 2A:6.
36   *Laws of Missouri, Passed at the Session of the Sixty-fifth General Assembly, Which Convened at the City of Jefferson, Wednesday, January 5, 1949* (Jefferson City, Mo., Mid-State Printing Co., 1949), pp. 150-153.
37   *Laws of Missouri, Passed at the Session of the Sixty-third General Assembly, Which Convened at the City of Jefferson, Wednesday, January 3, 1945*, pp. 1148-1154. Compiled by Wilson Bell, Secretary of State.
38   *State of Missouri, Official Manual for the Years Nineteen Forty-nine and Nineteen-fifty.* (Jefferson City, Mo., Mid-State Printing Co., 1949), p. 577.
39   *Ibid.*, p. 605.
40   *Ibid.*, p. 606.
41   "Tenth Biennial Report of the Board of Managers of the State Eleemosynary Institutions to the Sixty-first General Assembly of the State of Missouri for 1939 and 1940" ((Jefferson City, Mo., Midland Printing Co., 1941) pp. 8-9. Contained as Serial No. 27 in *Appendix to the House and Senate Journals of the Sixty-first General Assembly, State of Missouri* (Jefferson City, Mo., Midland Printing Co., 1941), Vol. 2.
42   *State of Missouri, Official Manual for the Years Nineteen Thirty-five and Nineteen Thirty-six* (Jefferson City, Mo., Midland Printing Co., 1935), p. 675.
43   General Assembly of the State of Missouri, Committee on Legislative Research, "The Mentally Ill: Their Care and Treatment in Missouri," Report No. 8 (Jefferson City, Mo., Mid-State Printing Co., 1948) pp. 15-18. Contained as Serial No. 28 in *Appendix ot the House and Senate Journals of the Sixty-fifth General Assembly of the State of Missouri, 1949* (Jefferson City, Mo., The Mid-state Printing Co., 1949), Vol. 2. Also Report of State Hospital No. 1, Fulton, Missouri, pp. 6-7, contained as section of Serial No. 27 in *Appendix to the House and Senate Journals of the Sixty-first General Assembly, State of Missouri* (Jefferson City, Mo., Midland Printing Co., 1941, Vol. 2.
44   Message of Governor Guy B. Park to the Fifty-eighth General Assembly of Missouri (Jefferson City, Mo., Midland Printing Co., 1935), p. 5. Contained in *Appendix to the House and Senate Journals of the Fifty-eighth General Assembly, State of Missouri* (Jefferson City, Mo., Midland Printing Co., 1935), Vol. I. Also State of Missouri, *Official Manual for the Years Nineteen Thirty-seven and Nineteen Thirty-eight* (Jefferson City, Mo., Midland Printing Co., 1937), p. 653.
45   General Assembly, Committee on Legislative Research, "The Mentally Ill," pp. 12-13, 28-34.
46   "Eighth Biennial Report of the Board of Managers of the State Eleemosynary Institutions to the Fifty-ninth General Assembly of the State of Missouri for 1935 and 1936," p. 28. Contained as Serial No. 27 in *Appendix to the House and Senate Journals of the Fifty-ninth General Assembly, State of Missouri* (Jefferson City, Mo., Midland Printing Co., 1937), Vol. 2.
47   St. Louis *Post-Dispatch*, Dec. 2, 1942, p. 3B:6-7.
48   *Ibid.*, June 17, 1943, p. 6B:4-5.
49   *Ibid.*, June 27, 1943, p. 3A:6-7.
50   *Idem.*
51   *Idem.*
52   *Ibid.*, Mar. 14, 1946, p. 1A:2-3.
53   Owen H. and Sarah D. Wangensteen, *The Rise of Surgery From Empiric Craft to Scientific Discipline* (Minneapolis, University of Minnesota Press, 1978), p. 314.
54   *Ibid.*, p. 286.
55   St. Louis *Post-Dispatch*, Jan. 4, 1921, p. 1A:5-6.
56   George W. Corner, *A History of the Rockefeller Institute 1901-1953* (New York City, The Rockefeller Institute Press, 1964), pp. 324-325.
57   St. Louis *Post-Dispatch*, Dec. 11, 1944, p. 3A:2-3.
58   *Idem.*
59   *Ibid.*, Oct. 23, 1947, p. 1A:6-7.
60   Paul Starr, *The Social Transformation of American Medicine* (New York, Basic Books, Inc., Publishers, 1983), pp. 260-261.
61   *Idem.*
62   "Bulletin of the St. Louis Medical Society," Vol. XXIX, No. 37, May 24, 1935, p. 580.
63   Starr, *opus cit.*, p. 265.
64   "Bulletin of the St. Louis Medical Society," Vol. XXVIII, No., 18, Jan. 12, 1934, p. 261.
65   *Ibid*, Vol. XXVII, No. 28, Mar. 24, 1933, p. 361.
66   *Ibid*, Vol. XXVIII, No. 3, Sept. 29, 1933, p. 45.
67   Starr, *opus cit.*, p. 305.
68   *Ibid*, p. 295.
69   "Bulletin of the St. Louis Medical Society," Vol. XXXII, No. 23, Feb. 18, 1938, p. 290.
70   *Ibid*, Vol. XXXIV, No. 3, Sept. 29, 1939, pp. 36-39.
71   St. Louis *Post-Dispatch*, Aug. 27, 1944, part II, p. 1:5-6.
72   *Ibid*, Dec. 17, 1944, p. 3A:2-3.
73   *Ibid*, May 11, 1947, p. 10A:4.
74   *Ibid*, May 19, 1946, p. 2D:2.
75   *Encyclopedia Americana*, 1961 edition, Vol. 25, pp. 186-188.
76   St. Louis *Post-Dispatch*, Nov. 11, 1920, part II, p. 1:2-3.
77   *Ibid*, Dec. 9, 1920, p. 20:1.
78   *Ibid*, Jan. 21, 1921, p. 1:2.
79   *Ibid*, Apr. 9, 1926, p. 1:1.
80   *Ibid*, Jan. 18, 1928, part II, p. 1:3.
81   St. Louis *City Ordinances, 1927-1928*, pp. 78854-78864.
82   St. Louis *Post-Dispatch*, July 27, 1933, p. 6A:3.
83   *Ibid*, Nov. 17, 1934, p. 8A:5.
84   *Ibid*, June 13, 1936, p. 5A:6.
85   *Ibid*, Nov. 14, 1936, p. 4A:2.
86   *Ibid*, Nov. 19, 1936, p. 3A:1.
87   *Ibid*, Nov. 14, 1936, p. 4A:2.
88   *Ibid*, Dec. 11, 1936, p. 1A:3.
89   *Ibid*, Aug. 24, 1938, p. 10A:3.
90   *Ibid*, Apr. 5, 1921, part II, p. 1:4; *ibid*, Dec. 13, 1921,

p. 3:3-4; *ibid.*, June 2, 1924, p. 1:1 (part II).
91 *Ibid.*, Sept. 8, 1921, p. 2:3.
92 *Ibid.*, Dec. 4, 1923, p. 16:4.
93 *Ibid.*, June 10, 1924, p. 15:4.
94 *Idem.*
95 *Ibid.*, Oct. 27, 1925, p. 14:3.
96 *Ibid.*, Sept. 19, 1926, part VII, p. 3:3.
97 *Ibid.*, Mar. 24, 1925, p. 1:4; *ibid.*, July 17, 1928, Part III,
    p. 1:5-6.
98 *Ibid.*, Mar. 24, 1925, p. 1:4.
99 *Ibid.*, June 3, 1931, p. 8A:4.
100 *Ibid.*, Feb. 7, 1937, p. 3C:1.
101 *Ibid.*, Dec. 15, 1928, p. 3:3; *ibid.*, Feb. 7, 1937, p. 3C:1.
102 *Ibid.*, Aug. 18, 1934, p. 5A:4-6; *ibid.*, Feb. 7, 1937, p. 3C:1.
103 *Ibid.*, Apr. 21, 1940, p. 2H:5; *ibid.*, Mar. 20, 1938,
    p. 6A:2-3.
104 *Ibid.*, Mar. 20, 1938, p. 6A:2-3.
105 *Ibid.*, June 4, 1939, pict. section p. 4.
106 *Ibid.*, Jan. 31, 1946, p. 3C:3.
107 *Idem.*
108 Starr, *opus cit.*, p. 348.
109 *Ibid.*, pp. 349-350.
110 St. Louis *Post-Dispatch*, Dec. 10, 1946, p. 5C:3.
111 *Ibid.*, Dec. 11, 1921, p. 5:2-6.
112 *Idem.*
113 *Ibid.*, Apr. 9, 1921, p. 2:3.
114 *Ibid.*, July 17, 1922, part II, p. 1:5.
115 *Ibid.*, Sept, 11, 1924, p. 22:2-3.
116 *Ibid.*, Nov. 24, 1928, p. 13:1-8.
117 *Ibid.*, Sept, 11, 1924, p. 22:2-3.
118 *Ibid.*, Jan. 4, 1929, p. 1:5.
119 St. Louis *Republic*, Mar. 2, 1904, p. 1:4.
120 St. Louis *Post-Dispatch*, Apr. 14, 1922, p. 17:4.
121 *Ibid.*, Nov. 15, 1922, p. 24:4.
122 *Idem.*
123 *Ibid.*, Sept. 4, 1923, part II, p. 1:4.
124 *Ibid.*, Sept, 7, 1923, p. 28:5.
125 *Ibid.*, Feb. 21, 1924, p. 36:4.
126 *Ibid.*, Apr. 25, 1925, part II, p. 1:4.
127 *Ibid.*, May 16, 1925, p. 3:2.
128 *Ibid.*, June 8, 1929, p. 1:5.
129 *Ibid.*, July 5, 1929, p. 14:4.
130 *Ibid.*, Feb. 24, 1930, p. 3:5.
131 *Ibid.*, Dec. 6, 1934, p. 6A:5.
132 *Idem.*
133 *Idem.*
134 *Ibid.*, Oct. 2, 1936, p. 6D:4.

Chapter 9

New Initiatives in Missouri's Health Care, 1950-1980

1. Major Administrative Changes

FOR THE DELIVERY of health services, Missouri, in the 1950s, was divided into five districts. The central offices of these five districts were located as follows: District No. 1, Cameron; District No. 2, Macon; District No. 3, Jefferson City; District No. 4, Poplar Bluff; District No. 5, Springfield.[1] By 1980, the number of offices had increased to seven. The staff of each office consisted of skilled professionals in the public health field, including physicians, nurses, educators, nutritionists, engineers and sanitarians.

Each county was authorized to establish either a mill-tax-supported health department governed by an elected board, or it could set up a health organization or nursing service directed by the county court. The role of the district offices was to support and amplify the work of the local health units.[2] Governments in the larger cities could set up their own health systems. The county units enforced state laws at the local level. They were responsible for protecting the health of children through maternity and baby clinics and other social services. They inspected and certified local businesses, which required licenses to operate.

The headquarters of the Division of Health in Jefferson City consisted, as of 1958, of four administrative sections, the responsibilities of which were as follows.[3]

Environmental Health Services, which consists of the bureau of public health engineering, and the bureau of food and drugs; Personal Health Services, which consists of bureau of dental health, bureau of mental hygiene, bureau of occupational health, bureau of cancer and chronic disease control, bureaus of communicable disease and tuberculosis control, and bureau of maternal and child health; Local Health Services, which consists of the bureau of public health education, bureau of public health nursing, and is charged with the responsibility of coordinating the public health activities within the six public health districts in Missouri; and General and Hospital Services, which consists of bureau of hospital facilities, bureau of hospital and nursing home licensure, bureau of laboratories, the Ellis Fischel State Cancer Hospital, and the Missouri State Sanatorium.

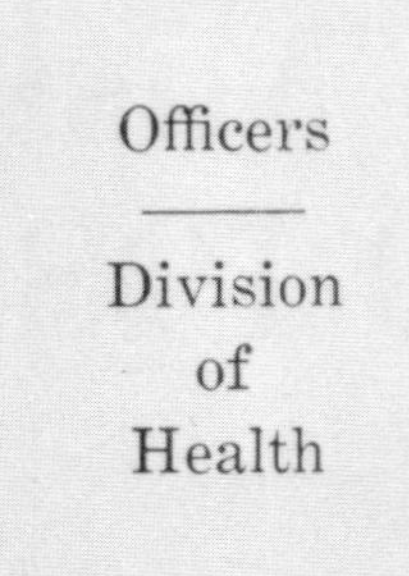

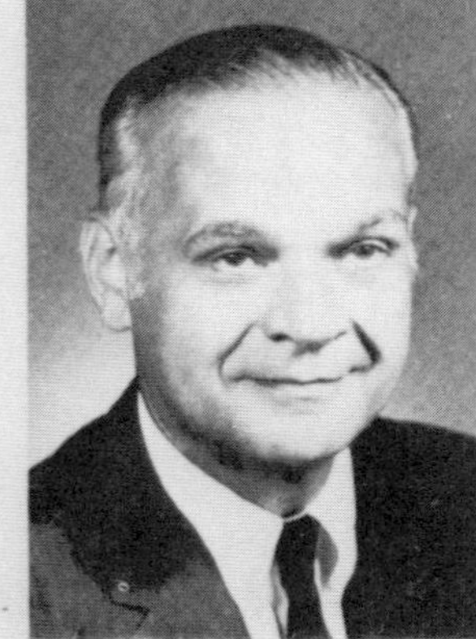

HERBERT R. DOMKE, M.D., Dr.P.H.
Director

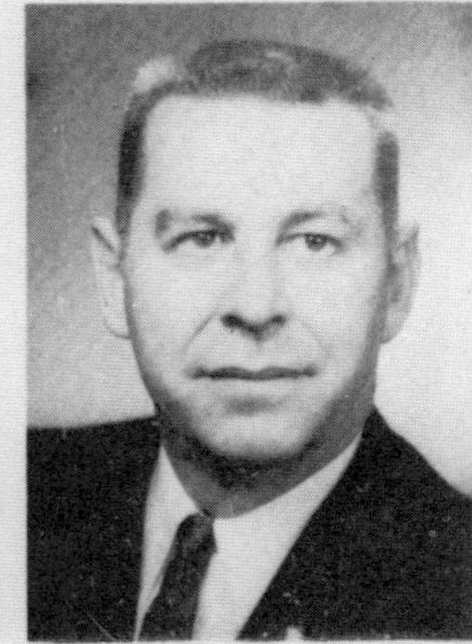

JOSEPH B. REICHART
Deputy Director

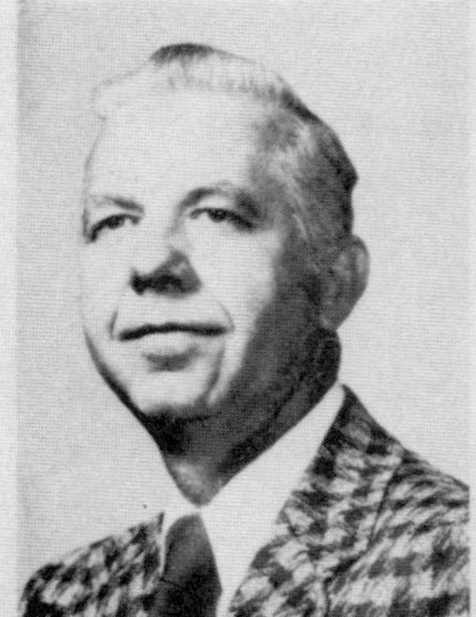

BILLY E. RIKARD
Section Director
Local Health Services

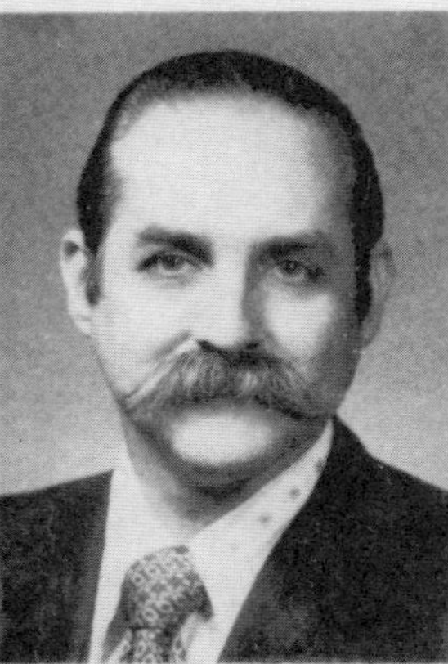

H. DENNY DONNELL JR., M.D.
Section Director Epidemiology
and Disease Surveillance

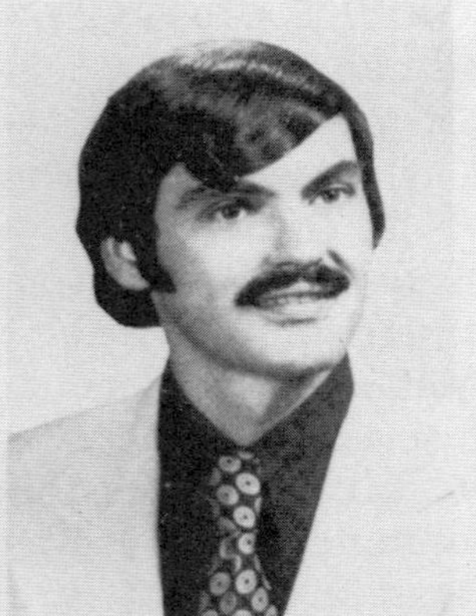

GARLAND LAND
Section Director
State Center for Health Statistics

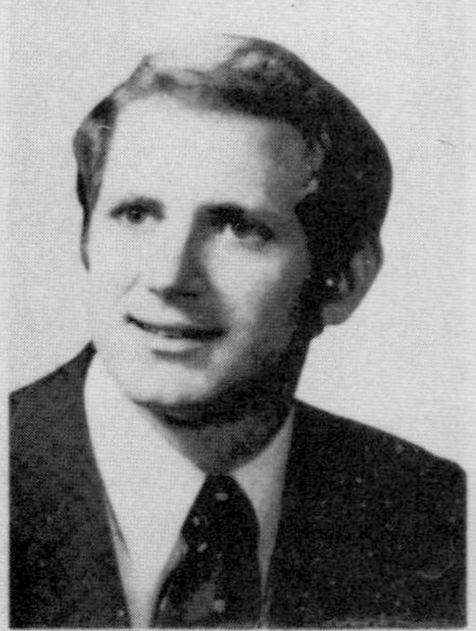

C. CHARLES STOKES JR.
Section Director
Management Services

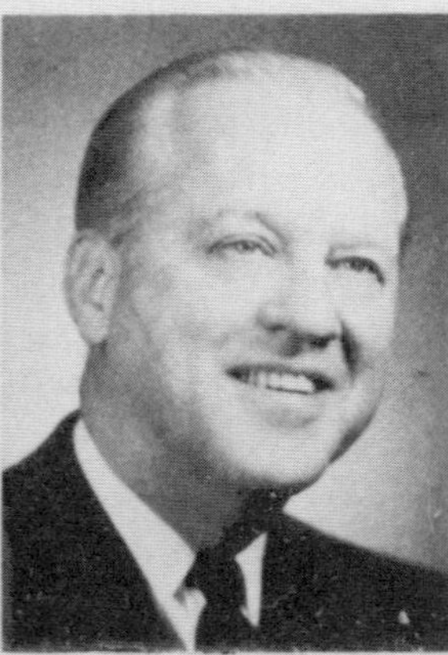

C. W. MEINERSHAGEN, M.D.
Acting Associate Director
Medical Care

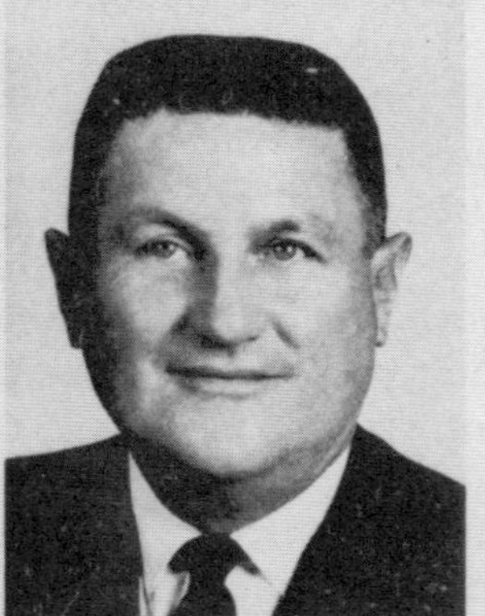

LYLE P. PARTIN, D.O.
Health Officer
District No. 2, Macon

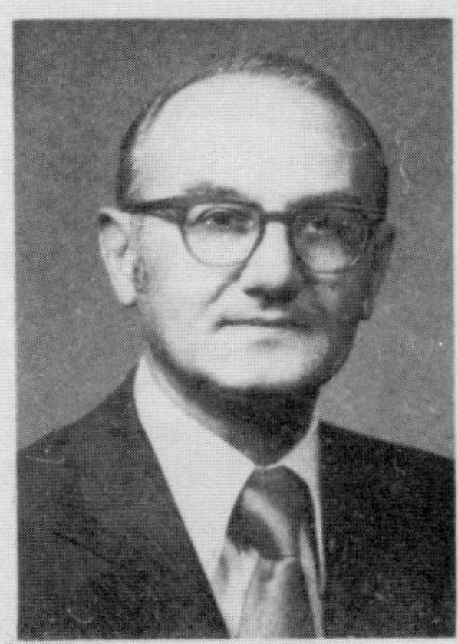

EUGENE VAN VRANKEN, M.D.
Health Officer
District No. 3, Jefferson City

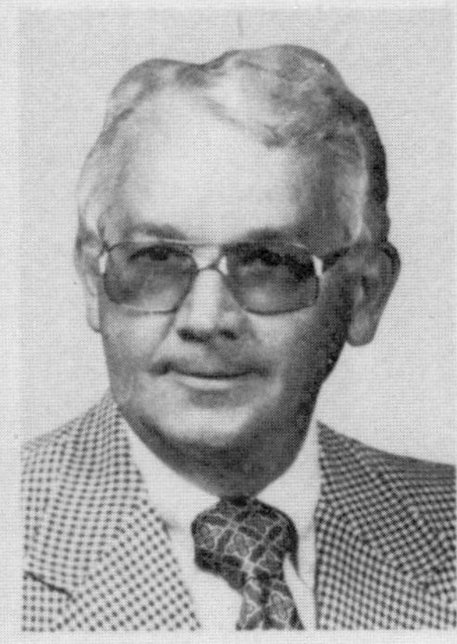

OLIN A. GRIFFEN, M.D.
Health Officer
District No. 5, Springfield

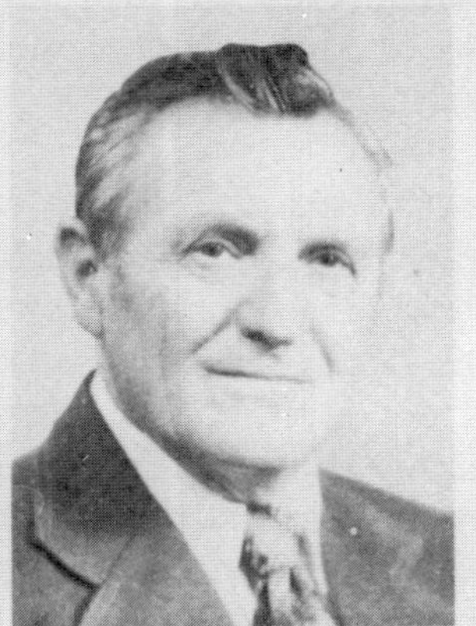

RICHARD F. JENKINS
Acting Administrator
District No. 1, Cameron

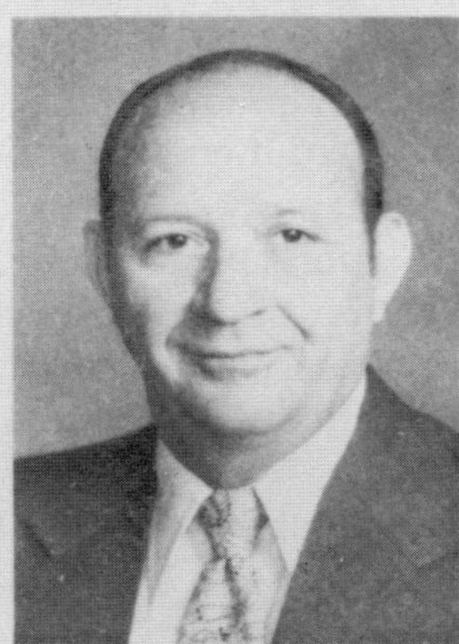

A. Z. TOMERLIN
Administrator
District No. 4, Poplar Bluff

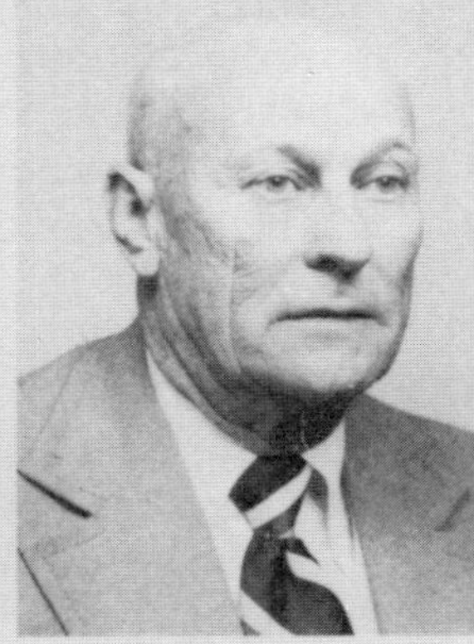

RICHARD BROWN
Administrator
District No. 6, Kansas City

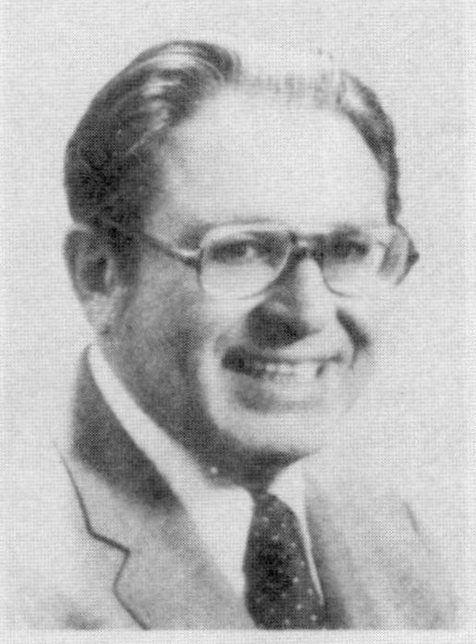

WILLIAM J. GOLDMAN
Administrator
District No. 7, Clayton

The important role played by the central office of the Division of Health is explained in the following quotation:[4]

> Basically the activities at the central office level in the field of public health are those of statewide planning, counseling, and finances. There are certain services rendered by the Division of Health which are so highly technical in nature that they cannot be decentralized to districts or local units. These include hospital construction, hospital licensing, highly exacting laboratory procedures, the control of water supplies in the larger cities and consultant services . . . .
>
> Highly trained public health personnel are maintained in the central office for consultation purposes. These persons deal with unusual problems in the field of communicable diseases, occupational health, dental health, veterinary public health, public health nursing, mental health, engineering and sanitation and health education. These consultants are responsible for the development of procedural manuals which guide the activities of personnel in district and local offices. Their services are available to both district and local units through the Section of Local Health Services.

On July 26, 1967, the general assembly passed legislation providing for the reestablishment of a State Board of Health, consisting of seven members appointed by the governor with senate approval. They were to serve four-year terms. Three of the members must be physicians and surgeons, licensed by the Missouri Board of Healing Arts. The other four, who were barred from being licensed doctors, were to be representative of those persons, professions and businesses supervised by the Division of Health and the State Board of Health.

The law specified that the State Board of Health should:[5] (1) appoint the director of the Division of Health; (2) be vested with all statutory responsibilities of the Division of Health other than those of an administrative nature; (3) formulate the budget for the Division of Health; (4) advise the director in the planning for and operation of the Division of Health.

It is noteworthy that the legislation, in order to minimize partisan political considerations, gave the authority to appoint the director to a commission, rather than to the governor. The law further provided that no more than four of the board members should be from the same political party.

The Omnibus State Reorganization Act of 1974 placed the Division of Health in the newly created Department of Social Services. The State Board of Health was retained with unchanged duties.

The reorganization act raised the Division of Mental Health (formerly the Division of Mental Diseases) to departmental status.[6] Within the department, three divisions were created: (1) the Division of Psychiatric Services; (2) the Division of Alcoholism and Drug Abuse; (3) the Division of Mental Retardation-Developmental Disabilities.

The purpose of the act was to provide a functional reorganization of the executive branch of state government. In the process, various boards and commissions, which had enjoyed a semi-independent existence, were assigned to one of the fourteen departments of the new structure. The Air Conservation Commission and the Clean Water Commission were transferred from a formal connection with the Division of Health to the new department of natural resources.[7]

2. *Nursing Homes and Ambulance Districts*

The fact that Missourians were living longer and that an increasing percentage of the population were senior citizens had important implications for the state's health care system. The major diseases of the second half of the twentieth century were of the chronic and degenerative type. For the year 1970, the ten leading causes of death in Missouri, with the number of deaths in the state for each ailment, were as follows: (1) heart disease, 19,400; (2) malignant neoplasms, 8,621; (3) cerebrovascular disease, 6,153; (4) accidents, 2,912; (5) influenza and pneumonia, 1,660; (6) diabetes, 1,115; (7) arteriosclerosis, 1,036; (8) diseases of early infancy, 927; (9) bronchitis, emphysema, 801; (10) cirrhosis of liver, 576; all other causes, 8,542; total deaths, 51,743, out of an estimated population of 4,676,501.[8]

The aging of the population created a demand for nursing homes to provide shelter and care for the elderly. The first nursing homes in Missouri were conducted in old buildings intended for other purposes, such as schools, colleges, hotels and other large structures. They were not designed for the quick and safe evacuation of bedridden or wheel chair patients in case of a fire.

Missouri, in 1941, enacted legislation requiring a person wishing to operate a nursing home to apply to the Division of Health for a license. The license would be granted if the premises occupied met standards of health and safety set by the Division of Health. Homes operated by religious and charitable organizations were exempted from complying with the law.[9] Lax enforcement at the local level reduced the effectiveness of the statute. As of February 1, 1957, it was reported that 7,627 patients were in licensed homes in Missouri, and 5,674 lived in unlicensed facilities.[10]

A tragic fire in the Katie Jane Memorial Nursing Home at Warrenton, Missouri, on Sunday February 17, 1957, killed seventy-two trapped patients. This event focused state and national attention upon the matter of providing greater security for these institutions.[11]

Investigations of the fire by local and state officials failed to discover the exact cause, but a number of contributing factors were revealed. The nursing home was conducted in the building that formerly housed the Central Wesleyan College. The two-story building, almost a century old, was of frame and brick construction. The floors, in the days when the building was in college use, were regularly oiled and polished. There were no outdoor fire escapes for inmates on the second floor. The fire occurred on Sunday when nursing homes are traditionally understaffed. If there were elevators, they were quickly disabled by the flames, leaving no escape possibility for the second floor residents. The old building lacked a sprinkler system. There were extinguishers, but the flames spread so rapidly that the nursing staff had no opportunity to organize a fire defense team. There was no evidence that the local fire department was immediately notified, so it arrived too late.[12]

Responding promptly to the tragedy, the general assembly, on March 13, 1957, passed a comprehensive new law governing nursing homes.[13] Operators of such homes were required to have a license, renewed each year. A fee of twenty-five dollars was charged for homes of fewer than fifty beds; establishments having fifty or more beds were assessed an annual charge of fifty dollars.

The law divided nursing homes into three classes: (1) those providing professional nursing care; (2) those furnishing only practical nursing care; (3) homes furnishing domiciliary or personal care exclusively. For each of these three categories of homes, the Division of Health was responsible for prescribing minimum standards in regard to the following features: (1) location and construction of the home; (2) number and qualifications of all personnel and hours of service; (3) all sanitary conditions within the home and surroundings; (4) diet related to the needs of each resident; (5) equipment, facilities and supplies essential to the care of the resident; (6) quality of patient care.

The new law applied to nursing homes operated by religious or charitable organizations, as well as to those managed by private or corporate parties. However, homes operated by the Christian Science denomination, although required to have licenses, could prescribe their own treatment programs based upon spiritual healing.

Anticipating that the new legislation would result in the closing of some of the weaker institutions, the general assembly passed a law authorizing counties to build and equip nursing homes, which would be leased to nonprofit organizations for their operation. The counties could issue general obligation bonds, with voter approval, to finance construction and equipment costs. They were permitted to seek federal assistance under the Hill-Burton Act to subsidize building expenses.[14]

An official of the U.S. Public Health Service defined the conditions that had to be met in order for a proposed nursing home to qualify for government grants:[15] (1) it must meet strict safety standards; (2) it must be operated as a nonprofit institution; (3) it must provide skilled nursing care; (4) its property must consist of new construction, not merely of a renovated building. It was estimated that the state needed new nursing homes for 5,000 patients.

By mid-August 1957, approximately 150 unsafe nursing homes had closed. Some of the displaced persons found better and more attractive quarters. Others had to move back with their families or friends. The majority probably went into unlicensed nursing homes which were the modern versions of poorhouses. The Department of Welfare payment of $110 a month for bedfast patients would not buy more adequate care.[16]

The nursing homes, built with federal subsidies, were a big improvement over the hodgepodge of quarters formerly occupied by nursing facilities. Most were on a single floor, usually in the suburbs where land costs were cheaper. They had sprinkler systems to contain fires. They were staffed to provide skilled nursing care. The major drawback was that only about eight percent of Missouri families could afford to patronize them.[17]

The financial deficiency of the average family was caused, in part, by the fact that Medicare paid the costs of patients discharged from hospitals to skilled nursing facilities for only a limited period, not for long-term care.[18] The duration of the stay in the nursing home was determined by a review board. If the patient was making little progress toward recovery in the skilled facility, his Medicare support would be withdrawn as being wasted. If he was making marked improvement, his stay in the skilled nursing facility would be terminated as no longer necessary. For patients requiring custodial care, Medicare paid nothing. It was feared that the policy of Medicare would place upon the hospitals an unacceptable burden of caring for chronic cases.[19]

On June 15, 1979, Governor Joseph P. Teasdale approved a comprehensive new nursing home law. Senator Harriett Woods and Representative Steve Vossmeyer played major roles in developing the bill and guiding it through their respective houses. Fortunately, the measure did not antagonize any important lobby. One of its opponents was Senator J. B. Banks of St. Louis, who feared that the strict standards of the law would force the closing of many of the marginal operations upon which poor families depended. Governor Teasdale had made nursing home reform one of his key campaign issues, so there was no risk of a gubernatorial veto.[20]

Diane E. Felix, a house staff member, in a careful summary, declared that the bill would:[21] "provide (1) for state regulation of boarding homes, for the first time; (2) limit licenses to one year, without automatic renewals; (3) establish minimum standards for patient care, diet, sanitation and fire safety; (4) provide for legal penalties, including damages and court injunctions sought by the state or private parties, where standards are violated; (5) provide for a nursing home patient 'bill of rights'; (6) require that operators who handle patients' private funds be bonded, establishing misuse of such funds Class A misdemeanors; (7) establish patient abuse and neglect as Class A misdemeanors, and failure to report abuse or neglect as a less serious infraction, punishable by a fine; (8) establish minimum training standards for nursing assistants; (9) provide grievance procedures for residents, with the Department of Social Services able to review complaints not settled by in-house grievance committees; (10) allow the state, residents, their families, or a home operator to file petitions in court forcing failing or unacceptable homes into receivership, under either the state or a private party, so that patient care does not suffer; (11) establish a special unit in the Department of Social Services to investigate the misuse of Medicaid by home operators or others connected with patient care."

The experience of the United States during World War II in getting wounded soldiers quickly to first aid stations and then to base hospitals furnished an example that was copied on the home front. Provisions were made to get badly injured passengers in car and boating accidents, persons suffering from heart attacks or strokes, and victims of severe burns or smoke inhalation to nearby hospitals by ambulance or other conveyances.

In order to supplement and improve the ambulance business carried on by funeral homes, the general assembly, on June 15, 1971, enacted legislation authorizing the establishment of public ambulance agencies. The first step was the organization of ambulance districts. Each district was divided into six areas, approximately equal in population. In each subdivision, an ambulance district director was elected. The local board, consisting of the six ambulance district directors, was given the following powers: (1) to establish and maintain an ambulance service; (2) to acquire land and other property; (3) to operate the business; (4) to charge reasonable fees; (5) to borrow money and issue certificates of indebtedness; (6) to employ the necessary professional workers and services.[22]

Two years later, another law was passed dealing with the qualifications of the ambulance attendants. These were divided into four classes: (1) apprentices; (2) attendants; (3) attendant-drivers; (4) mobile emergency technicians. Workers in each category had to be licensed. A candidate for a license had to demonstrate physical fitness for the job sought, moral integrity, freedom from drug and alcohol abuse, and a clean police record. Attendants and attendant-drivers must have successfully completed a training schedule equal to the advanced course in first aid given by the American Red Cross or the U.S. Bureau of Mines. Besides, they must hold a current valid chauffeur's license from the state of Missouri. Applicants for a mobile emergency medical technician's license, in addition to satisfying the general licensing requirements, "must have successfully completed an emergency service training program consisting of a minimum of two hundred (200) hours of training including, but not limited to, didactic and clinical experience in a cardiac care unit and in an emergency vehicle unit."[23]

Mobile emergency medical technicians were authorized to perform the following procedures at the scene of an accident in an ambulance or at the emergency room of a licensed hospital: (1) render rescue, first aid and resuscitation services; (2) perform cardiopulmonary resuscitation and defibrillation in a pulseless, nonbreathing patient. When direct communication with a doctor was maintained, the mobile emergency technician was empowered to take the following action: (1) administer intravenous saline or glucose solutions; (2) perform gastric suction by intubation; (3) perform endotracheal intubation; (4) administer parenteral injection of a list of emergency drugs.[24]

3. Warnings Against Future Disaster

During the 1960s, warnings began to appear in the St. Louis press regarding the destruction, which modern industrial society was wreaking, on the environment — its air, water, forests and other resources. The new awareness apparently was connected with the successful voyaging of American astronauts to the moon. This enterprise acquainted the public with the concept of the earth as a spaceship, with a limited envelope of sustainable oxygen and an irreplaceable store of natural resources. The fantasy that other planets, if this world became uninhabitable, might be colonized by earth citizens was exposed as without foundation by later interplanetary probes.

An exposition of one aspect of the earth's degradation was presented in an article in the *St. Louis Post-Dispatch* of April 24, 1968, entitled "The Effluent Society; Our Poisoned Water," by Alton Blakeslee, Associated Press Science Editor. Recalling that of all the planets, only the earth has an abundant supply of water, covering 70 percent of its surface, Blakeslee regretted that "earth's water is becoming increasingly befouled, smelly, and repulsive through man's carelessness, disdain, greed, or innocence of consequences of his actions upon the balances of nature." Among major sources of water pollution, he lists raw or poorly treated human sewage or industrial wastes, oil from ship spillage or sinkings, pesticides, detergents, dirt washed from farms and heat from nuclear power plants.[25]

Fortunately, the federal government was beginning to turn its attention to the problem. The Water Quality Act of 1965 created the Federal Water Pollution Control Administration and started a program enjoining the states to establish quality standards for interstate waters within their boundaries. The Clean Water Restoration Act of 1966 authorized 3.9 billion dollars for grants to the states to help build sewage treatment plants, for research and for other water pollution control programs.[26]

Severe air pollution, caused by motor vehicles, factories, homes, and power plants, afflicts our industrial cities. Medical authorities blame this condition for producing some lung cancers and for exacerbating asthma, emphysema, tuberculosis and congestive heart failure.

Beginning in the 1960s, the Congress inaugurated a series of progressively more stringent controls of the exhaust emissions of motor vehicles. Under the Clean Air Act of 1963 and subsequent amendments, Congress provided funds for air pollution abatement; also matching funds to the states for research, training of personnel and experimental programs to demonstrate methods of lowering air pollution. The budget of the Department of Health, Education and Welfare for 1967 for all such programs was $64,000,000. The Air Quality Act of 1967 increased spending to $428,300,000 over a three-year period. Health, Education and Welfare was empowered to establish standards, designate air quality regions and enforce the standards.[27]

During the last week of March 1969, Elvis J. Stahr, president of the National Audubon Society, was in St. Louis to assist in planning for the society's national convention, to be held in the city April 25-29.[28] Stahr had achieved a distinguished career in political and collegiate administration before he resigned the presidency of Indiana University to become the nation's No. 1 bird watcher. A graduate in law at Oxford University, secretary of the army under President John F. Kennedy, dean of the University of Kentucky's law school, vice chancellor of the University of Pittsburgh, and president of the University of West Virginia as well as president of Indiana University, Stahr was convinced that his role as head of one of the nation's major conservation societies offered him an unrivaled opportunity to render public service.

Stahr was particularly concerned over the sociological effects of overcrowding and living under blighted conditions:

If you jam people up, the irritations and tensions which come from crowded city living make humans selfish. They race to be first in line to catch a cab or get on a subway. They are ungracious in department stores. It is hard to measure the effects of overcrowding, but that does not mean they are unreal.

Ugliness has a very depressing and oppressing effect on people who are trapped in it. Dirty streets, sidewalks, trash, broken windows, paucity of growing things and lack of parks give children and adults a warped idea of the city surrounding them. Such an environment is like being in jail. All these people see is what their fellow men have done to mess up their environment. They have no stake in beauty.

Regarding the challenge of his new job, Stahr, in an interview with a reporter of the *St. Louis Post-Dispatch*, said:

People tend to think of conservationists as wild-eyed, impractical persons, standing in the path of progress. But I think conservationists are almost harshly realistic. They are facing up to forces that we ignore at our peril. To me, conservation is as practical, as important as Mother Earth herself!

The *Post-Dispatch* used the national celebration of Earth Day, April 22, 1970, as an occasion for recounting what our industrial society is doing to the environment and to suggest a method of ameliorating the destructive practices:[29]

From California to the New York island, this land is cluttered with no-return bottles, bedsprings and abandoned automobiles. From the waving wheat fields and the golden valleys there is a run-off of deadly pesticides and herbicides that infest plants, fish, birds and wildlife and find their way into the milk we drink and the meat we eat. The ribbons of highway threaten to merge into a gigantic concrete raceway, and the endless sky too often disappears in a brown pall. From the depleted redwood forests to the oil-covered Gulf stream waters, this land is sacrificing its most precious resources to the heedless march of technology . . . .

The magnificent technology which is causing the environmental crisis is doing so not because it is a failure but because it is a success. Agricultural pesticides are an example. They are intended to exterminate pests that destroy crops, and they do. But in the process some also kill other pests and predators which assure a balance in insect populations, and they drain into the streams and end up in our food supply.

But does this mean environmental preservation can be attained only through the destruction of technology? That is both unacceptable and unnecessary. What is required, it seems to us, is a re-examination of technological progress in terms of all its consequences, not simply the immediate ones. To this end the true economic costs of technology must be identified and properly assigned, and we ought to modify any legal bias that has the effect of giving the polluter a prior right.

At the United Nations Conference on the Human Environment, held in Stockholm June 8, 1972, a fundamental difference was exposed between the viewpoints of the industrialized and the undeveloped nations of Asia, Africa and South America.[30] While the developed nations were displaying alarm over the damage being done to the environment by unrestrained industrial growth, the major concern of the Third World countries was to raise the living standard of their impoverished populations by the introduction of technology, with less regard for the environmental impact.

Robert S. McNamara, head of the World Bank which was financing many of the Third World development projects, told the conference "the wealthy nations could afford to combine rising environmental protection at home with increased development assistance to the poor countries." As a basis for decision making, he called for more research into the impact of development on the environment.

Responding to this suggestion, the conference agreed to set up 110 specially equipped stations to monitor changes in the world's climate and the levels of air pollution at various points around the world. Ten of the stations, in isolated parts of the globe, were to watch for changes in the volume of dust in the atmosphere, the gradually increasing carbon dioxide content of the air and the depletion of the ozone shield.[31]

A study conducted by a group of scientists from six nations, working at the Massachusetts Institute of Technology during 1972, warned that:[32]

If present rates of world population growth, food production, industrialization, pollution and depletion of resources continue . . . the most probable result will be "a sudden and uncontrollable decline in both population and industrial capacity."

The study calls for urgent efforts to create a new lower-keyed "world of non-growth, that would insure that human society can survive indefinitely on earth with an enriching existence for all."

4. *Missouri's Problems With Water and Air Pollution*

St. Louis, Kansas City and St. Joseph are located on two of the nation's major waterways. Thus, nature has provided them with a convenient and inexpensive sewer system, of which they took advantage much to the discomfort and damage to their down-stream neighbors:[33]

The Kansas Cities discharged so much waste into the Missouri that it adversely affected the water supplies of Lexington, Boonville, Jefferson City, St. Charles and even St. Louis on the other side of the state. The cities downstream had to take special measures, including extra chlorination, to make water from the river palatable and to guard against bacterial contamination . . . .

St. Louis has been a major offender, discharging untreated sewage into the Mississippi. Industries on both sides of the river have been doing the same with their wastes. More than 450 tons a day have been dumped into the river here, sending oily scum, sewage, garbage and other trash downstream. Federal authorities asserted that the St. Louis area produced the worst river pollution in the United States.

The City of St. Louis grinds garbage before flushing it into the Mississippi, a practice it defended as preventing chunks

from being discharged; but federal and state officials report that large pieces of garbage have been floating down river as far as 150 miles of here.

Kansas City and St. Louis were not the only offenders:[34]

Thousands of gallons of treated sewage flow into the James River near Springfield each day. Runoff from lead mines causes slime and algae growth in the Black River and Huzzah Creek.

Discharges from a municipal waste treatment plant at Lebanon disappear underground and reappear in the Niangua River. Gravel operations muddy the Meramec River. A poultry processing plant and city treatment plant at Anderson disgorge wastes into Indian Creek.

Cabool and Fort Leonard Wood dump thousands of gallons of inadequately treated wastes into the Big Piney River daily, causing excessive and unsightly weed growth that could lead to serious pollution problems.

The first well-planned attack on the pollution of the Missouri River was launched in August 1959 by Arthur S. Flemming, secretary of Health, Education and Welfare in the Eisenhower administration. Under the authority of the federal Water Pollution Control Act of 1956, he ordered the city of St. Joseph and its industrial and meat packing firms to cease discharging untreated wastes into the river. He charged that their action created a serious health hazard. He also directed the city and its industrial firms to "install and place in operation by June 1, 1963 proper, adequate and effective municipal and industrial sewage and waste collection, treatment and disposal facilities."[35]

On July 1, 1960, Flemming issued a similar clean-up order to Kansas City, Missouri, and Kansas City, Kansas. Earlier the Kansas City, Missouri, city council had defied an order of the Missouri Water Pollution Board to grant no more permits to home builders for additions to the sewer system until the city took definite action to halt river pollution.[36]

The metropolitan St. Louis sewer district had made an agreement with the federal government to construct, by 1967, a system of interceptor sewers and treatment plants, at an estimated cost of $100,000,000. By its voluntary compliance, St. Louis avoided a clean-up order from Secretary Flemming.[37]

The federal government used the carrot as well as the stick to get balky cities to halt river pollution. The Clean Water Restoration Act of 1966 had authorized 3.9 billion dollars for grants to build sewer facilities and for other pollution control measures. But the competing demands of the Vietnam War prevented a large part of the funding from reaching the states. Congress authorized $450,000,000 for anti-pollution work in fiscal 1968 but President Lyndon Johnson used only $200,000,000 for its stated purpose.[38]

It was not until the early 1970s that federal subsidization of anti-pollution work was put on an orderly and dependable basis. On October 18, 1972, Congress, over the veto of President Richard Nixon, passed a 24.6 billion dollar bill for cleaning up the nation's waters. Of this total, 18 billion dollars was allocated for "paying 75 per cent as the federal share of the cost of waste treatment plants. States and municipalities would pay the rest."[39]

Missouri's share over the three-year period would be $298,134,000. In addition, "St. Louis stood to receive an extra $13,000,000 and Kansas City an extra $9,300,000 in funds that will be reimbursed to them for investments made when the full federal matching share was not available."[40]

The question of how much pollution, if any, would be allowed in the nation's waters was answered in the following statement accompanying the law:[41]

Congress under the new amendments declared it to be a national goal that the discharge of pollutants into navigable waters be eliminated by 1985. An interim goal for 1983 calls for achieving water quality to protect fish and wildlife and provide for recreation.

Missouri, in its first anti-pollution law enacted July 6, 1957, affirmed the determination of the state "to act in the public interest to restore and maintain a reasonable degree of purity in the waters of the state, and to require, where necessary, reasonable treatment of sewage, industrial wastes and other wastes prior to their discharge into the waters of the state."[42]

To carry out this policy, a water pollution board of six members, appointed by the governor, was created. Each member would represent a special interest. One member would sponsor agricultural concerns; one industrial interests; one municipal constituents; one mining companies; one recreational, fish and wildlife interests; and the sixth member would represent the public at large. The theory was that through the interplay of special interests in the committee the public interest would be served.[43]

Any person planning action that would result in water pollution had first to secure a permit from the board. A person not satisfied with any order of the board or any decision regarding a permit had the right to call for a public hearing before the board. Upon the basis of the evidence produced at the hearing, the board would make its decision and issue its order. The order would be final unless a dissatisfied party chose to appeal to the local circuit court.

The board was responsible for preparing a comprehensive plan for the prevention of future pollution and the reduction of existing pollution in the state's waters. The board also was enjoined to establish "standards of water purity for any of the waters of the state, which specify the maximum degree of pollution permissible in accordance with public interest in water supply, the conservation of fish, game and aquatic life, and agricultural, industrial and recreational uses."[44] Violations of any provisions of the act or orders of the board were punishable by a fine of not less than $25 and not more than $500 or by imprisonment for not more than ninety days.

The compromised position taken on water purity, the representation of special interests on the board with a potential majority favoring pollution, and the light fines for violators indicated that the state legislature was not yet ready to take a strong stand for clean water. Fortunately, the people of the state were ahead of the legislature in this matter. On October 5, 1971, they approved a $150,000,000 bond issue to pay the state's share of federal clean water programs.[45]

The citizens of St. Louis, embarrassed by their city's reputation as one of the nation's major polluters, on November 6, 1962, approved a $95,000,000 clean water bond issue. The firm of Horner and Shifrin, consulting engineers, recommended to the St. Louis metropolitan sewer district that two large sewage treatment plants be built for the St. Louis area. This plan was accepted.[46]

Sites on the Mississippi River, one in the northern part of the city and the other in the south, were selected. The northern location was the abandoned Bissell's Point pumping station, located at East Grand Avenue and Ferry Street. The southern site was in Lemay, south of the River des Peres and east of South Broadway.[47]

A 23-mile interceptor sewer system tunnelled through solid limestone at the depth of 75-100 feet and running alongside the river, was planned to connect the two treatment plants. The creeks and sewers of St. Louis and part of St. Louis County would discharge their human and industrial wastes into the interceptor system en route to the treatment plants.[48]

At the plants, the wastes "will be given primary treatment, which will remove a high percentage of solids and a smaller amount of dissolved matter. After removing up to 80 per cent of the solids and 50 per cent of the dissolved matter, the plants will discharge the effluent into the river."[49] The St. Louis primary sewage treatment system was completed in December 1970.

Kansas City accomplished the first phase of its sewage treatment program on April 16, 1967, utilizing funds from a $75,000,000 bond issue approved in 1960. The system comprises five treatment plants, eleven pumping stations and a network of sewers thirty miles from north to south. "Primary treatment is being given to 99.7 per cent of the city's waste water discharges. Sludge from the sewage is pumped to an incinerator and burned."[50]

The halting of air pollution has proved more difficult and baffling than the abatement of the contamination of inland waterways. The restoration of clean air is an international problem. Air currents and pollutants recognize no man-made boundaries. Sulfur dioxide, as acid rain from midwestern power plants, destroys the lakes and forests of the Adirondacks and Eastern Canada. The technology for halting contamination from power plants and industrial establishments is expensive and not conclusively satisfactory. In some cases, the halting of pollution would mean the closing of factories, the loss of jobs and the end of urban growth.

The roots of the present crisis go back, in the United States, to the 1920s and 1930s, when the opportunity to build systems of public transportation was passed up in favor of allowing individual workers to drive their own vehicles to their jobs. The motor car became a necessity of employment and, after working hours, a major means of recreation. The introduction of labor-saving equipment in the home and the lighting of our big cities on a 24-hour a day basis required ever-increasing amounts of electricity and giant plants to produce it. The changes that took place in the United States occurred in Europe, Asia and South America also as the standard of living increased and the vast oil resources of the Middle East became available.

The apparent warming of the earth's atmosphere from the greenhouse effect, the thinning of the ozone shield that protects the earth from ultraviolet radiation, the destruction of the Brazilian rain forests, the increasing frequency and intensity of oceanic disturbances have revived and intensified the concern of environmentalists regarding the dangers and disasters that might result from the dislocation of the delicate balance of our planet's envelope of various gases.

The state of Missouri, in 1965, established the Air Conservation Commission, as part of the Division of Health. The commission consisted of the director of the Division of Health and six other members, chosen from the fields of industry, labor, agriculture, municipal or county government, and the general public. The member, or members, representing industry must be persons knowledgeable in the area of air pollution. The aim of the law, thus, was explained:[51]

> It is the intent and purpose of this act to maintain purity of the air resources of the state to protect the health, general welfare and physical property of the people, maximum employment and the full industrial development of the state. The commission shall seek the accomplishment of this objective through the prevention, abatement and control of air pollution by all practical and economically feasible methods.

The law provided for the appointment of an executive secretary to conduct the business of the commission in the periods between meetings, subject to the oversight of the full commission.

Among the powers and duties of the commission were the following:[52]

> After holding public hearings . . . establish areas of the state and prescribe air quality standards for such areas giving due recognition to variations, if any, in the characteristics of different areas of the state which may be deemed by the commission to be relevant . . . .

> Enter such order or determination as may be necessary to effectuate the purposes of this act. In making its orders and determinations hereunder, the Commission shall exercise a sound discretion in weighing the equities involved and the advantages and disadvantages to the person involved and to those affected

by air contaminants emitted by such person . . . .

The act declared that it was not intended to monopolize the field of pollution abatement and that the various political subdivisions could pass appropriate legislation provided their enactments were at least as stringent as those of the state. Political subdivisions were authorized to make agreements and form organizations among themselves to effectuate the purpose of pollution control.

The federal Clean Air Act of 1967 required the secretary of Health, Education and Welfare to designate air quality control regions, each of which shared common characteristics and problems. These regions were the major cities with their suburban extensions. For these regions, the secretary published air quality criteria for various pollutants. The criteria specified the lowest level of pollution at which adverse effects on human health could be expected. The sulfur oxide criterion, for example, concluded that an accumulation of .10 parts per million of sulfur oxide or .20 parts per million in a 24-hour period was the lowest level at which adverse health effects might occur.[53] Using the criteria as guides, it was the responsibility of the states in the various designated regions to establish supervision of pollution sources to assure that the criteria levels were not exceeded. These regulations would involve the kind of fuels burned, the sulfur content of the coal or oil used, and the emission controls in place at plants and factories.

Regulations issued by the Missouri Air Conservation Commission limited the sulfur content of coal burned in the winter months to 2 percent, in plants with a capacity of less than two billion British thermal units per hour. The installations affected were most fuel users, except the large electric utilities.

The regulations also specified that after three years the electric utilities would be required to burn coal of 1.4 percent or less of sulfur content or install special equipment to reduce emission levels.[54]

In response to state and federal regulations, St. Louis industries made various changes. Some shifted to low sulfur coal or to oil or gas. Union Electric built higher smoke stacks which spread the pollutants over a wider area. A number installed special emission control devices. By 1976, St. Louis air, which had been one of the dirtiest and most foul-smelling in the nation, was much improved.

The *St. Louis Post-Dispatch*, in a feature article of August 30, 1976, summarized some of the changes:[55]

With a few major exceptions, such as Granite City Steel, Union Electric Co. and N. L. Industries, most major industries have complied with tough regulations adopted in 1967. Airborne concentrations of carbon monoxide, sulfur dioxide and dust, soot and fly ash (known collectively as particulate matter) have been greatly reduced, in some instances to half their former levels.

The overall war against pollution has profited from the passage, in 1969, of the National Environmental Policy Act. This act requires "federal agencies to evaluate the environmental impacts of their projects and to set out the expected consequences in detailed statements."[56] The law had two important results:[57]

First, because the environmental impact statements are public information and must incorporate the concerns of lay persons and groups, the law has given

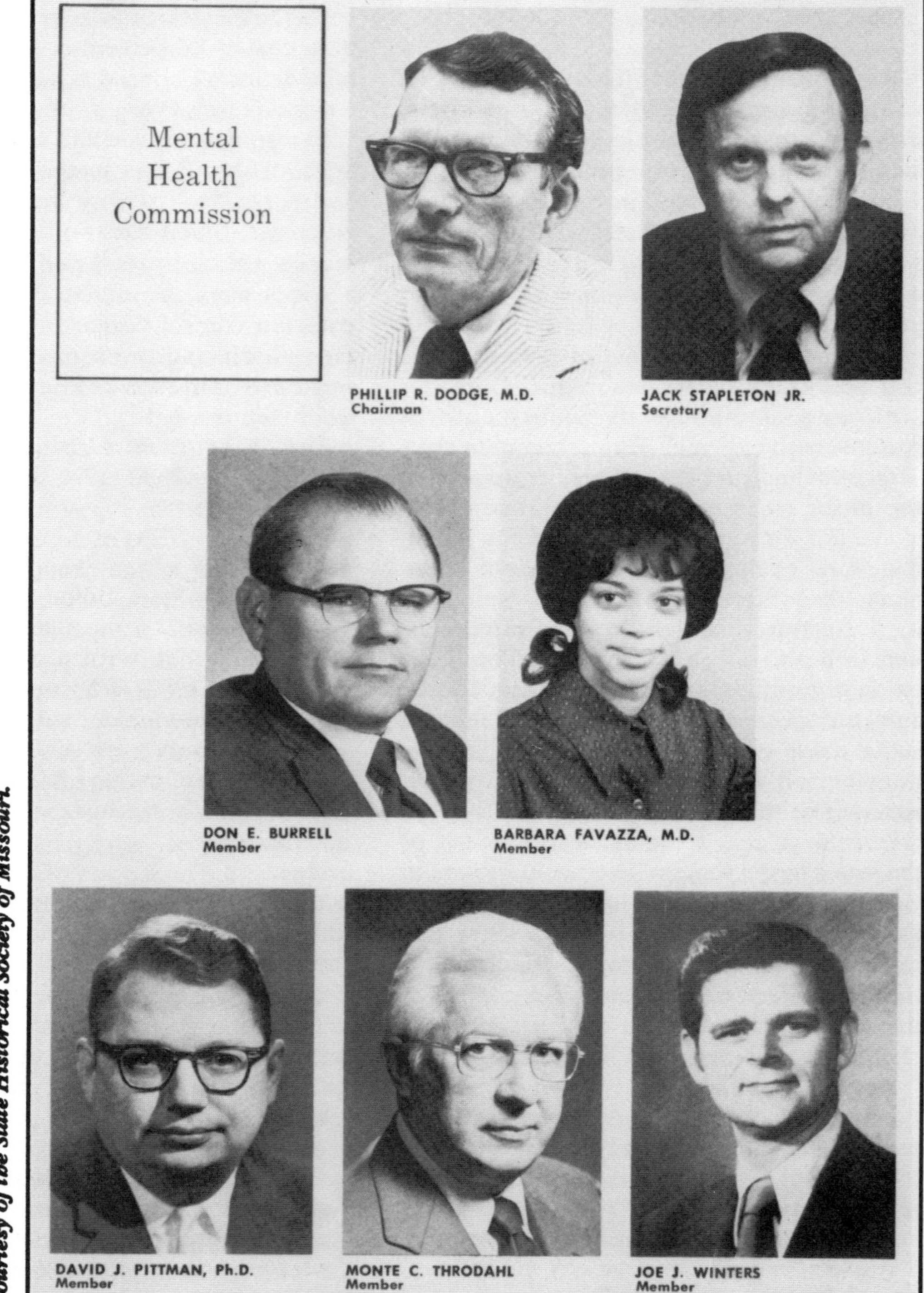

PHILLIP R. DODGE, M.D.
Chairman

JACK STAPLETON JR.
Secretary

DON E. BURRELL
Member

BARBARA FAVAZZA, M.D.
Member

DAVID J. PITTMAN, Ph.D.
Member

MONTE C. THRODAHL
Member

JOE J. WINTERS
Member

the public a toehold in the inner sanctum of agency planning . . . .

Second, because the adequacy of environmental impact statements may be challenged, the National Environmental Policy Act has thrown the brunt of controversy into the courts. More than 160 federal projects and programs have been challenged with some notable effect.

Although the law applies exclusively to federal projects, many cities and counties today are considering the environmental impact of their own public undertakings as well as the effect of prospective business enterprises wishing to locate with them.

5. Efforts to Improve Mental Health Care

As a result of an investigation by a special senate mental health study committee, the general assembly, in 1957, created a Mental Health Commission of five members, three of which were required to be skilled in the treatment of mental diseases. The commission, rather than the governor, was empowered to select the director of the Division of Mental Diseases. The establishment of the commission was a major element of Governor James T. Blair's legislative program, which also included an expanded role for the division's headquarters as thus described:[58]

Complete reorganization of the division office, with a staff of experts replacing a small, non-professional administrative section, was the key objective of legislation passed in 1957 creating the State Mental Health Commission and the new job of executive director.

The division in addition to regulating activities at the mental hospitals, also will seek to co-ordinate mental health endeavors of all kinds, private as well as public, throughout the state.

The commission chose as executive director Dr. Addison M. Duval, assistant superintendent of St. Elizabeth's Hospital, Washington, D.C. and an expert in public mental hospital work. Duval's first undertaking was to prepare a ten-year plan for the improvement of Missouri's institutions, with specific objectives for each of the biennial periods from 1961 through 1971.

Duval's plan was a compromise that preserved many features of the old system of mental care, while a new, more efficient program was in process of development. It called for expansion and improvement of staffs at the state's mental schools and hospitals; also for rehabilitation of the buildings at state hospitals. But it did not suggest any new construction at the five adult mental centers. Among new proposals were the release of qualified patients for continued care in nursing homes or boardinghouses; the establishment of community treatment centers; the subsidization of psychiatric care in general hospitals; the expansion of outpatient service at the state's mental health centers; and the education and involvement of the public in mental health matters.[59]

The Duval plan was indorsed unanimously by 150 representatives of forty-seven organizations attending the first Mental Health Conference meeting in St. Louis, September 8-9, 1960. It called for increased expenditures of at least $8,500,000 during the coming biennium. A resolution was adopted creating five committees to promote public and legislative support for the proposal and to advise the State Mental Health Commission regarding legislative matters to be submitted to the general assembly.[60]

The ten-year plan was adopted by the legislature and Governor John Dalton. Dalton, for 1961-1963, had budgeted an increase of $6,300,000 for the mental hospitals building restoration fund. The legislature added $2,400,000 to make possible a five percent salary increase for employees of the Division of Mental Diseases along with other state workers.[61] Thus, the program got started in an upbeat fashion. But not for long!

Without warning, and apparently without justification, Governor Dalton, in mid-November 1961, replaced the entire Mental Health Commission with his own appointees and then had a subservient board fire Dr. Duval. The *St. Louis Post-Dispatch*, in an editorial of November 16, 1961, commented bitterly:[62]

> Missouri is left in consequence, without a functioning independent commission to safeguard professional leadership even if that leadership could be re-established. The progress accomplished in more than six years of effort such as Missouri had never experienced before has been essentially wiped out.

> When this effort started, the director of the state's mental hospitals was a political hack. Missouri was among the five most backward states in mental health, and doing nothing about it. The unfortunates in its mental institutions were getting custodial care and little more.

One can only speculate on the reasons for Governor Dalton's action. It is obvious that he did not approve the decision of the legislature denying him the power to appoint the director of the Division of Mental Diseases. Governors zealously protect against encroach-

ment their administrative domains. The fact that Dr. Duval's program was developed during the administration of Dalton's predecessor may have undermined his early support. Dalton apparently preferred a program on which he could put his own signature. Finally, there is a possibility hinted in the press that he and Dr. Duval did not see eye to eye on the critical issue of financing the ten-year plan on a generous basis.

On November 20, 1961, Dr. George A. Ulett was named by the Missouri Mental Health Commission as acting director of the State Division of Mental Diseases; he was later advanced to full director. Dr. Ulett, at the time of his appointment, was serving as medical chief of Malcolm Bliss Mental Health Center in St. Louis and as professor of psychiatry at Washington University. He announced that he would place major emphasis on research and teaching in developing a strong mental program for Missouri.[63]

In a speech before the Kansas City Mental Health Association on April 30, 1962, Dr. Ulett proposed the establishment of three intensive care hospitals in Missouri. According to his plan, all patients would "enter the state hospital system through one of the intensive care or admitting hospitals. In this way patients would receive early in their illnesses the latest and most effective treatment." The three hospitals would be located in the Malcolm Bliss Mental Health Center in St. Louis, the Psychiatric Receiving Center in Kansas City, and in a proposed new structure to be built in Columbia. Dr. Ulett predicted that in the new centers, with a ratio of one psychiatrist for eight patients, the average stay would be reduced to one month, in comparison with the usual eight months treatment period in the older state hospitals.[64] The new installations would have inpatient services, day centers, outpatient clinics, spe-

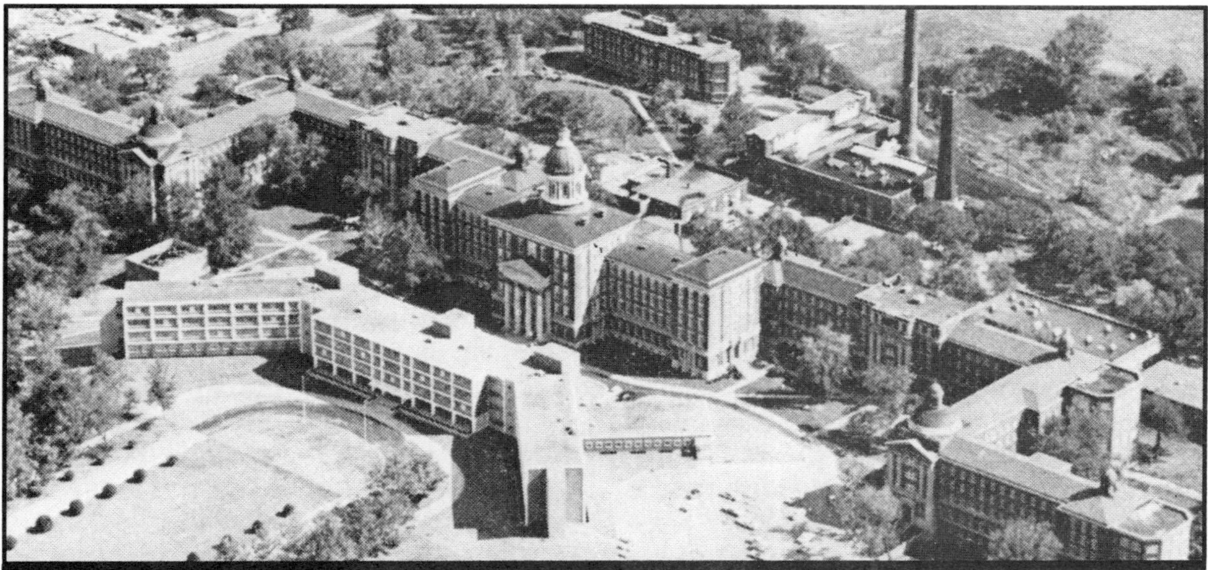

St. Louis State Hospital. Courtesy of the State Historical Society of Missouri.

cial units for alcohol and drug abuse, and units for the treatment of children. Dr. Ulett's proposal was indorsed by the legislature and Governor Dalton and became the central feature of the state's mental care system.

Governor Dalton, on August 30, 1962, announced the establishment of the Missouri Institute of Psychiatry. The institute would be housed in a new building on the grounds of the St. Louis State Hospital and would provide beds for 250 patients transferred there from state hospitals while undergoing special treatment and observation. Dr. Max Fink, in charge of experimental psychiatry at Hillside Hospital in New York City, was chosen as the first director. He outlined, as follows, the goals of the new institute:[65]

(1) Broad research to determine which patients fail to respond to a variety of treatment and why.

(2) Study of what treatment methods appear to work best in specific cases and evaluation of new concepts in mental illness therapy.

(3) Classification of the physiological, biochemical and sociological causes of mental illness.

(4) Training of specialists in hospital psychiatry, psychologists, social workers and eventual assumption of responsibility for a nurses' training program in which the St. Louis State Hospital prepares 1500 nurses a year for service in a five-state area.

In addition to the five mental hospitals and the three intensive care centers for adult patients, the state maintains a separate program for mentally retarded and developmentally disadvantaged youths. Residential treatment for such individuals is provided at the St. Louis State School-Hospital, Marshall State School-Hospital, Nevada State School-Hospital, St. Louis Developmental Disabilities Treatment Center, and the Higginsville State School-Hospital. Diagnostic and treatment services are available at centers operated in the following communities: Hannibal,

Kirksville, Albany, Kansas City, Joplin, Springfield, Marshall, Rolla, Poplar Bluff, Sikeston and St. Louis.[66]

Dr. Ulett, on January 17, 1967, in order to provide more effective and better care, instituted a new organizational scheme for the state's five mental hospitals, according to which the population of each hospital would be divided into several treatment groups:[67]

> The new plan calls for the establishment of a geographic section plan under which each hospital will be divided into smaller administrative units. Each unit will be operated by a mental health team and will be composed of patients from one small geographic area who will stay in a particular section of the hospital.
>
> Each team, headed by a psychiatrist, will be responsible for the admission, diagnosis, treatment, discharge and follow-up care of the patients in its section . . . .
>
> The system will replace the traditional type of state hospital organization in which several professional departments in each hospital are responsible for a particular phase of the care of many patients who are spread throughout the institution.

The story of Unit One of the St. Louis State Hospital on Arsenal Street illustrates how the new system worked in actual practice.[68] When in 1968 Dr. M. B. Ahmed, a Pakistani who had secured his psychiatric training in Scotland, took charge, Unit One had approximately 500 patients, all suffering from psychiatric disorders. The unit was responsible for providing mental health services to a major portion of St. Louis County with 445,000 persons. Some of the patients had been confined for more than fifty years and had completely lost touch with the outside world. To reestablish the contacts of the patients with their former communities, Dr. Ahmed took drastic action:

> In an effort to achieve this, early in 1968 Ahmed sent about a third of his original 500 patients to nursing homes, thereby getting them out of Unit One and putting them an important step closer to ordinary life. Another third was discharged within a few months after Ahmed's arrival — their only problem, he insists, was that no one had ever told them they were ready to go home. The others, though not ready for release, were told that they would be permitted to go home as soon as possible.

Since Unit One served St. Louis County, Ahmed, in 1969, took over the administration of the psychiatric services in the St. Louis County Hospital and made it part of Unit One administratively. The county hospital's psychiatric unit had beds for 25 patients, facilities for day patients and outpatients, and 24-hour emergency service. It provided everything available at the Arsenal Street establishment — but without the stigma of a mental institution.

In November 1970, Ahmed opened a mental health clinic at the Kinloch Community Center in north St. Louis County. He explained that this was "an effort to bring psychiatric care to the people, instead of taking people out of the community, when they need help, and the emphasis is on preventive psychiatry." He described his patients in Unit One as ordinary people who became "depressed, anxious, frightened, unable to cope with the job or cope with the family." The Kinloch community clinic was designed to detect such problems before they became so acute that hospitalization was necessary.

Dr. Ahmed maintained that psychiatric services should be an accepted part of "comprehensive community health care" and that his staff of three doctors, six social workers, two psychologists, one occupational therapist, and two vocational rehabilitation specialists operated in full cooperation with the other local health agencies.

Important advances were made in hospital treatment therapies, comparable to the introduction of hydrotherapy in the 1920s and electro-shock and insulin therapy in the 1930s. The revolutionary new agents were the tranquilizers, such as chlorpromazine and reserpine, the latter derived from an old snakeroot remedy used in India for many centuries. Although it has not been scientifically established just how these drugs work, they apparently "reduce the activity of the hypothalamus in the brain — the source of emotional energy — without impairing the functions of the brain's cortex, or 'thinking' part. This has the effect of quieting severely disturbed mental patients and making them amenable to psychotherapy and rehabilitative programs."[69] These drugs were important supplements to the wide range of activities employed in Missouri's mental institutions, including music therapy, recreational therapy, individual and group psycho-therapy, motivational therapy, and educational and vocational therapy. To prepare patients to cope with the problems of the outside world, the hospitals instituted general educational programs leading to high school degrees and also vocational programs in such fields as commerce, home economics, auto mechanics, machine and metal work, custodial and building maintenance, building trades, and small engine repair. Selected patients were permitted to live in self-governing group houses in which they had to make decisions and do things for themselves.

Provided with a budget of $73,000,000 a year, the Ulett program was making good progress, with funds available for treatment, research and training of professional personnel. But because of a lag in revenue collections, State Comptroller John C. Vaughn, in early April 1971, announced that he would be forced to cut back budget allotments 15 percent for all state agencies during the final quarter of the fiscal year ending in June 1971. As a consequence, the State Division of Mental Health began making plans to lay off as many as 2,200 employees in its twenty-one institutions. To help adjust to the budget cut, 2,000 of the division's 9,000 workers offered to take unpaid leaves of absence for the months of May and June. Dr. Ulett instituted a sharp curtailment of admissions at all state hospitals; and as many patients as could be sent home without danger to themselves or to others would be temporarily discharged.[70]

The financial crisis shattered the unified support for Dr. Ulett's program. The Missouri Institute of Psychiatry became the target of angry criticism. Numerous employees expressed the opinion that they were not opposed to research, but when it came to the division spending money on research or patient care, they thought priority should be given to patient care. Another criticism was that regular staff members needed at the St. Louis Hospital were being transferred to the institute to work on research projects, and also that treatment projects at the hospital were being disrupted by the movement of patients to the institute.[71]

In defense of the institute's usefulness, Dr. Ulett cited the high rate of return to health and their homes of participants in the institute's programs. He also mentioned the administrative benefits which would accrue from a computer system being developed and installed, which would provide the following data:[72]

> information on the number of patients in the various institutions, their case histories, the number and kind of employes [sic], operational costs at individual hospitals and other statistical data was being centralized, organized, and could be used by the division and institution directors to upgrade internal management.

He called attention to the growing use of the computer in diagnosing patient illnesses, analyzing clinical data noted on cards by the doctor or psychiatrist at bedside.

Ulett's arguments were not persuasive to the legislature, which instituted a sharp cut in funds and severe restrictions on the type of research the institute could conduct. Ulett, who had led the division during ten years of constructive growth and in the process been accused of being an empire builder and an incompetent administrator, submitted his resignation in September 1972.[73] One by one staff members of the institute, sensing that there was no professional future for them, also resigned.

The final blow to the institute was the failure of the Missouri School of Medicine and the Missouri Division of Mental Health, which jointly operated the institute, to agree on the terms of a new research contract. The proposed contract, drawn up at the order of the state Office of Administration, "would have required that the university pay the salaries of employes [sic] and purchase equipment. But the authority over what was purchased and who was hired at the institute would have been the responsibility of the St. Louis State Hospital purchasing and personnel depart-

ments."[74] The university considered that such a contract would have meant too much interference by the St. Louis State Hospital and the Division of Mental Health in the operation of the institute's research program.

The United States Supreme Court, in 1974, established the principle that persons confined in mental institutions were entitled to fundamental constitutional guarantees.[75] To vindicate these rights, a program of legal assistance for patients at Malcolm Bliss Mental Health Center was established under the guidance of Jesse Goldner, assistant professor of law and psychiatry at St. Louis University. Four advanced law students kept regular office hours at the hospital. Although most cases concerned matters such as divorces, business transactions and landlord-tenant relationships, there also were cases of unjustified hospital confinement. One such case involved a young woman, picked up by police in a bus station because she seemed lost and confused. While being examined by doctors regarding her sanity, she stated that "Arthur Brown and the Fire Gods" were her deity. The doctors adjudged her as suffering from schizophrenia, not realizing that her alleged deity was a California rock band. Her case was heard in probate court with student legal assistance, and she was released from confinement.[76]

In 1975, the bar association of metropolitan St. Louis began an inquiry regarding the services of court-appointed attorneys in psychiatric commitment and guardianship cases in St. Louis and St. Louis County probate courts. Missouri law provided that persons allegedly suffering from mental illnesses can be temporarily detained in a hospital, but if they do not agree to stay for treatment, a commitment order must be obtained through the probate court to keep them. Counsel is appointed for such persons when they do not retain their own attorney.[77]

The *St. Louis Post-Dispatch*, upon investigation, found that the current court-appointed lawyer, a local Democratic politician, in nearly all psychiatric commitment cases in the St. Louis probate court "had failed routinely to discuss commitment cases with medical personnel, examine medical records or spend appreciable time with clients." In only one out of 375 cases, in which he served as court-appointed attorney, had he been able to secure the release of his client.[78]

A class action suit regarding patients' rights was filed in 1972 with the United States district court in Jefferson City by two St. Louis area lawyers, Richard Boardman of the Legal Aid Society and Stanley Goldstein, a member of a University City law firm. The purpose of the suit was to obtain "remedies in behalf of more than 350 state hospital inmates who, it is claimed, are confined in grossly inadequate facilities with inadequate medical and psychiatric treatment, many of whom were assigned to a maximum security building without a hearing in which the state might have been required to show the necessity for such confinement."[79]

The suit alleged that inmates of the maximum security Biggs Building of State Hospital No. 1 at Fulton, Missouri, were receiving "mere custodial care rather than treatment, are excessively drugged, are forced to do hospital jobs in the name of therapy and finally wind up, without hearings or review of their case, being incarcerated for much longer than they would have been if they had been sent to prison in the first place."[80]

Following a long delay, United States District Judge Elmo Hunter, on August 11, 1979, issued a ruling upholding the right of mentally ill criminals to livable quarters and adequate medical treatment. Judge Hunter's pronouncement cited the need for certain building improvements at the Biggs center to assure greater comfort and privacy. His opinion pointed out several areas in which Biggs needed additional staff members. Representative Wayne Goode, chairman of the House Appropriations Committee, promised that the ruling would mean a higher priority for the criminally insane unit in the following legislative session.[81]

The capstone of the reform movement was a comprehensive patients' "bill of rights" enacted by the legislature on June 12, 1978. The law made a major change in the basis for involuntary commitment. The previous statute required only that a patient be mentally ill and in need of hospital care. The new statute specified that it must be established that a patient was suffering from a mental disorder and "presents a likelihood of serious physical harm to himself or to others."[82]

The law set up a regular schedule of hearings and examinations in cases of involuntary commitment:[83]

Such persons could be held only four days before being given a hearing and only 14 more days before a second hearing. If their involuntary detention is to continue, they are entitled to another hearing within three months, a case review each successive six months and recommitment proceedings each year.

The procedure had important benefits for the patient as well as for the hospital. The patient was guaranteed against the nightmare of being locked up and forgotten. At regular intervals, he had the opportunity to present evidence to justify his discharge. So he had every reason to cooperate with the authorities in expediting his recovery. To the hospital staff, it was a major means of alleviating

Officers

——

Department
of
Mental
Health

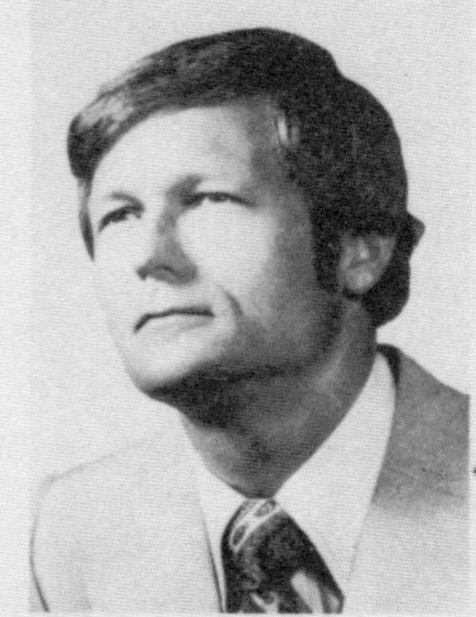

C. DUANE HENSLEY, Ph.D.
Director

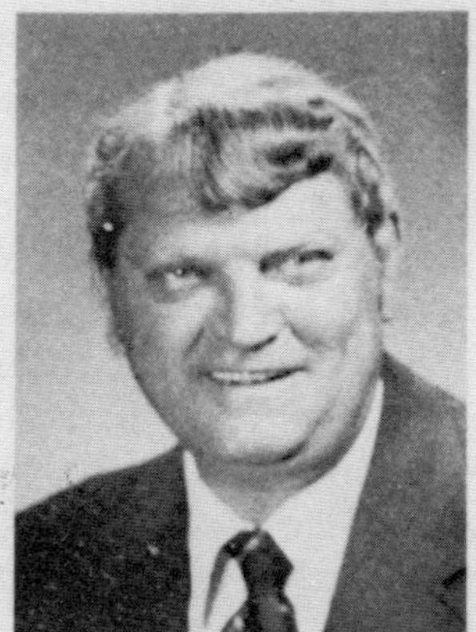

DAVID L. ROBERTS
Deputy Director
Administration

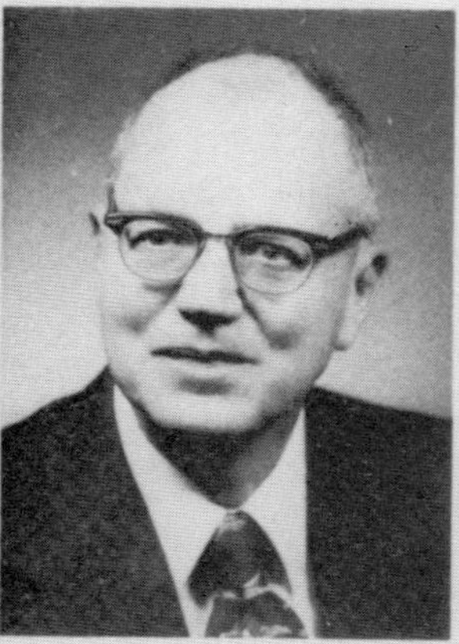

HENRY V. GUHLEMAN, JR., M.D.
Chief Psychiatric Consultant,
Acting Director
Psychiatric Services

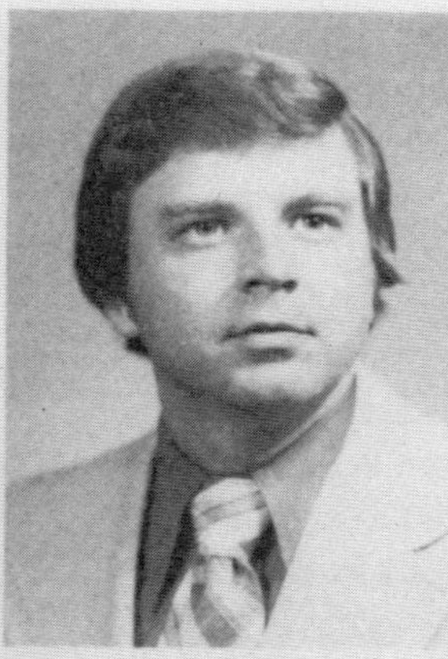

JOHN G. SOLOMON
Director, Division of
Mental Retardation—
Developmental Disabilities

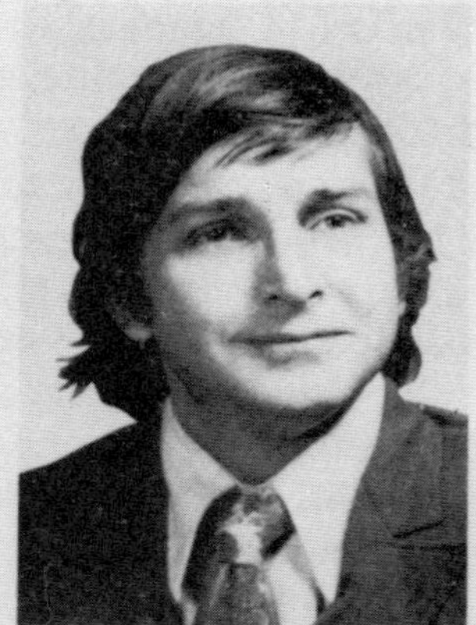

WILLIAM LERNER, M.D.
Director, Division of
Alcoholism, Drug Abuse

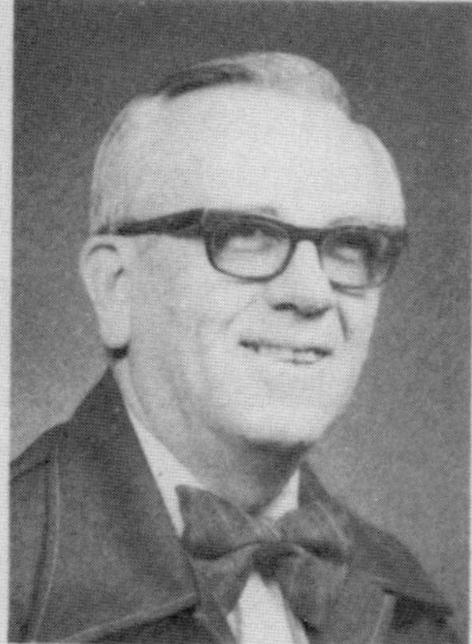

WALTER J. CONWAY
Director, Community
Mental Health Services

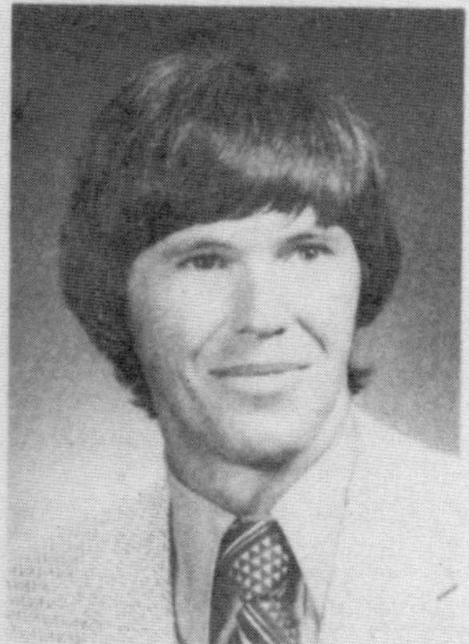

JOHN MAYFIELD
Assistant to Director

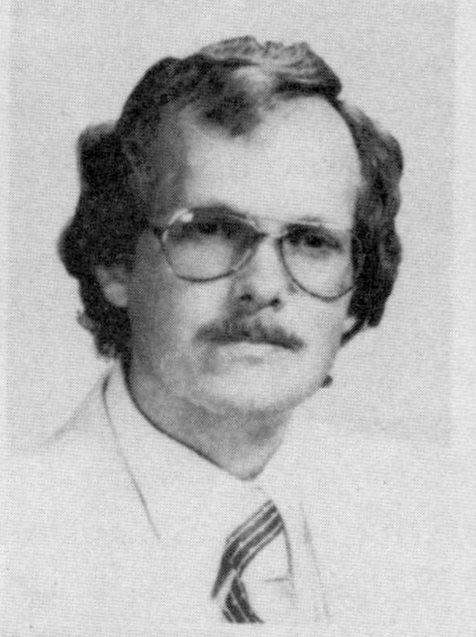

DeVON J. HARDY
Coordinator, Children and
Youth Services

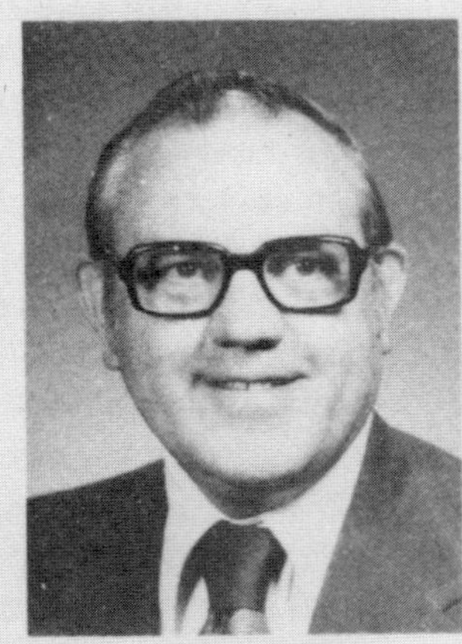

LAWSON B. MONTGOMERY
Personnel Officer

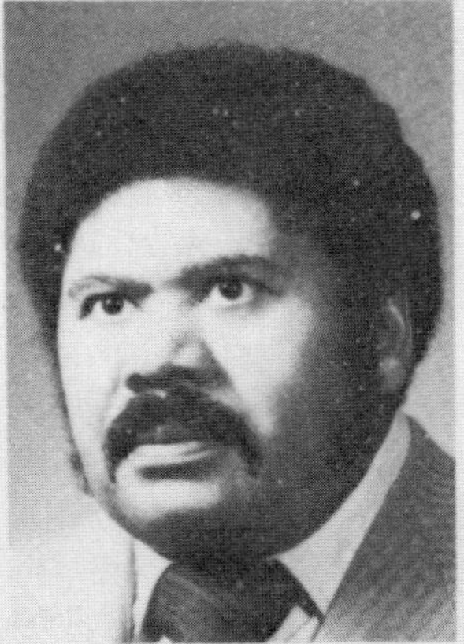

DAVID BRENT
Chief Human Relations
Officer

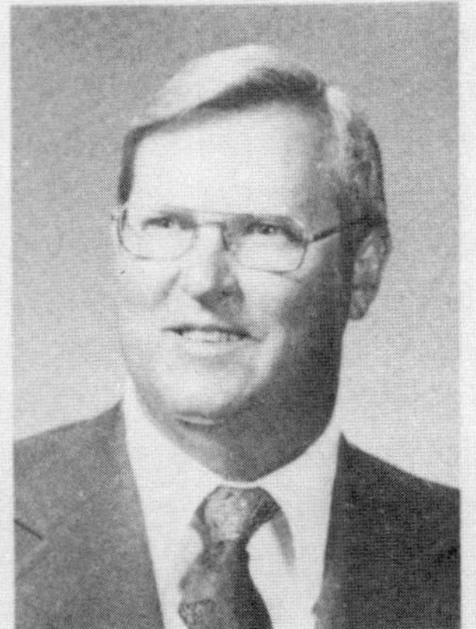

HOWARD DERRIEUX
Capitol Improvements
Coordinator

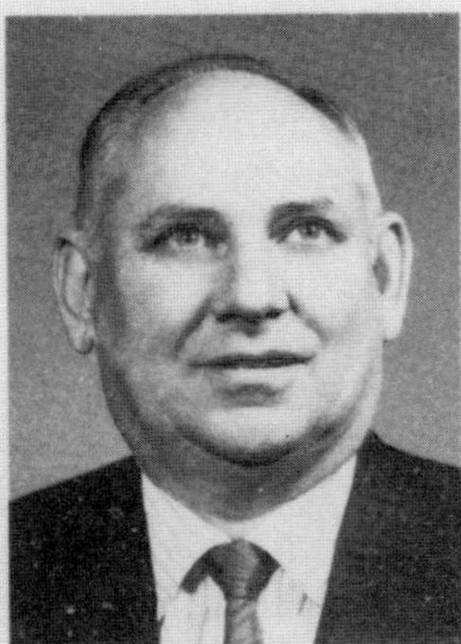

MARVIN E. NEBEL
Research Analyst

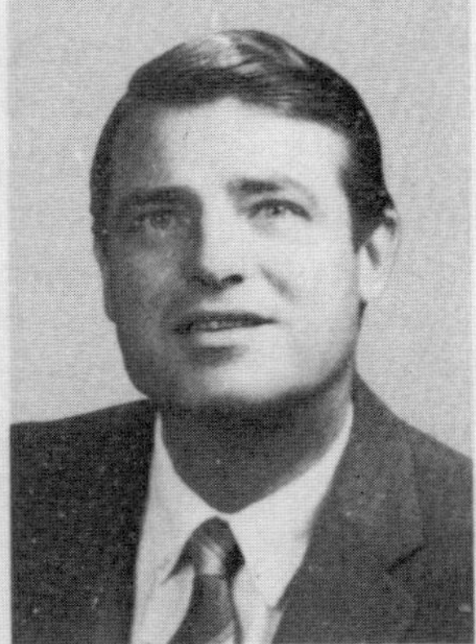

EDWARD L. DAVIS
Director, Patient Placement

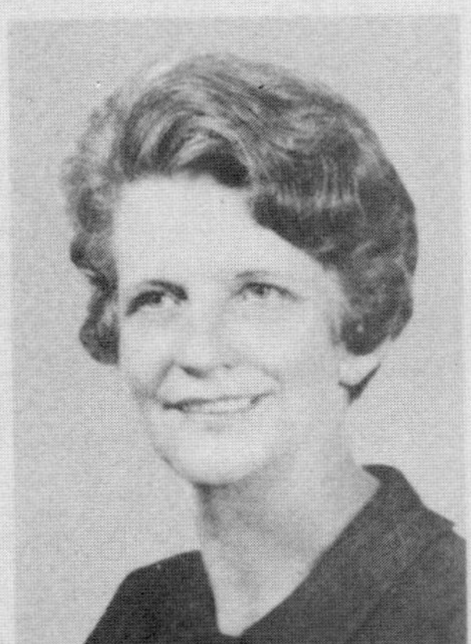

HELENE LANDBERG
Dietary Consultant

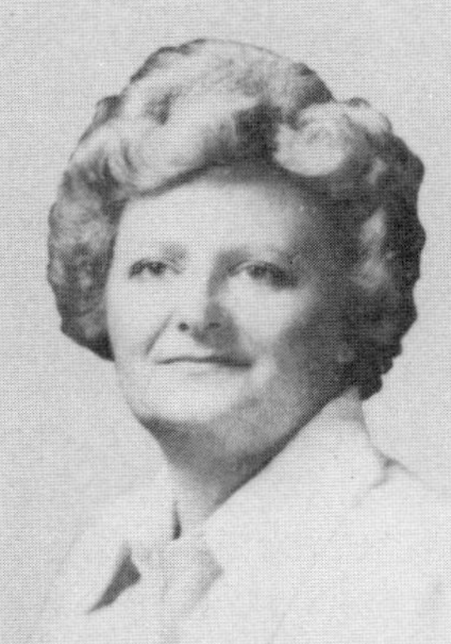

ANNA MAE BLEDSUE
Administrative Assistant

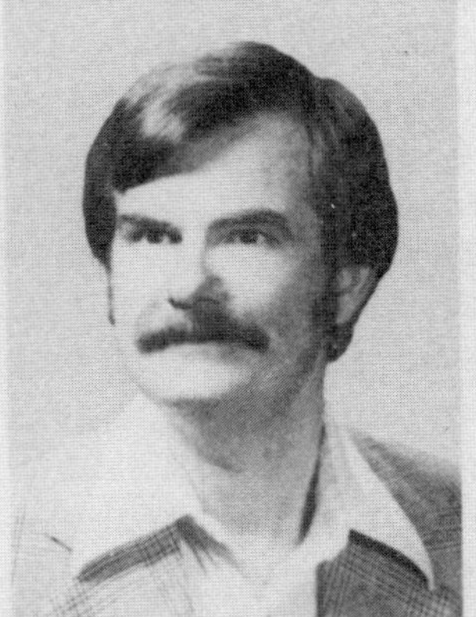

LAWRENCE DOSS, M.D.
Consultant, Community
Mental Health

overcrowding. Periodically, they could take a careful look at their patient census and discharge those ready for the change.

The law incorporated the principle of the gradual release of patients to the least restrictive environment possible,[84] such as licensed boarding houses, licensed nursing homes or family homes, with continuing responsibility being retained by the state hospitals. It spelled out specific privileges to which the patient was entitled, including:[85]

> a right to his own clothes and possessions; to hold small amounts of money for minor purchases; to communicate confidentially by sealed mail or telephone; to have access to current newspapers, magazines, radio and television; to a balanced diet, exercise and outdoor recreation; and to unrestricted visits with his attorney, physician or clergyman.

The law also provided that all patients, whether voluntary or involuntary, had the right to refuse the convulsive electro-shock treatment, unless it is ordered by a court following a comprehensive hearing.

The general assembly, in 1957, passed legislation transforming the small administrative headquarters of the Division of Mental Health into a staff of medical experts. The new staff, as illustrated by its composition as of 1977, was geared to the problems and requirements of community based mental health care. The organization was headed by a director and a deputy director; the latter had special responsibility for administration. Under the director were the chiefs of the three major divisions of the organization: Comprehensive Psychiatric Services, Mental Retardation-Developmental Disabilities, and Alcoholism and Drug Abuse. Trained specialists headed the various functional sections, including Community Mental Health Services, Children and Youth Services, Personnel, Human Relations, Capital Improvements, Research, Patient Placement, and Dietary Management.[86]

An important feature of the departmental organization was the system of advisory councils. At the state level, there was an advisory council to the director of the Division of Comprehensive Psychiatric Services, one to the director of the Division of Alcoholism and Drug Abuse, and another to the director of the Division of Mental Retardation-Developmental Disabilities. Finally, there were eight Regional Advisory Councils reporting to each state council, e.g., the State Advisory Council on Comprehensive Psychiatric Services. There was a two-way flow of communication in each of the three main branches of the department, e.g., from the director of Comprehensive Psychiatric Services to the State Advisory Council on Comprehensive Psychiatric Services and finally to the eight regional councils, and in reverse from the eight regional advisory councils through the State Advisory Council to the director of the division. The system enabled the director of each of the three branches to get from the state and regional councils their reactions to existing policies and to proposed changes.

Two programs were developed for bringing psychiatric care to the mentally ill in their own communities. Under the Community Mental Health Centers Act of 1975, federal funds became available for the construction of nonstate community treatment centers. In Missouri, as of 1977, centers had been built in the following communities: Joplin, Mexico, North Kansas City, Lee's Summit, Cape Girardeau, Independence, Hannibal and Springfield. Since these centers were not state operated or funded, they probably had to contract with local doctors for providing professional services and upon various local funding means, e.g., United Way, for their operation.[87]

The second method was to establish satellite or outreach centers in which psychiatric teams from Missouri's mental hospitals would hold clinics, usually once a month on a scheduled basis. Farmington State Hospital was a pioneer in the development of traveling clinics and served Cape Girardeau, Dexter and Marble Hill. Fulton dispatched traveling teams to Hermann, Hannibal and Rolla. St. Louis State Hospital held clinics in Jefferson, Pike, Franklin and Lincoln counties. Teams from the Mid-Missouri Mental Health Center in Columbia visited Moberly, Bethany, Boonville, California, Carrollton, Fayette, Keytesville, Marshall, Sedalia and Versailles.

The teams would ordinarily include a psychiatrist, social workers, psychologists, occupational therapists and vocational rehabilitation specialists. Much of the patronage of the visiting teams consisted of former patients, who were being provided continuing treatment and counseling away from their former hospital. They also did diagnostic work and early treatment of new patients.

As of 1977, there were "approximately 8,450 Department of Mental Health clients placed in community facilities such as licensed professional nursing homes, licensed practical nursing homes, licensed domiciliary nursing homes, licensed boarding homes, certified foster care homes, licensed group care homes, licensed residential centers and in their own natural homes as part of a continuing treatment program by the Department."[88]

Deinstitutionalization was not merely a Missouri phenomenon, but a national practice prompted by United States Supreme Court decisions requiring that mental patients be treated in the least restrictive environment, by state-enacted "bills of rights" for patients, and by the recommendations of many leading members of the national psychiatric profession. Under the influence of this procedure, the attendance in mental institutions in the United States dropped from 560,000 to 170,000 in the period from 1955 to 1979.[89]

Though the intent was benevolent, the result in many cases was tragic. Community treatment centers were not constructed in the expected numbers. High quality nursing homes were too expensive for the states to afford. County poorhouses had long been abandoned in many communities. For thousands, the price of their new freedom was life in temporary shelters, jails and in other makeshift quarters, including public streets.

What went wrong? Although the new treatment system was basically sound, it was swamped by the sheer numbers of the mentally and physically handicapped persons. Dr. C. Duane Hensley, director of the Department of Mental Health, in 1977, gave this estimate of the magnitude of Missouri's problem:[90]

In Missouri, there are estimated to be between 7,000 and 12,000 opiate addicts and 75,000 poly drug users (often including alcohol). Abuse of legally prescribed drugs is widespread and generally untreated. One person in ten is presumed to be emotionally disturbed or mentally ill. At least two percent of the population is mentally retarded and in need of services. The array of developmental disabilities included in mental health care would perhaps account for another two percent of the population.

These separate estimates of the persons needing various kinds of mental health care, made by the organizations concerned with their treatment, roughly correspond to Langner and Michael's estimate of 25% of the population. Using 1975 population figures, these estimates total 1,190,750 Missourians.

Although 25% of Missouri's population may be in need of treatment in varying degrees, resources, motivation and opportunity generally preclude that only about 8% of those in need of treatment are receiving it. Many persons are treated privately and through community mental health centers but such statistics are difficult to gather. In summary, approximately 1,094,927 Missouri citizens estimated to be in need of mental health services are not receiving them from the Department of Mental Health.

6. An Enlarged Role for the Mt. Vernon Sanatorium

The changing incidence of disease and the advance of medical science enabled the state sanatorium at Mt. Vernon to expand its role in Missouri's system of health care. Established in 1907, its original function was to combat tuberculosis, which as late as 1911 caused 5,113 deaths in the state. Patients were housed in cottages, where they would have the maximum exposure to fresh air and sunshine; these along with a nourishing diet and extended bed rest, were the main factors in a lengthy treatment program which might last a year or more.

The development of antibiotics, which were effective in treating tuberculosis and the general improvements in living standards reduced the number of deaths in Missouri to 144 in 1970. At the same time, however, new pulmonary diseases were increasing due principally to smoking and to breathing the air of cities contaminated by industrial fumes and motor car emissions.

The name of the institution was changed to Missouri State Chest Hospital in 1971, and patients with a broader range of ailments began to be admitted. Today, it is recognized as one of the world's finest chest centers, "treating not only tuberculosis, but all pulmonary disease with emphasis on fungus disease, carcinoma, bronchiectasis, emphysema and asthma." Approximately half of the sanatorium's patients have diseases other than tuberculosis.[91]

The hospital provides "specialized diagnostic, medical, surgical, nursing and physiotherapy services for patients with chest diseases." Its outpatient care includes laboratory and X-ray examinations and the supply of therapeutic drugs to former patients and to persons reacting positively to tuberculin skin tests. It serves as headquarters for statewide tuberculosis prevention programs.[92]

In 1960, two wings, named for a longtime superintendent, Dr. Charles A. Brasher, were added, providing space for laboratory work and outpatient services. Ten years later, the six-story, 220-bed Warren E. Hearnes Chest Clinic and Research Pavilion was completed. This constituted a modern, centralized hospital complex, which made possible the abandonment for treatment purposes of the former scattered cottages.[93]

The hospital operates an on-site educational program for its staff, in order to keep them informed and proficient in the newest theories and methods of treating respiratory diseases. For its youthful patients, it offers elementary and high school courses with accredited graduation, also a commercial course. For older patients, looking to re-entry in the business world, rehabilitation and social services assistance are available.[94]

The average stay in the hospital has been reduced each year since 1947, and the rate of recovery has gone up steadily. As of 1969-1970, approximately 1,800 patients a year were being treated.

Entrance to the hospital is limited to citizens of Missouri. Patients are of two classes: free patients, who are certified by their home counties as unable to pay for their treatment. For these the home county pays $7.50 a month. Patients, who are financially able to do so, pay $50 a month.[95]

7. Present Status of the Nursing Profession

Patricia Rice, in a feature story in the *St. Louis Post-Dispatch* of May 2, 1977, thus summarized the status of the nursing profession in Missouri:[96]

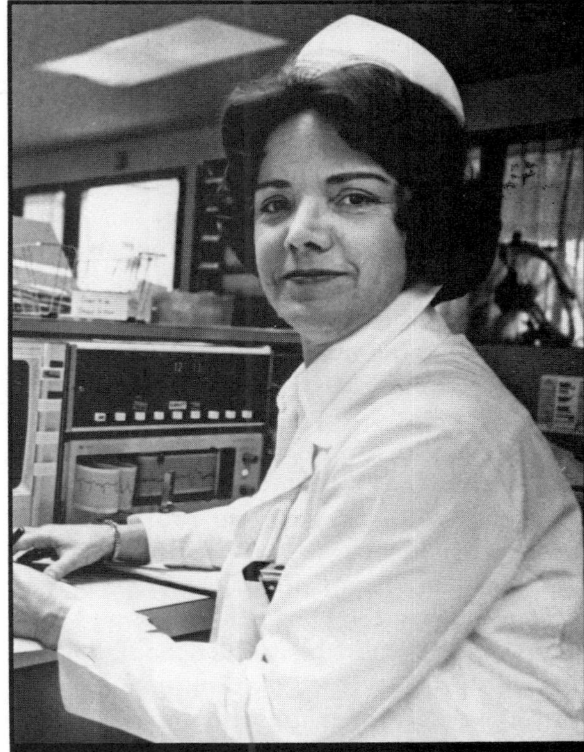

Nurse at a monitoring station at the University of Missouri Hospital. Courtesy of the State Historical Society of Missouri.

The role of the nurse is changing. Nurses are upgrading their skills and broadening the scientific horizons of their health-care vocation while reminding one another not to forget that their bedside manner, warmth and compassion is vital to the patient's health.

More and more nurses are acquiring their Ph. D. degrees. The doctoral degree is valuable, even essential, for nurses who direct or instruct in university schools of nursing, or who head a large hospital or nursing home. These tasks require not only professional medical skills but also administrative and public relations talents.

The relation of nurse and doctor was also undergoing a transformation:[97]

It has been an easy out for nurses to say that if something is not written on the chart "there is no order," rather than to question the doctor about a new possibility, urge the patient to discuss it with the doctor or, in non-medical situations, take the initiative and responsibility to use their own judgment.

The crucial role of the nurse in the administration of drug therapy has long been recognized:[98]

Nurses for years have called the doctor and reported a particular reaction or lack of results and suggested he might change his directions . . . . Today that procedure is going further. The expression, "nursing diagnosis," is being used by doctors as well as nurses and nursing schools. That diagnosis is one of several that a hospital team uses in evaluating a patient's health.

While the number of women entering medical schools and becoming physicians has been increasing dramatically, there is a parallel growth in the number of men entering the field of nursing. Historically, nursing was a men's profession in the United States until near the end of the nineteenth century. During the Civil War, most nurses were convalescent soldiers, awaiting return to their units. The reasons for the present influx are complex. Some male nursing students may be drop-outs from the exhausting pace and stringent requirements of medical school. For others, the profession of nursing may be their first choice. There is the assurance of a competitive demand for their services when they graduate. They can begin earning top pay after three or four years in school, rather than the eight or nine years necessary for a doctor. They will not have to enter their professional field with a debt of possibly $200,000-$300,000 to pay off. They can avoid the lean years of getting started, equipping an office and building a satisfactory patronage. They do not have to worry seriously about malpractice suits. In nursing school, the male student meets hundreds of attractive women of marriageable age. He can marry earlier with the prospect of establishing, with a two-wage earner team, a satisfactory level of income, unencumbered by the indebtedness that would have been incurred in becoming a M.D.

Prenatal care is a field of special opportunity for nurses. Routine checkups, basic tests and all of prenatal supervision for normal, low-risk mothers could be handled by nurses. The nurse is the key staff member in nursing homes, few of which have a resident doctor. She can perform most of the regular medical tests. Since the nurse is able to observe and get to know the patients, she is apt to notice problems that the doctor on his infrequent visits may miss.

Many nurses, after finishing the basic training, specialize in such fields as surgery, dietetics, gerontology, burns, pediatrics and sports medicine. Nurses work with computers and with the latest diagnostic technology, such as CAT scanners, magnetic resonance imaging and ultra sound photography for cancer detection.[99]

Nursing is one of Missouri's important professions in terms of employment. As of 1975, there were 6,017 practicing registered nurses in the St. Louis area and 2,126 actively employed licensed practical nurses. The number of nurses aides in the area as of that date is not known, but it would probably equal the total of the two higher groups. There were 15,527 registered nurses in Missouri, who were working full or part-time, and 6,783 licensed practical nurses. Again the figures do not include nurses aides. They also exclude nurses who were not occupied with patient care, such as those in administrative positions in local health departments and nurses in research work.[100]

Chapter IX
New Initiatives in Missouri's Health Care, 1950-1980

1   State of Missouri, *Official Manual 1959-1960*. Edited by Walter H. Toberman, Secretary of State, pp. 612-613.
2   *Idem.*
3   State of Missouri, *Official Manual 1957-1958*. Edited by Walter H. Toberman, Secretary of State, p. 579.
4   State of Missouri, *Official Manual 1959-1960*. Edited by Walter H. Toberman, Secretary of State, p. 613.
5   *Laws of Missouri, Passed at the Regular, First and Second Extra Sessions of the Seventy-Fourth General Assembly. Regular Session Which Convened at the City of Jefferson, Wednesday, January 4, 1967*. Issued by the Committee on Legislative Research, General Assembly of Missouri, pp. 284-285.
6   Missouri Department of Mental Health, "Special Legislative Report on Mental Health Services January 1977." (Jefferson City, Mo. 1977) p. 4.
7   *Laws of Missouri Passed at the First Regular, First Extra, Second Regular and Second Extra Sessions of the Seventy-Fourth General Assembly. First Regular Session Which Convened at the City of Jefferson, Wednesday, January 3, 1973*. Edited by James C. Kirkpatrick, Secretary of State, pp. 530, 546.
8   Missouri Division of Health, Department of Public Health and Welfare, "Missouri Public Health Statistics, Vital Statistics, 1970, Table 9. Department of Public Health and Welfare of Missouri. (Jefferson City, Mo. 1971)
9   *St. Louis Post-Dispatch*, February 19, 1957, p. 1:5.
10 *Ibid.*, p. 10:6.
11 *Ibid.*, p. 1:8.
12 *Idem.*
13 *Laws of Missouri Passed at the Regular and First Extra Session of the Sixty-Ninth General Assembly. Regular Session Which Convened at the City of Jefferson, Wednesday January 2, 1957*. Edited by Walter H. Toberman, Secretary of State, pp. 666-672.
14 *St. Louis Post-Dispatch*, May 15, 1957, p. 16A:1.
15 *Ibid.*, February 21, 1957, p. 6B:3-4.
16 *Ibid.*, Aug. 18, 1957, p. 3A:2-5; *ibid.*, Sept. 15, 1966, p. 3A:2-5.
17 *Ibid.*, June 14, 1965, p. 1:3.
18 *Ibid.*, Dec. 11, 1969, p. 1C:1-2.
19 *Ibid.*, July 9, 1970, p. 3A:5-8.
20 *Ibid.*, June 7, 1979, p. 1A:1-2.
21 *Ibid.*, June 9, 1979, p. 1A:5-6.
22 *Laws of Missouri Passed at the First Regular, Second Regular and First Extra Sessions of the Seventy-Sixth General Assembly. First Regular Session Which Convened at the City of Jefferson, Wednesday, January 6, 1971*. Edited by James C. Kirkpatrick, Secretary of State, pp. 231-234.
23 *Laws of Missouri Passed at the First Regular, First Extra, Second Regular and Second Extra Sessions of the Seventy-Fourth General Assembly Which Convened at the City of Jefferson, Wednesday January 3, 1973*. Edited by James C. Kirkpatrick, Secretary of State. pp. 307-313.
24 *Ibid.*, p. 312.
25 *St. Louis Post-Dispatch*, Apr. 24, 1968, p. 2H:2-3.
26 *Ibid.*, p. 2H:3-4.
27 *Ibid.*, Apr. 23, 1968, p. 3D:2-7.
28 *Ibid.*, Mar. 30, 1969, p. 3G:2-7.
29 *Ibid.*, Apr. 22, 1970, p. 2B:2-3.
30 *Ibid.*, June 8, 1972, p. 2A:1-2.
31 *Ibid.*, p. 2A:4.
32 *Ibid.*, Mar. 19, 1972, p. 6C:1.
33 *Ibid.*, Aug. 28, 1966, p. 1B:8.
34 *Ibid.*, Mar. 2, 1971, p. 1C:1-2.
35 *Ibid.*, Aug. 13, 1959, p. 6A:1.
36 *Ibid.*, July 1, 1960, p. 3A:5.
37 *Idem.*
38 *Ibid.*, Apr. 26, 1967, p. 13A:2-3.
39 *Ibid.*, Oct. 19, 1972, p. 16A:1.
40 *Ibid.*, p. 16A:1-2. The three years provided for were 1973, 1974, and 1975.
41 *Ibid.*, p. 16A:2.
42 *Laws of Missouri, Passed at the Regular and First Extra Session of the Sixty-Ninth General Assembly, Session Which Convened at the City of Jefferson Wednesday, January 2, 1957 and Adjourned Tuesday, May 31, 1957*. Edited by Walter H. Toberman, Secretary of State, p. 660.
43 *Ibid.*, p. 663.
44 *Ibid.*, p. 664.
45 *St. Louis Post-Dispatch*, Oct. 6, 1971, p. 1A:6-8.
46 *Ibid.*, Apr. 22, 1962, p. 3A:1.
47 *Ibid.*, Sept. 11, 1964, p. 3A:6-7; *ibid.*, Jan. 25, 1970, p. 45E:1-3.
48 *Ibid.*, July 21, 1965, p. 3A:2-4.
49 *Ibid.*, Jan. 25, 1970, p. 45E:1; *ibid.*, Dec. 2, 1970, p. 28D:1.
50 *Ibid.*, Apr. 17, 1967, p. 3A:8.
51 *Laws of Missouri Passed at the Regular, First and Second Extra Sessions of the Seventy-Third General Assembly. Regular Session Which Convened at the City of Jefferson, Wednesday, January 6, 1965*. Issued by the Committee on Legislative Research, General Assembly of Missouri, p. 336.
52 *Ibid.*, p. 337.
53 *St. Louis Post-Dispatch*, Jan. 29, 1969, p. 6A:2.
54 *Ibid.*, Aug. 23, 1967, p. 1A:4.
55 *Ibid.*, Aug. 30, 1976, p. 3B:2.
56 *Ibid.*, Nov. 21, 1972, p. 10A:1-2.
57 *Idem.*
58 *Ibid.*, Jan. 18, 1959, p. 1A:1.
59 *Ibid.*, Sept. 8, 1960, p. 1A:3; *ibid.*, Sept. 10, 1960, p. 3A:1.
60 *Ibid.*, Sept. 10, 1960, p. 3A:1.
61 *Ibid.*, June 22, 1961, p. 2B:2.
62 *Ibid.*, Nov. 16, 1961, p. 2B:2.
63 Ibid., Nov. 21, 1961, p. 1A:1.
64 Ibid., May 1, 1962, p. 3A:1.
65 Ibid., Oct. 7, 1962, p. 32D:2-3.
66 Missouri Department of Mental Health, "Toward a Client-Oriented Service Delivery System." November 1977. Jefferson City, Mo., 1977. pp. 2-3.
67 *St. Louis Post-Dispatch*, Jan. 17, 1967, p. 3A:1.
68 *Ibid.*, Mar. 28, 1971, p. 1G:2-7.
69 *Ibid.*, May 27, 1956, p. 3A:5-6.
70 Ibid., *Apr. 7, 1971, p. 1A:1.*
71 *Ibid.*, Apr. 22, 1971, p. 4E:1-2.
72 *Idem.*

73 *Ibid.,* Sept. 17, 1972, p. 18A:1-3.
74 *Ibid.,* Jan. 11, 1974, p. 1A:4-6.
75 *Ibid.,* Sept. 29, 1975, p. 5A:1-3.
76 *Ibid.,* Dec. 30, 1974, p. 4S:1-3.
77 *Ibid.,* Oct. 5, 1975, p. 1A:5-6.
78 *Ibid.,* p. 5A:7-8.
79 *Ibid.,* June 3, 1972, p. 4A:2-3.
80 *Idem.*
81 *Ibid.,* Aug. 14, 1979, p. 3A:1-4.
82 *Laws of Missouri, Passed at the Second Regular Session of the Seventy-Ninth General Assembly, Second Regular Session Which Convened at the City of Jefferson, Wednesday, January 4, 1978.* James C. Kirkpatrick, Secretary of State, p. 516.
83 *St. Louis Post-Dispatch,* Apr. 26, 1978, p. 12A:1-2.
84 *Laws of Missouri, 1978,* p. 525.
85 *St. Louis Post-Dispatch,* Apr. 26, 1978, p. 12A:1-2.
86 *State of Missouri, Official Manual 1977-1978.* Edited by James C. Kirkpatrick, pp. 752-753.
87 Missouri Department of Mental Health, Toward a Client-Oriented Service Delivery System," pp. 5-6.
88 *Ibid,* p. 6.
89 *St. Louis Post-Dispatch,* May 20, 1979, p. 4B:1-3.
90 Missouri Department of Mental Health, "Special Legislative Report on Mental Health Services, January 1977, Jefferson City, Mo., 1977, p. 15.
91 *State of Missouri, Official Manual 1971-1972,* Edited by James C. Kirkpatrick, Secretary of State, p. 767.
92 *State of Missouri, Official Manual 1977-1978.* Edited by James C. Kirkpatrick, Secretary of State, pp. 1115-1116.
93 *State of Missouri, Official Manual 1971-1972,* pp. 767-768.
94 *Ibid.,* p. 768.
95 *State of Missouri, Official Manual 1969-1970,* Edited by James C. Kirkpatrick, Secretary of State, p. 757.
96 *St. Louis Post-Dispatch,* May 2, 1977, p. 2D:1.
97 *Idem.*
98 *Idem.*
99 *Ibid,* May 2, 1977, p. 2D:3.
100 *Ibid,* May 2, 1977, p. 2D:5.

Index

A

B

C